# TUMOR MARKERS RESEARCH FOCUS

# TUMOR MARKERS RESEARCH FOCUS

DEBORAH H. CHANG
EDITOR

**Nova Biomedical Books**
*New York*

For permission to use material from this book please contact us:
Telephone 631-231-7269; Fax 631-231-8175
Web Site: http://www.novapublishers.com



Library of Congress Cataloging-in-Publication Data
Tumor markers research focus / Deborah H. Chang, editor.
p. ; cm.
Includes bibliographical references and index.
ISBN-13: 978-1-60021-544-5 (hardcover)
ISBN-10: 1-60021-544-0 (hardcover)
1. Tumor markers. I. Chang, Deborah.
[DNLM: 1. Tumor Markers, Biological. 2. Neoplasms--diagnosis. QZ 241 T9257 2006]
RC270.3.T84T88 2006
616.99'40072--dc22

2006101244

--

*Published by Nova Science Publishers, Inc. ✦New York*

# Contents

# Preface

Tumor markers are molecules occurring in blood or tissue that are associated with cancer, and whose measurement or identification is useful in patient diagnosis or clinical management. This book analyses potential signals of cancerous tumors, otherwise known as markers or indicators. This includes, direct and rapid determination of cancer antigen, potential tumor markers for cholangiocarcinoma, melanoma inhibitory activity, metastatic uveal melanoma, measurement of tumor oxygenation, bladder cancer markers, epithelial cell adhesion and progresion markers in prostate tumors.

Chapter I - Osteolytic bone disease is a frequent complication of multiple myeloma, resulting in skeletal complications that are a significant cause of morbidity and mortality. A characteristic feature of myeloma bone disease is that the lesions rarely heal and bone scans are often negative in myeloma patients who have extensive lytic lesions, offering very little in the follow-up of bone disease. X-rays are also of limited value in monitoring bone destruction during anti-myeloma or anti-resorptive treatment. Biochemical markers of bone turnover, such as N- and C-terminal cross-linking telopeptide of type I collagen (NTX, CTX/ICTP, respectively), bone specific alkaline phosphatase, osteocalcin, and newer ones such as the tartrate resistant acid phosphatase isoform 5b, and bone sialoprotein provide information on bone dynamics that in turn may reflect disease activity in bone. Several studies have shown bone markers to be elevated in myeloma patients and reflect the extent of bone disease, while in some of them bone resorption markers correlate with survival. These markers may also be helpful in identifying those patients likely to respond to bisphosphonate treatment, and monitoring the effectiveness of bisphosphonate therapy in the management of myeloma bone disease. Anti-myeloma therapy including autologous stem cell transplantation seems to normalize abnormal bone remodelling by reducing bone resorption markers and increasing bone formation indices. This chapter attempts to summarize the existing data for the role of markers of bone remodelling in assessing the extent of bone destruction in myeloma and monitoring bone turnover during specific anti-myeloma treatment. The authors also discuss some novel markers that may be of particular interest in the near future.

Chapter II - Hepatoma-derived growth factor (HDGF), unrelated to hepatocyte growth factor, is a heparin-binding protein originally purified from human hepatoma HuH-7 cells. Through nuclear targeting in an autocrine or a paracrine manner, HDGF exhibits a mitogenic activity in certain hepatoma cells, fibroblasts and vascular smooth muscle cells (VSMCs), as well as an angiogenic activiy. To date, however, it is unknown if the exogenous mitogenic effect of HDGF is mediated by a cell surface receptor or the protein uptake. Recently, HDGF was found to exert a mitogenic effect on lung epithelial cells *in vitro* and *in vivo*. These findings suggest that HDGF may play a critical role in the development and progression of lung cancer. HDGF expression was analyzed using a rabbit polyclonal antibody raised against the C-terminus of the human HDGF sequence. Weak staining of VSMCs was used as the internal positive control. Then, the authors investigated the relationship between HDGF expression and clinicopathological variables in 102 patients subjected to complete resection of non-small-cell lung cancer (NSCLC: 70 adenocarcinomas and 32 squamous cell carcinomas). Follow-up of the 102 patients ranged from 4.1 to 150.0 (median 65.8) months; 59 patients (57.8%) died of recurrence of lung cancer during follow-up. HDGF expression was strongly detected in the nucleus of cancer cells; the HDGF-labeling index (LI) was 20—95 (median 64.5)%. There was no significant association between HDGF-expression level and clinicopathological variables. Patients with NSCLC showing a high HDGF-LI (≥65%) had significantly worse overall survival than patients with NSCLC showing a low HDGF-LI. Multivariate analysis showed that pathological stage and HDGF-expression level were significant independent prognostic factors for overall survival, and that HDGF was associated with a higher risk ratio than pathological stage for overall survival (2.572 versus 2.061). Moreover, the Ki-67-LI and the intratumor CD31-positive microvessels density in patients expressing high levels of HDGF were significantly higher than in those expressing low levels of HDGF. The authors consider HDGF is a useful prognostic marker in patients who have undergone complete resection of NSCLC and may play a critical role in the pathobiology of lung cancer through its mitogenic and angiogenic activities. Moreover, the authors demonstrated that HDGF expression was higher in malignant pleural mesothelioma cells than in benign mesothelial cells and that many of the thymoma tumor cells highly expressed HDGF but not non-neoplastic lymphocytes. Although the molecular characteristics and biological functions of HDGF warrant further investigation, this factor may be a new tumor marker and a target molecule for the treatment of thoracic malignancy.

Chapter III - The Minichromosome Maintenance (MCM) Proteins constitute a family of 6 related proteins that participate in the initiation of DNA replication during the cell cycle. These proteins are essential components of proliferating eukaryotic cells. Although the MCM proteins are detected in normal proliferating cells, they are not detected in differentiated cells or cells that have exited the cell cycle. In cancer, the high proliferation state of these cells is associated with an increased expression of MCM proteins that can be detected in both the malignant precursor lesions and carcinomas. In cervical neoplasia, the detection of the MCM proteins is commonly observed in squamous cell carcinoma, adenocarcinoma and cervical intraepithelial neoplasia (i.e., precancerous lesions). The specific detection of MCM proteins in cervical neoplasia has been described in both cervical histology specimens and cervical cytology specimens. In cervical neoplasia, this increased expression of the MCM genes has been described at both the mRNA level and the protein level. Recent investigations have suggested that a semi-quantitative difference in MCM protein expression in cervical disease is associated with more advanced cervical dysplasia. In addition to the detection of proliferating cells, the use of MCM over-expression can be used to distinguish between mild dysplasia and moderate/severe dysplasia. During the pathogenesis of cervical neoplasia, the over-expression of the MCM genes appears to be a direct consequence of oncogenic HPV alteration of the cell cycle and specific activation of the E2F-1 transcription factor. This constitutive activation of E2F-1, independent of cell cycle regulation, leads to aberrant entry of the infected cells into the S-phase of the cell cycle. Increased expression of many S-phase genes occurs in response to this effect of high risk HPV on aberrant S-phase entry, but the MCM proteins appear most useful in terms of stable and reproducible detection within these abnormal cells. Continued research into the MCM proteins is anticipated to further define the clinical utility of the MCM proteins for improved detection and diagnosis of high-grade cervical disease.

Chapter IV - Tumour markers are either sent into the blood, urine or tissues by the tumour itself, or by the body in response to the tumour. With the advent of sophisticated technologies more sensitive tumour markers have been reported in the last few years. One of the major cancers being investigated for serum tumour markers is for gynaecological cancers, especially cancer of the ovary. In this report the authors will focus on the new developments after the discovery of cancer antigen-125. Broadly the approaches leading to tumour marker discovery could be classified into three (1) biomarker discovery using proteomic approaches (2) using genomic approaches and (3) more recently using metabolomics approaches. And there is another entirely different approach using mass spectrometry based pattern profiling for cancer diagnosis. Using proteomics approach more than 30 serum markers have been evaluated alone and in combination with CA-125 by different investigators. Some of the promising markers include: HE4, mesothelin, M-CSF, osteopontin, kallikrein(s), soluble EGF receptor, serum amyloid A1, bikunin, leptin, prolactin, osteopontin, and insulin-like growth factor-II. Serum secretory leukocyte protease inhibitor levels as well as creatine kinase B are some other promising serum markers identified for ovarian cancer. Currently the focus is on the development of multiplex platforms for simultaneous assay of several markers with small volumes of serum. A more recent advance is to use immune system as a biosensor where serum immunoglobulins from cancer patients could be used as bait for detecting cancer specific antigens. This global approach to antigenic profiling, epitomics, has applications to cancer diagnostics. Molecular genetic markers for ovarian cancer include BRCA-1, BRCA-2, Ras oncogenes, C-erb2 proto-oncogene, p53 suppressor gene and Bcl-2 oncogene. Using rigorous genomic approaches, whole transcriptome have been investigated for biomarker discovery. Interrogation of the entire transcriptome in human cancers and normal tissues, coupled with refined methods for sequence motif searching, and biological methods for enrichment are likely to yield many more tumour marker candidates. The other novel approaches developed from the above platform technologies include use of (1) anti-tumor antibodies which have the potential as cancer biomarkers were the anti-tumor response tends to be confined to individuals with ovarian cancer (2) another approach is to use a multianalyte cytokine panel profiling technology for simultaneous measurement of concentrations of 24 cytokines (cytokines/chemokines, growth, and angiogenic factors) in combination with CA-125. Using mass spectrometry approaches, pattern based recognition has reported higher sensitivity and specificity. The same technology has helped in the identification of 3 biomarkers (a) apolipoprotein A1 (down-regulated in cancer); (b) a truncated form of transthyretin (down-regulated); and (c) a cleavage fragment of inter-alpha-trypsin inhibitor heavy chain H4 (up-regulated). The other promising technology is to use metabolites as markers for cancer. One of the first markers identified using metabolites, lysophophatidic acid, happens to be a marker for ovarian cancer. Recently a new potential marker, Carcinoma cell-specific Mig7, have been identified for circulating and migrating cancer cells. This would form the next generation of imaging techniques which would play key role in the noninvasive screening for early detection of cancer.

Chapter IV A - Ovarian cancer is characterized by a lack of clinical symptoms, presentation in advanced stages and poor survival. Despite major research development leading to an increased comprehension of the pathophysiology of this disease, advances in successful therapeutics have lagged. It is the most frequent cause of death by gynecological cancer. To date, new strategies have been considered in order to improve the early diagnosis of the disease by means of image techniques, tumor marker assays, proteomics and gene-expression microarrays. Tumor markers will be discussed in this review as an alternative to the early diagnosis, follow-up of patients already undergone treatment and in the differentiation between benign and malignant ovarian masses, with intent to optimize and amplify the benefits of treatment. CA 125 is the most frequent tumor marker for ovarian tumors, but due to the difficulties in the differentiation between benign and malignant tumors, it has been associated to other biomarkers such as CA 15.3, CA 19.9 and CA 72.4 to improve the accuracy of the method in the screening of ovarian cancer. Besides, serial measurements of CA 15.3, CA 19.9 and CA 72.4 constitute an alternative to patients with negative CA 125. In mucinous tumors, measurements of CA 72.4 are recommended in the differentiation between benign and malignant tumors, although the positivity rate of CA 72.4 has been found to be significantly lower than CA 125 in patients with borderline tumor. The tumor markers ß-human chorionic gonadotropin and alpha-fetoprotein are useful in the diagnosis and follow-up in women with ovarian tumor of germinal origin. The serum levels of inhibin and estrogen can be increased in tumors of the sex cord and from stromal origin. However, it will also be emphasized that the detection of tumor markers in diseases other than cancer, reflecting its heterogeneity, has turned difficult its use as an isolated method, being necessary new discoveries to optimize its use in ovarian tumors. Despite the new advances, the diagnosis of ovarian cancer is late and the treatment in advanced stages is still based on surgery of cytoreduction and chemotherapy. Combination of transvaginal ultrasound, Doppler and quantification of serum tumor markers is a good strategy for the diagnosis of ovarian neoplasia.

Chapter IV B - Phyllodes tumors of the breast are biphasic lesions characterized by leaf like pattern arising from stromal expansion, with the stroma showing variable degree of cellularity and even sarcomatous changes. While most phyllodes tumors are benign, some may recur or metastasize, behaving in a malignant fashion. Conventionally, histological parameters of stromal cellularity, nuclear pleomorphism, stromal overgrowth, mitotic activity and margin configuration are used for grading, but to date, these criteria are not definitive. Recently, attempts have been made to evaluate the overexpression of various protein markers that have been proven to be useful in other human malignancies. p53 is a tumor suppressor gene located on 17p13, implicated in cell growth and division regulation, DNA repair and apoptosis. In phyllodes tumors, there is increased p53 protein expression in higher grade lesions compared to lower grade lesions. Hormonal receptor expression in phyllodes tumors is not well known. Estrogen and progesterone receptor expression was more common in the epithelial than the stromal component, and the epithelial expression decreased with increasing grade of the phyllodes tumors. Ki67 is a non histone nuclear protein that is present throughout the cell cycle, but it reaches a peak value during the G2M phase. It was reported that the Ki67 (proliferation) index increased progressively form benign to malignant phyllodes tumors. Furthermore, flow cytometry showed that benign phyllodes tumors were diploid, and aneuploidy was identified in some of the higher grade phyllodes tumors, paralleled by an S phase fraction increase from benign to malignant phyllodes tumors. Tumor angiogenesis assessed by microvessel density has been extensively investigated for carcinoma of the breast, and has been proposed as a prognostic factor in breast cancer. In phyllodes tumors, a progressive increase in microvessel density with increasing grade of phyllodes tumours has been demonstrated. Interestingly, this increase was independent of other traditional histologic criteria, suggesting that angiogenesis may be an important independent predictor for malignancy. c-kit (CD117) is a proto-oncogene that encodes a tyrosine kinase receptor and is now considered a diagnostic marker for gastrointestinal stromal tumors (GIST). It has been shown that there is a progressive increase in c-kit expression from benign to malignant phyllodes. The underlying mechanism for this differential c-kit expression remains uncertain, and is probably distinct from that of GIST. The potential of tyrosine kinase inhibitor as a treatment modality in malignant phyllodes tumors remains to be explored.

Chapter V – Estradiol (E2) plays a key role in the development and progression of breast cancer. While in postmenopausal women systemic E2 levels are greatly diminished, intratumoral sex steroid concentrations remain high thus providing an estrogenic environment that is favourable for tumor growth. The local estrogen E2 concentration is essentially mediated by the concerted action of the four enzymes aromatase, 17□ hydroxysteriod dehydrogenase type 1 (17□HSD1), estrogen sulfotransferase (EST) and steroid sulfatase (STS). While the enzymatic activity of aromatase and STS results in an increase of bioactive estradiol, 17□HSD2 and EST reduce local E2 levels by converting the hormone into biologically inactive estrogen sulfates or less active metabolites. The importance of aromatase has been identified early and has lead to extensive studies investigating the predictive and prognostic value of this enzyme. Considerably less is, however, is known about the other three enzymes. This is especially remarkable since it has been suggested that STS activity, which transforms estrone sulfates into the biologically active unconjugated E2, is in general 100-500 times higher than aromatase activity, which converts androgens into estrogens. Several new compounds, such as dydrogesterone, sulfamates and tibolone, have been developed which are potent sulfatase inhibitors. In this article the authors describe the action and relevance of modulators of local E2 in breast cancer. The authors also discuss the prognostic value of intratumoral enzyme expression pattern and their potential use as predictors of response to endocrine antineoplastic therapies.

Chapter VI - The American Cancer Society estimates that in the United States, 234,460 new cases of prostate cancer will be diagnosed in 2006. Although 80% of diagnosed patients will eventually die from an unrelated reason, prostate cancer still accounts for the second highest cause of cancer-related deaths in men in the United States, with 27,350 deaths estimated for 2006. This has produced much interest in the early diagnosis and treatment of clinically pertinent cases in which the length or quality of life would be greatly impacted by the natural course of prostate cancer.

From 1988 to the present, the availability of clinically practical screening tests has been limited to the digital rectal exam (DRE), the serum prostate specific antigen (PSA) test, and transrectal ultrasound (TRUS)-guided prostate biopsy. Early in the PSA era, which revolutionized the diagnosis of prostate cancer, many prostate biopsies were performed simply for elevated values. These patients yielded many positive pathologic findings and went on to receive treatment by way of radical prostatectomy, radiation therapy, and hormone suppression therapy. However, with the knowledge that upwards of 80% of patients diagnosed with prostate cancer will eventually die of a cause unrelated to their slowly progressive cancer, interest was turned to detection of more “clinically relevant” cancers, those cancers that would potentially impact the quality and length of a patient’s life. More sensitive methods of detecting serum PSA levels and extrapolative derivatives of this biomarker such as PSA doubling time (PSA DT), PSA velocity (PSAV), PSA density (PSAD), percentage free PSA, and the use of the PSA nadir after primary treatment have progressively furnished superior detection and treatment modalities of prostate cancer. The Surveillance, Epidemiology, and End Results (SEER) program has demonstrated that advances in screening and detection of prostate cancer over the past 20 years have yielded diagnosis at progressively lower levels of prognostic risk. For many patients, this has afforded curative treatment and a decrease in prostate cancer specific mortality. The proportion of patients with low-risk disease defined as those with a PSA≤10 ng/mL, Gleason pathologic grade less than 7 (without any grade 4 or 5 component), and clinical stage T1 or T2a disease has increased from 31% of patients in 1990 to 47% of patients in 2001. In contrast, the high-risk diagnoses (PSA>20ng/mL, Gleason sum > 7, or clinical stage T3 or T4) has decreased from 41% to 15% of prostate cancer diagnoses [2]. The American Cancer Society estimates that this downward risk migration with earlier treatment is the reason for the 3.5% yearly decrease in the death rate noted in recent years. This positive news is contrasted by the unfortunate fact that some patients may be subjected to unnecessary invasive procedures with their numerous possible complications. Efforts are being directed to develop algorithms and screening tests with greater sensitivity and specificity for clinically relevant prostate cancer to decrease unnecessary biopsies and treatment and to also decrease overall healthcare costs.

Modern advances in the fields of genomics and microarray technology have allowed the medical community to embrace the possibility of diagnosis and treatment of diseases even before their clinical presentations. This is of immense clinical interest in oncology, as the ability to effect change on tumor biology at a cellular level would revolutionize the treatment of all types of cancer. These advances are beginning to elucidate biomarkers that could potentially be used to diagnose, as well as follow current treatment in numerous types of cancer, including prostate cancer.

Chapter VII - *Aim*: To assess the validity of free to total (F/T) prostate specific antigen ratio as a predictor of prostate biopsy outcome, and its usefulness in improving biopsy positive predictive value.

Material and methods: A consecutive series of 1,093 prostate biopsies performed during 2002-2005 was considered. Variables tested as possible predictors were age, findings at palpation (DRE) and ultrasonography (TRUS), total PSA, and F/T. Association to biopsy outcome (cancer vs non-cancer) was investigated by univariate and multivariate analysis.

*Results:* All tested variables showed a statistically significant and independent association to biopsy outcome, either at univariate or multivariate analysis. Nevertheless, no variable had a good performance as a biopsy indicator: depending on the considered variable, from 3.4 to 7 cancers would be missed to spare 10 benign biopsies. Using 0.12, 0.15 or 0.20 cut off for F/T would spare 77.3, 64.4 or 43.1% of benign biopsies but would miss 54.0, 35.6 or 21.0 % of cancers, respectively. Cost-benefit ratio was slightly better, though still clinically unacceptable, among random biopsies with negative DRE and TRUS, in the 4-10 ng/ml total PSA range: missed cancers varied from 2 to 1.2 per 10 spared benign biopsies, depending on F/T cut off value.

*Conclusion:* Although it may contribute to diagnostic suspicion, F/T should neither discount a biopsy indicated for suspicious DRE or TRUS, nor determine random biopsies prompted by PSA elevation.

Chapter VIII - Despite advances in our cellular and molecular knowledge, hepatocellular carcinoma (HCC) remains one of the major public health problems throughout the world. It is now known to be highly heterogeneous: it encompasses various pathological entities and a wide range of clinical behaviors, and is underpinned by a complex array of gene alterations that affect supra-molecular processes. Surgical resection is currently the most effective treatment strategy, but many cases are unsuitable for surgery because of the presence of intrahepatic or distant metastases at the time of diagnosis, and so it is therefore extremely important to recognize the disease and any recurrence as early as possible.

Four categories of HCC tumour markers have been proposed: a) onco-fetal and glycoprotein antigens; b) enzymes and iso-enzymes; c) cytokines and d) genes. A family of tumour-associated antigens called cancer-testis (CT) antigens has recently been identified and their encoding genes have been extensively investigated. CT antigens are expressed in a limited number of normal tissues as well as in malignant tumors of unrelated histological origin (including the liver), and are being vigorously pursued as targets for therapeutic cancer vaccines. They are also being evaluated because of their role in oncogenesis and the recapitulation of portions of the germ line gene-expression programme, which might contribute characteristic features to the neoplastic phenotype such as immortality, invasiveness, immune evasion, hypomethylation and metastatic capacity. Given that cancers are being recognized as increasingly complex (an intrinsic property of every human neoplasia), the authors here review the role of CT antigens as liver tumour biomarkers and their validation process, and discuss why they may improve the effectiveness of screening HCC patients and help in determining the risk of developing HCC.

Chapter IX - Urine pregnancy test is a basic laboratory investigation at present. It is widely used for detection of pregnancy in suspected female cases. Basically, this test used the immunological reaction for detection of human choriogonadotropin (hCG). The hCG is a hormone that is used as a tumor marker. Here, the author reports the application of urine pregnancy test as a tumor marker for male from a tertiary hospital laboratory. It was found that there are some applications of urine pregnancy test as a tumor marker in lung cancer. This application can be an alternative and inexpensive tool in diagnosis and following up the patient with lung cancer.

Chapter X - In this chapter the authors demonstrate that short seven-amino acid residue motifs with high degree of similarity to the sequence LDKYACN (residues 26-32) of human epidermal growth factor (EGF) are characteristic for a number of tumor-associated fetal proteins including alpha-fetoprotein (AFP) and growth factors of EGF family and transforming growth factor (TGF-β) superfamily. Besides, the EGF motifs were found in proteins involved cell adhesion and migration. In multi-modular proteins such motifs are localized within their EGF-like modules. An EGF-like motif LDSYQCT of human AFP (residues 14-20) has been obtained as isolated peptidic fragment using solid phase chemistry and tested for biological activity. Ability of this peptide to regulate cell proliferation and apoptosis has been experimentally demonstrated. Here the authors suppose that the short EGF-like motifs are responsible for common functions of the proteins and may be considered as a signature of their participation in regulation of embryonic and tumor cell proliferation, differentiation, migration and survival.

Chapter X A - A biological marker is a substance, a structure or a process that entails a cellular, biochemical, molecular or genetic alteration, measurable qualitatively or quantitatively in biological samples from tissue, cells or bodily fluids and that can determine or predict the current status or outcome of a disease.

The detection of tumor-specific DNA changes, such as promoter gene hypermethylation, seems to be a more advantageous strategy than the techniques based on protein or RNA detection because DNA is more stable than RNA and, in contrast to proteins, DNA is amplifiable, which results in a heightened sensitivity to protein detection.

Aberrant methylation of the promoter gene regions has been identified early in the tumor genesis process, with it being presented in preneoplastic lesions and in preinvasive carcinomas. This enables the detection of these changes in DNA isolated in bodily fluids or from gastrointestinal washings. Recently, it has been reported that patients with infiltrating tumors present free-circulating DNA in the plasma that originates predominantly from necrotic or apoptotic tumor cells. This facilitates the development of diagnostic or plasmatic screening methods by means of the identification of typical genetic patterns for each tumor or group of tumors.

The frequency of these alterations, the earliness of their appearance and the development of decision sensitive and efficient mechanisms for the detection of DNA methylation by means of methylation-specific PCR techniques convert into hypermethylation of the gene promoter areas in a biological marker of risk states that could enable the development of a screening method for the early diagnosis of neoplasias.

Chapter X B - Cholangiocarcinoma, a malignancy of the biliary duct system, tends to grow slowly and to infiltrate the walls of the ducts, dissecting along tissue planes and leading to biliary tract obstruction. Surgery remains the only curative treatment option for cholangiocarcinoma. Currently, the diagnosis is still hard and the specific tumor marker for cholangiocarcinoma is not available. Several serum and bile markers for the diagnosis of cholangiocarcinoma have been mentioned including fast liver alkaline phosphatase, carbohydrate antigen (CA) 19-9, interleukin-6, lactate, trypsinogen-2, pancreatic polypeptide, p53 mutations, p16 (INK4a), p14 (ARF) promoter hypermethylation. In this article, these new potential tumor markers for cholangiocarcinoma will be reviewed.

Chapter XI - Hepatoma is a common gastrointestinal malignancy in viral hepatitis cases which is difficult to detect in early stages. The two important viral hepatitis associated with hepatoma are hepatitis B and hepatitis C viruses. Alpha fetoprotein (AFP) is a tumor marker which has been introduced for screening but in the settings where the rate of hepatitis B and hepatitis C seropositivity is very high, the diagnostic benefit is still doubtful. Here, a metanalysis on the previous reports is conducted and the conclusion that serum AFP can not be recommended for viral hepatitis carriers over standard tests is set.

Chapter XII - Hepatocellular carcinoma (HCC) is one of the most common and aggressive malignant tumor and recently ranked the third leading cause of cancer death worldwide. The incidence of HCC has been steadily increasing; and the major etiologic factors such as alcoholism and chronic hepatitis virus infection are the causative agents. Currently, there is no definite cure available and surgery is the primary treatment modality. Regardless of the advanced surgical technique, the prognosis is still poor, owing to the high rate of cancer recurrence and late diagnosis when the tumor becomes practically unresectable. Today, the liver cancer surveillance program relies on the detection of serum alfa-fetoprotein (AFP) and ultrasound imaging, which however, has limited sensitivity and specificity, and often operator dependent, respectively. Thus, identification of new biomarkers for better diagnosis of HCC is of great interest and high clinical priorities. Recent efforts on genomic and proteomic research have led to the discovery of panel diagnostic and prognostic markers for HCC. These include fucosylated fraction of AFP, heat shock proteins, glypican-3, and other biomarkers. Some of these markers are being evaluated in multi-center trials under the auspice of Early Detection Research Network. Besides, there have been significant efforts on unearthing a handful of biomarkers that are correlated with different clinical situations of liver diseases as in the cases of cirrhosis and tumor metastasis. In the foreseeable future, at-risk patients (viral hepatitis and cirrhosis) would benefit from earlier intervention and better treatment options for liver cancer that is made possible as a result of cancer biomarker discovery.

Chapter XIII - Tissue tumor markers play important role in diagnosis of variety neoplasms. This review aims to summarize: 1/ diagnostic and prognostic difficulties in thyroid and colorectal cancer; 2/ currently available thyroid and colorectal tumor markers; 3/ role of galectin-3 in diagnosis and/or prognosis of these tumors. Results of the authors current related studies will be also presented.

Thyroid tumors of follicular cell origin represent diagnostically and prognostically difficult group of neoplasms. Namely differentiation between follicular adenoma and carcinoma or between follicular tumor and follicular variant of papillocarcinoma desires additional methods of evaluation, such as immunohistochemical examination of tumor markers (proliferative markers, thyroid peroxidase (TPO), cytokeratin 19 (CK-19), galectin-3 etc).

Colorectal carcinoma is the common cancer in the industrial countries with the high mortality. The main task at the time of pathologist´s diagnosis consists in assessment of metastatic potential of colorectal cancer using tumor markers such as metalloproteinases (MMP), tissue inhibitors of metalloproteinases (TIMPS), mucins, and galectin-3 as well.

Galectin-3 (endogenous ß-galactoside-binding protein) as a member of widely distributed carbohydrate-binding proteins that have beeen implicated in the spectrum physiological and pathobiological processes including malignant transformation. Galectin-3 was proven to be expressed in variety cancer cells, mainly of thyroid and colorectal cancer. Its expression in above mentioned tumors has been intensively studied in respects of diagnostic and prognostic role of this tumor marker.

In conclusion, plenty of prognostic and diagnostic thyroid and colorectal tumor markers has been so far studied. However, the ideal specific marker occuring solely within malignant tumor and reliably predicting its biological behavior does not exist. Galectin-3 seems to be promising diagnostic marker in malignant thyroid tumors of follicular cell origin as well as prognostic marker predicting metastases in colorectal carcinomas. Based on the authors research results and literary experience the authors recommend to add this marker to the list of significant thyroid and colorectal tissue tumor markers.

Chapter XIV - Uncontrolled cell proliferation is one of the major features of tumor cells. The rate of cell proliferation determines the biologic behavior and, in many cases, the clinical course of a neoplasm. Thus, proliferative indices provide valuable prognostic information in this setting. However, in the case of aggressive human lymphoid tumors, there is an admixture of normal (reactive) cells in all organs infiltrated by neoplastic cells. To ascertain the influence of reactive cell on proliferative index measurements, an approach for detection of tumor cell subpopulation in large cell lymphomas has been developed. The results suggest that proliferative indices calculated for lymphoid neoplasms depend not only on the proliferative activity of the tumor cells, but also on the percentage of cells that are neoplastic. 'Tumor cell proliferative indices' can differ significantly from proliferative indices for the corresponding overall cell populations. The authors propose that the use of tumor cell proliferative indices results in more accurate assessment of disease prognosis. Also, it seems that the use of different features of cell populations can give valuable information concerning biological behavior of human neoplasms. The complex digital image analysis approach allows the authors to describe peculiarities in nuclear size distributions (e.g., histogram form, descriptive statistics of overall populations and subpopulations, etc.), morphologic characteristics of cells in different subpopulations, and proliferative rates of cells in overall cell population and different subpopulations. Taken together, these characteristics are referred to as 'the cell population structure'. The significance of the cell population structure investigations for lymphoma diagnostics is discussed.

Chapter XV - Presently, tumor marker is a group of laboratory investigation used in medical laboratory. Laboratory medicine principle is also applied for the tumor marker investigation. Here, the author reports two case studies on aberration of tumor marker test in laboratory medicine. The first case is a female patient with post operative ovarian clear cell carcinoma presented with the unexpected and unexplained high CA125 level due to the immunological alteration from medication. The second case is a male patient with chronic hepatitis B infection presented with abnormal high AFP level due to the macromolecule phenomenon. These two cases are good examples in tumor marker determination in laboratory medicine.

Chapter XVI - Epithelial (E-) cadherin has a major role in the maintenance of intercellular junction between epithelial cells. The association of the catenins (α-, β- and γ-) to E-cadherin in the formation of the E-cadherin-catenin complex unit (ECCU) is a key step in the function of intact adhesion complexes at the *adherens* junction. Alterations in E-cadherin or any one of the catenin molecules may lead to reduced cell-cell adhesion resulting in tumour cell invasion. In our previous studies, loss and reduced expression of E-cadherin and β-catenin was associated with poor tumour differentiation, peritoneal metastasis, advanced tumour stage, and poor patient prognosis.

*Purpose*: the immunohistochemical expression of E-cadherin and the catenins was examined in a selected group of Epithelial Ovarian Tumours (EOT) in an attempt to evaluate the inter relationship between each of these proteins essential in the formation of the ECCU, and their role in ovarian carcinogenesis.

*Patients and methods*: The series of this study includes 5 borderline tumours and 19 carcinomas selected from a previous studies based on the observation that these tumours showed negative expression for either E-cadherin or β-catenin.

*Results*: Disruption of the E-cadherin–catenin complex was noted in terms of both E-cadherin and catenin loss. Negative expression of E-cadherin and the catenins α-, β-, and γ- was observed in the majority of the EOT. Some tumours continued to express E-cadherin at the cell membrane, yet showed loss of the catenins, implying that the necessary components to directly interact and associate with E-cadherin are absent and as a result a functional ECCU cannot be formed.

*Conclusion:* Accepting the limitation of our sample size, our results show that loss of E-cadherin or the catenins necessary for strong cell-to-cell adhesion occur in borderline and malignant tumours, implying that the normal function of these molecules is disrupted. Disturbance of the E-cadherin-catenin complex by loss of E-cadherin, or β-catenin, to α-catenin may play a role in ovarian carcinogenesis, since cell movement, proliferation, and tumour cell invasion are key events that would require loss of tight cell-cell adhesion.

Chapter XVII - To attain a goal of personalized medicine, the authors need to improve our understanding of cancer at the molecular level to implement effective primary and secondary prophylaxis, early diagnosis, and optimize drug treatment for each individual. With help from biomedical sciences the authors can start answering vital questions regarding inheritance of cancer risk, biology and treatment of individual patient: Am I at risk for cancer? Is family history an important factor? Have I inherited and/or can I pass my predisposition to cancer? Is there anything I can do to alter the risk? If the cancer already exists, the authors want to know if it responds to a particular therapy and whether it will respond over time. Genomic (DNA), transcriptional (RNA) and translational (protein) research alone will not be sufficient to provide answers to these questions, which are likely to come from concerted efforts in these disciplines with a focus on early stages of cancer. Proteomics has potential for discovering new practical biomarkers for primary prophylaxis (avoidance of risk factors), secondary prophylaxis (mass screening), and early detection. Emerging tools for sensitive, high resolution and high throughput proteomic analysis including protein arrays, multiplexed immunoassays and mass spectral body fluids (blood, cerebrospinal fluid, urine) and tissue analyses are now yielding new putative proteomic biomarkers and protein signature patterns that need to be validated in the clinic. Recently discovered dramatic gender-specific differences in expression of thousands of genes further underline needs for analysis of the proteome in health and disease. These novel approaches to prophylaxis, early detection and therapy are expected to change the ways how cancer is diagnosed and treated.

In: Tumor Markers Research Focus
Editor: Deborah H. Chang, pp. 1
ISBN: 978-1-60021-544-5


*Expert Commentary A*

# Tumor Markers in Prostrate Cancer

***Edward N. Rampersaud, Leon Sun and Judd W. Moul***

Increased sensitivity of testing, decreased morbidity associated with diagnosis, and effective treatment are the pillars of today's medical practice. As such, advances in prostate cancer screening and detection are of principal interest. Primary treatment of prostate cancer at present includes four focal modalities: prostatectomy, radiation therapy, cryotherapy and watchful waiting. Much of the basic science research of late has been directed at the molecular targeting of prostate cancer cells, yielding the main arm of current clinical research which is focused on chemotherapeutic and hormonal treatment of those who fail our current primary treatment armamentarium. Data analyses from numerous prostate cancer databases across the United States are becoming increasingly successful in predicting those that would most likely fail current primary therapy and benefit from pre-emptive adjunctive treatments. Many of these studies have been focused on the use of peri-treatment PSA and its derivatives (PSA velocity, PSA doubling-time, PSA nadir, etc.) combined with screening pathology data to predict post-treatment failure as well as predicting prognosis. Other studies have been analyzing data concerning tumor biopsy and the potential to lend insight regarding total tumor characteristics and behavior. In regards to cancer detection, biomolecular testing and microarray technology are proving to be promising innovations that may one day serve to augment the diagnostic arsenal available. The discovery and application of novel biomarkers may pave the road to earlier diagnosis with greater sensitivity than current methods.

All of these various research endeavors must continue so that earlier detection, combined with a better understanding of cancer biology can produce increasingly better outcomes with decreased morbidity. The future holds the true means of cancer eradication in the prevention of initial disease development and progression. Whereas the imagination can see the day of genomic identification and intervention of those bound to develop prostate cancer, today we yield to the tools available: namely the PSA test and its derivatives, digital rectal examination, clinical history, and prostate biopsy.

In: Tumor Markers Research Focus
Editor: Deborah H. Chang, pp. 3-31
ISBN: 978-1-60021-544-5


*Chapter I*

# Biochemical Markers of Bone Remodelling for Multiple Myeloma

***Evangelos Terpos[1,2] and John Meletis[3]***
[1]Department of Haematology and Medical Research, General Airforce Hospital, Athens, Greece
[2]Department of Haematology, Faculty of Medicine Imperial College London, London, UK
[3]First Department of Internal Medicine, University of Athens School of Medicine, Laikon General Hospital, Athens, Greece

## Abstract

Osteolytic bone disease is a frequent complication of multiple myeloma, resulting in skeletal complications that are a significant cause of morbidity and mortality. A characteristic feature of myeloma bone disease is that the lesions rarely heal and bone scans are often negative in myeloma patients who have extensive lytic lesions, offering very little in the follow-up of bone disease. X-rays are also of limited value in monitoring bone destruction during anti-myeloma or anti-resorptive treatment. Biochemical markers of bone turnover, such as N- and C-terminal cross-linking telopeptide of type I collagen (NTX, CTX/ICTP, respectively), bone specific alkaline phosphatase, osteocalcin, and newer ones such as the tartrate resistant acid phosphatase isoform 5b, and bone sialoprotein provide information on bone dynamics that in turn may reflect disease activity in bone. Several studies have shown bone markers to be elevated in myeloma patients and reflect the extent of bone disease, while in some of them bone resorption markers correlate with survival. These markers may also be helpful in identifying those patients likely to respond to bisphosphonate treatment, and monitoring the effectiveness of bisphosphonate therapy in the management of myeloma bone disease. Anti-myeloma therapy including autologous stem cell transplantation seems to normalize abnormal bone remodelling by reducing bone resorption markers and increasing bone formation indices. This chapter attempts to summarize the existing data for the role of markers of bone remodelling in assessing the extent of bone destruction in myeloma and monitoring bone turnover during specific anti-myeloma treatment. We also discuss some novel markers that may be of particular interest in the near future.

# Introduction

Multiple Myeloma (MM) is a clonal plasma cell disorder characterized by bone destruction, immunodeficiency, and renal impairment. Nearly 3,500 people in the UK are diagnosed with MM each year. This accounts for 10% of blood cancers and 1% of all cancers. More than 55% of patients who present with MM are aged 60 or older, while less than 3% of MM occurs in patients younger than 40 years; median survival ranges between 3.5-5 years [1, 2]. A cure in MM appears to be achievable only by allogeneic transplantation, which is not the treatment of choice for the majority of patients due to high rate of transplant-related mortality [3]. A major clinical feature of MM is the presence of osteolytic bone disease and generalized osteoporosis, which can lead to severe bone pain, pathologic fractures, spinal cord compression, and hypercalcemia. Over 85% of myeloma patients have bone disease. It thus represents a major cause of morbidity and mortality [4]. Progression of skeletal disease is often not affected by chemotherapy even in responding patients [5]. The mechanisms of bone destruction appear to be related to increased osteoclastic bone resorption, which is not accompanied by a comparable increase in bone formation [6]. Thus, a characteristic feature of myeloma bone disease is that the lesions rarely heal even when the patients are in complete remission [7]. This finding is in keeping with the observation that bone scans are often negative in myeloma patients who have extensive lytic lesions, and offer very little in the follow-up of bone disease in these patients [8]. Furthermore, sequential measurement of bone mineral density (BMD) using DEXA-scans produced heterogeneous local BMD changes and the available data do not support routine use of sequential DEXA-scans in MM [9]. The bone disease in MM is usually assessed by X-rays of the skeleton. X-rays are useful in the diagnosis of osteolytic lesions, but do not give any dynamic information on the ongoing bone resorption. In contrast, biochemical markers of bone metabolism specifically reflect bone resorption or bone formation rates and are strongly affected by the processes active in myeloma bone disease. Therefore, biochemical markers of bone remodelling are used more often nowadays in an attempt to improve monitoring of bone destruction in MM.

In addition, strategies that target osteoclast activation and proliferation represent an important approach to the management of myeloma bone disease. Bisphosphonates consist of a heterogeneous group of agents that affect bone metabolism and regulation of calcium homeostasis, mainly through an inhibitory effect on osteoclasts [10]. Several studies have demonstrated their efficacy in myeloma bone disease and therefore they are included in all therapeutic regimens for stage II/III myeloma patients [11, 12]. Biochemical markers of bone resorption and formation have also been used to follow up myeloma bone disease during bisphosphonates administration. This chapter attempts to summarize the existing data for the role of markers of bone remodelling in assessing the extent of bone destruction in myeloma and monitoring bone turnover during specific anti-myeloma chemotherapy or bisphosphonates administration.

# Pathogenesis of Bone Disease in Multiple Myeloma

Although the mechanisms responsible for the development of myeloma bone disease currently remain unclear, several studies have begun to shed new light on this process. Histomorphometric studies have demonstrated that myeloma bone destruction is related to increased osteoclastic activity, which is not accompanied by a comparable increase in osteoblast formation. This uncoupling of resorption and formation leads to rapid bone loss [13]. A number of cytokines and growth factors that are produced either by myeloma cells or by stromal cells, due to interactions between them, have been implicated in the increase in osteoclast formation and activity in MM. The adherence of myeloma cells to bone marrow stromal cells results in enhanced production of cytokines, such as interleukin-6 (IL-6), interleukin 1-beta (IL-1β), interleukin 11 (IL-11), tumor necrosis factors alpha and beta (TNFα, TNFβ), basic fibroblast growth factor (bFGF), macrophage-colony stimulating factor (M-CSF), which stimulate human osteoclast formation [4]. IL-6 also acts as a survival factor for myeloma cells [14]. Furthermore, stromal cells also produce receptor activator of nuclear factor kappa-B ligand (RANKL), a member of the tumor necrosis factor (TNF) gene family. Following activation of the cellular receptor RANK on osteoclasts by its ligand, RANKL, differentiation, proliferation, and survival of osteoclasts is enhanced, osteoclast fusion and activation is promoted, and osteoclastic apoptosis is suppressed, leading to a dramatic increase of the number and activity of osteoclasts [15, 16]. In addition, production of osteoprotegerin (OPG), a soluble decoy receptor of RANKL produced by marrow stromal cells, is suppressed through the above interactions and has been found to be reduced in patients with MM [17-19]. The mechanisms through which OPG levels are decreased have not been clearly defined yet, but a study by Standal et al has shown that OPG is bound, internalized, and degraded by the myeloma cells through CD138 [20]. The ratio RANKL/OPG is reversed in myeloma, leading to osteoclast activation and bone destruction [15, 19, 21-24]. Several reports have suggested that myeloma cells also produce RANKL and that the expression of RANKL by human myeloma cells mediates osteoclast formation *in vitro* and correlates with bone destruction *in vivo* [25-27]. However, other investigators have not been able to detect RANKL expression on myeloma cells [21]. The amount of RANKL produced by myeloma cells is rather small to stimulate osteoclast formation by itself and it may be sufficient only to prevent osteoclast apoptosis [4, 28]. Several cytokines produced by both myeloma and stromal cells, such as IL-3, IL-6, IL-11 exerts their effect through RANKL/RANK/OPG pathway, inducing osteoclastogenesis [4, 10, 29, 30].

Myeloma cells also produce large amounts of macrophage inflammatory protein-1 alpha (MIP-1α), which is a low molecular weight chemokine that belongs to the RANTES family, and activates the osteoclasts directly [31-34]. MIP-1α levels are elevated in both bone marrow plasma and serum of patients with active MM and correlate with the presence of lytic lesions [35, 36]. High concentrations of MIP-1α were mainly found in patients with advanced and active disease. Furthermore, MIP-1α has also been shown to increase RANKL expression on bone marrow stromal cells, thus inducing further bone destruction [33]. The major role of both RANK/RANKL and MIP-1α pathways in myeloma bone disease has been established in murine models. The inhibition of RANKL and MIP-1α activity results in markedly decreased bone destruction and a significant reduction in tumor burden [37-40].

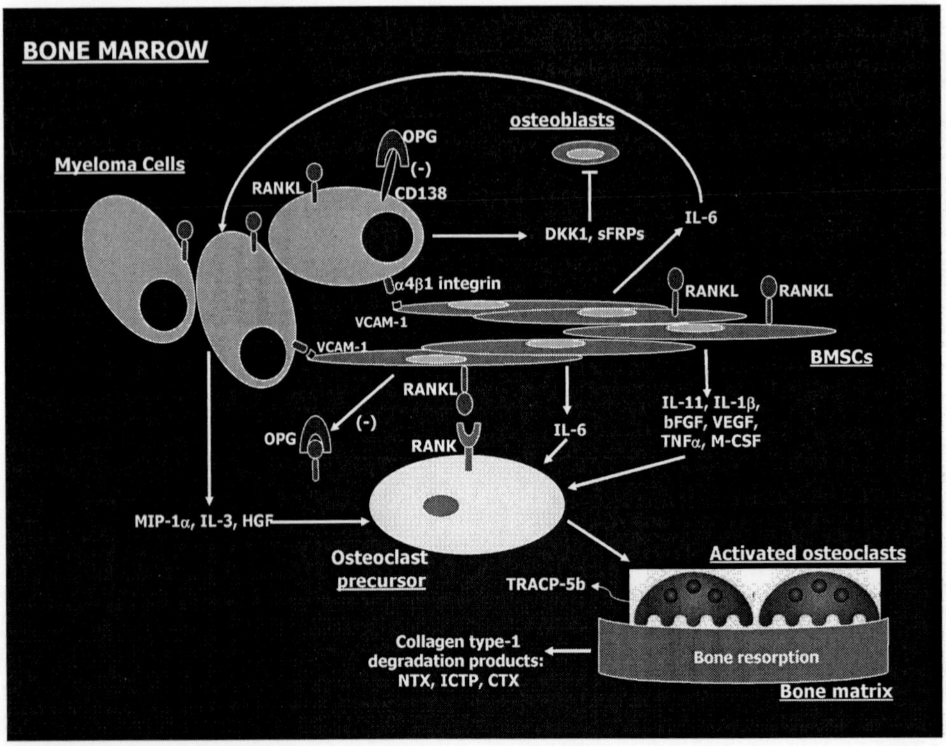


Figure 1. The adherence of MM cells to bone marrow stromal cells (BMSC)/osteoblasts enhances the production of RANKL, M-CSF, and other cytokines with OAF activity (IL-6, IL-1β, TNFs, bFGF, IGFs), while it suppresses the production of OPG (the decoy receptor of RANKL). The above cytokines also modify the bone marrow microenvironment, up-regulating the RANKL expression and secretion by both BMSC and osteoblasts. Furthermore, myeloma cells produce MIP-1α, HGF, and VEGF that enhance the proliferation and differentiation of osteoclast precursors, while myeloma cells express both transmembrane and soluble RANKL. OPG binds both surface and soluble RANKL inhibiting osteoclast development and bone resorption. Syndecan 1 (CD138) expressed on the surface of, and secreted from, the myeloma cells can bind soluble OPG, thus preventing its inhibitory effect on RANKL function. Therefore the ratio of RANKL/OPG is increased, leading to osteoclast differentiation, proliferation and activation. Myeloma cells also produce Dkk-1 protein and sFRP-2 that inhibit stromal cell differentiation to osteoblasts, thereby decreasing bone formation. These interactions result in increased bone resorption, as depicted by the increased levels of bone resorption markers (NTX, ICTP, CTX, TRACP-5b).

As mentioned above, in MM the increased bone formation is accompanied by suppression in osteoblast function. Osteoblasts in active myeloma are functionally exhausted and promptly undergo apoptosis in the presence of myeloma cells from patients with severe bone disease [41]. Tian et al reported that myeloma cells produce dickkopf 1 (Dkk-1) protein, an inhibitor of *Wnt* signalling pathway, which is crucial for osteoblast differentiation. In this study, marrow plasma from patients with MM that contained >12 ng/ml of Dkk-1 inhibited osteoblast differentiation, while gene expression levels of Dkk-1 correlated with the extent of bone disease [42]. Another recent study showed that most malignant plasma cells from patients with advanced bone destructive lesions also expressed secreted Frizzled-related protein 2 (sFRP-2) another antagonist of *Wnt* signalling. Furthermore, exogenous sFRP-2 suppressed osteoblast differentiation induced by bone morphogenic protein-2, and immunodepletion of sFRP-2 significantly restored mineralized nodule formation *in vitro*, suggesting a predominant role for MM cell-derived sFRP-2 in the impairment of bone formation by MM [43]. Thus, in addition to enhanced osteolysis, MM cells also suppress bone formation at least in part through an inhibition of the canonical *Wnt* pathway by secreting sFRP-2 and Dkk-1. The presence of soluble factors produced by myeloma cells that suppresses osteoblast differentiation is a very important finding, which, however, does not entirely explain why myeloma bone lesions do not heal when the patients are in complete remission. There may possibly be a more long-lasting change in the marrow microenvironment that results in an inability of osteoblast precursors to differentiate, even in the absence of myeloma cells. However, this hypothesis remains to be proven.

Figure 1 summarizes the currently available data on osteoclast activation and osteoblast suppression in MM reflecting the role of myeloma microenvironment in the development of myeloma-related bone disease.

## Markers of Bone Remodelling

Throughout life bone undergoes continuous remodelling with removal of old bone and replacement with new bone. Bone turnover is always initiated by osteoclasts eroding a mineralized surface. This process is followed by the recruitment of successive teams of osteoblasts to the outer edge of the erosion cavity that secrete new bone matrix and gradually fill in the resorption cavity [44]. Resorption of old bone and formation of new bone are balanced under normal conditions. In MM, there is a pronounced imbalance in these processes: increased activation of osteoclasts and suppression of osteoblast function. Over the past two decades, the isolation and characterization of cellular and extracellular components of the skeletal matrix have resulted in the development of biochemical markers that specifically reflect either bone formation or bone resorption. Most of the traditional and new markers of bone resorption measure the collagen degradation products from osteoclast activity and include urinary hydroxyproline, hydroxylysine glycosides, total or free pyridinoline cross-links, and cross-linked N- or C-telopeptides [45]. A novel marker, serum tartrate resistant acid phosphatase isoform type 5b (TRACP-5b) which is an enzyme secreted by activated osteoclasts and bone sialoprotein (BSP), a non-collagenous protein have been demonstrated to reflect bone resorptive processes [46, 47]. The formation markers are direct or indirect products of active osteoblasts that enter into the circulation (Figure 2). These include serum bone-specific alkaline phosphatase, osteocalcin and type-I procollagen peptides [48]. All the above markers are depicted in tables 1 and 2. Fasting urinary calcium, used by some investigators to measure bone resorption, is not discussed here as it has been found to be of limited value in MM [49].

**Table 1. Markers of bone resorption**

| Marker | Abbreviation* | Tissue of origin | Analytical Method | Analytical specimen |
|---|---|---|---|---|
| Hydroxyproline | Hyp | All tissues and all genetic types of collagen | Colorimetric, assay, HPLC | Urine |
| Hydroxylysine | Hyl | All tissues and all genetic types of collagen | Reversed-phase HPLC | Urine |
| Galactosyl- hydroxylysine<br>Glucosyl- galactosyl- hydroxylysine | Gal-Hyl<br>Glc-Gal-Hyl | Both Gal-Hyl and Glc-Gal-Hyl appears to be specific for bone collagen degradation | Reversed-phase HPLC | Urine |
| Pyridinoline | PYD | Bone, cartilage, tendon, blood vessels | HPLC, ELISA | Urine |
| Deoxypyridinoline | DPD | Bone, dentin | RIA | Urine (free DPD can be also measured in serum or plasma) |
| N-terminal cross-linking telopeptide of type-I collagen | NTX | All tissues containing type-I collagen | ELISA, RIA | Urine, serum |
| C-terminal cross-linking telopeptide of type-I collagen | CTX | All tissues containing type-I collagen | ELISA, RIA | Urine, serum (β-form only) |
| C-terminal cross-linking telopeptide of type-I collagen generated by MMPs | CTX-MMP or ICTP | All tissues containing type-I collagen | RIA | Serum |
| Tartrate resistant acid phosphatase isoform 5b | TRACP-5b | Bone (osteoclasts) | Colorimetric RIA, ELISA | Serum, plasma |
| Bone sialoprotein | BSP | Bone, dentin, hypertrophic cartilage, carcer cells | RIA, ELISA | Serum |

*According to the Bone Marker Nomenclature by the Committee of Scientific Advisors of the International Osteoporosis Foundation (121)

**Table 2. Markers of bone formation**

| Marker | Abbreviation* | Tissue of origin | Analytical Method | Analytical specimen |
|---|---|---|---|---|
| Osteocalcin (or bone gla-protein) | OC | Bone, platelets | RIA, ELISA, IRMA | Serum |
| Bone alkaline phosphatase | Bone ALP | Bone | ELISA, IRMA, colorimetric assay | Serum |
| Procollagen type-I N propeprtide | PINP | Bone, soft tissue, skin | RIA, ELISA | Serum |
| Procollagen type I C-propeptide | PICP | Bone, soft tissue, skin | RIA, ELISA | Serum |

*According to the Bone Marker Nomenclature by the Committee of Scientific Advisors of the International Osteoporosis Foundation (121)

**Table 3. Studies describing the levels of markers of bone remodelling in MM patients and correlation with clinical data**

| Authors-year | No of patients | Parameter studied | Comparison with controls (symbol refers to MM patients) | Correlation with extent of bone disease | Correlation with survival |
|---|---|---|---|---|---|
| Nawawi et al, 1996[86] | 17 | DPD | ↑* | NA | NA |
| | | TRACP | NS | | |
| | | OC | NS | | |
| | | bALP | NS | | |
| | | PICP | NS | | |
| Abildgaard et al, 1997[87] | 109 | ICTP | ↑* | NA | Yes |
| | | OC | NS | | Yes |
| | | bALP | ↑* | | No |
| | | PICP | NS | | No |
| | | PIIINP | ↑* | | No |
| Withold et al, 1998[88] | 15 | DPD, PYD | ↑* | NA | NA |
| | | bALP, PICP | ↓* | | |
| | 73 | DPD | | | |

**Table 3. (Continued)**

| Authors-year | No of patients | Parameter studied | Comparison with controls (symbol refers to MM patients) | Correlation with extent of bone disease | Correlation with survival |
|---|---|---|---|---|---|
| Carlson et al, 1999[89] | | ICTP<br>OC<br>PICP | ↑*<br>↑*<br>NS<br>NS | Yes<br>Yes<br>No<br>No | No<br>Yes<br>No<br>No |
| Woitge et al, 1999[67] | 18 | PYD<br>DPD<br>NTX<br>CTX<br>BSP | ↑*<br>↑*<br>↑*<br>↑*<br>↑* | NA | NA |
| Fonseca et al, 2000[90] | 313 | ICTP<br>TRACP<br>OC<br>bALP<br>PICP | ↑*<br>↑*<br>↓*<br>NS<br>NS | Yes<br>No<br>No<br>Yes<br>No | Yes<br>No<br>No<br>No<br>No |
| Terpos et al, 2000[91] | 62 | NTX<br>OC<br>bALP | ↑*<br>↓*<br>↓* | NA | NA |
| Woitge et al, 2001[104] | 43 | OC<br>bALP | NS<br>↓* | NA | NA |
| Corso et al, 2001[92] | 52 | DPD<br>OC<br>bALP | ↑* | Yes<br>No | NA |

**Table 3. (Continued)**

| Authors-year | No of patients | Parameter studied | Comparison with controls (symbol refers to MM patients) | Correlation with extent of bone disease | Correlation with survival |
|---|---|---|---|---|---|
| | 57 | DPD | ↓* | No | |
| Jakob et al, 2002[93]** | | NTX | NS | Yes | No |
| | | ICTP | ↑* | No | p=0.05 |
| | | | NS | Yes | Yes |
| Alexandrakis et al, 2002[94] | 38 | PYD | ↑* | | |
| | | DPD | | Yes | NA |
| | | NTX | ↑* | Yes | |
| | | OC | ↑* | Yes | |
| | | bALP | ↑* | No | |
| Abildgaard et al, 2003[95] | | | ↑* | No | |
| | 34 | PYD | NS | | |
| | | DPD | | Yes | NA |
| | | ICTP | ↑* | Yes | |
| | | NTX | ↑* | Yes | |
| Terpos et al, 2003[19] | | | ↑* | Yes | |
| | 121 | NTX | ↑* | | |
| | | TRACP-5b | | Yes | No |
| | | OC | | Yes | No |
| | | bALP | ↑* | Yes | No |
| | | sRANKL/OPG | ↑* | No | No |
| | | | ↓* | Yes | Yes |
| | | | ↓* | | |
| | | | ↑* | | |

*Statistically significant ($p<0.05$)
**MM compared with MGUS patients
NS: non significant
NA: not assessed

Biochemical markers of bone remodelling are noninvasive, comparatively inexpensive, and, when applied and interpreted correctly, helpful tools in the assessment of bone diseases. However, factors that affect the markers' levels, including circadian rhythmicity, diet, age, gender, renal function and drugs, should be clearly defined and appropriately adjusted whenever possible. Another important issue is that biochemical indices reflect the total bone turnover and give little information about the function of individual groups of osteoclasts. All these issues are discussed below.

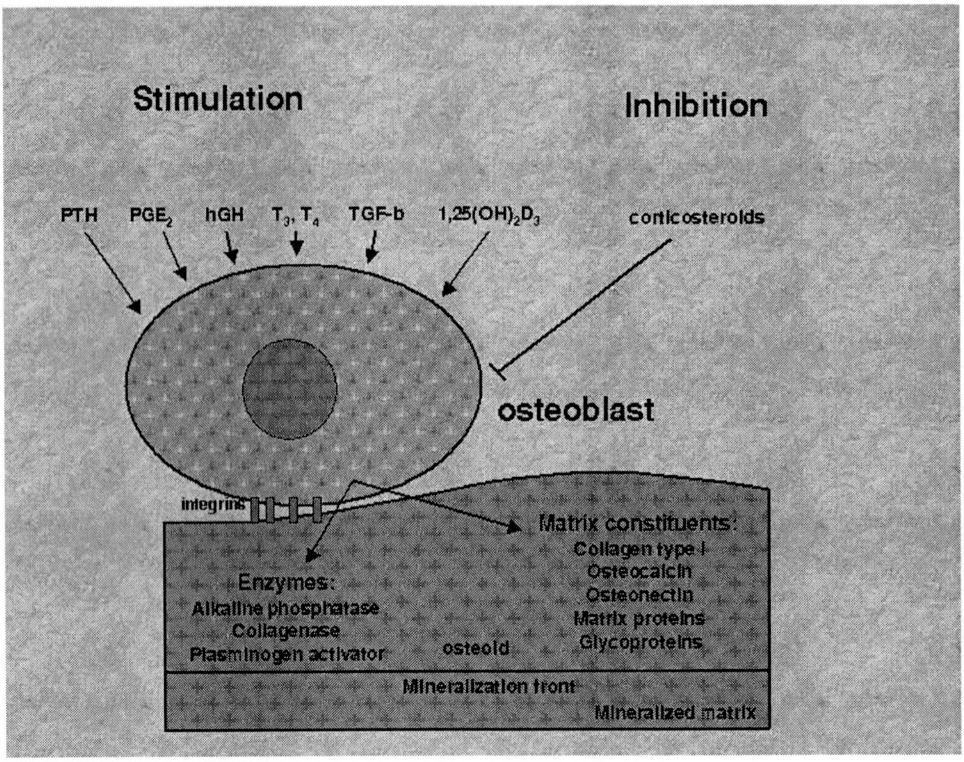


Figure 2. Osteoblast activation: Through stimulators, the osteoblasts produce enzymes, such as ALP and matrix constituents, such as collagen type I and osteocalcin. Bone ALP, osteocalcin, and degradation products of collagen type I can be measured in urine and serum.

# Biochemistry

## Resorption Markers

***Hydroxyproline and Hydroxylysine:*** Hydroxyproline (Hyp) is formed in the cell from the posttranslational hydroxylation of proline. Hyp is the predominant amino acid of collagens, comprising about 13% of these proteins. Hydroxylysine (Hyl) is another amino acid essentially unique to collagenous proteins. Bone is the primary store of collagen in the body, but both Hyp and Hyl are present in essentially all tissues and all genetic types of collagen. The Hyp released during collagen degradation is primarily metabolized in the liver and subsequently excreted in the urine. However, only about 10% of Hyp-containing products from collagen breakdown are excreted in the urine [44]. The small pool of urinary Hyp originates from the N-propeptide of type I collagen. Normal ingestion of gelatin or collagen-rich foods such as meat can increase the level of urinary Hyp, and the urinary peptides containing Hyp from endogenous collagen breakdown are indistinguishable from the dietary peptides [50, 51]. This is a major disadvantage for the use of this marker as a specific index of bone resorption.

Hyl is glycosylated and two glycosides are formed, galactosyl hydroxylysine (Gal-Hyl) and glucosyl galactosyl hydroxylysine (Glc-Gal-Hyl), which also appear in the urine [52]. While Hyl and its glycosides are less abundant than Hyp in bone collagen, certain properties make Hyl theoretically a better marker of bone turnover than urinary Hyp. Gal-Hyl is not metabolized and not influenced by dietary factors [53]. In normal urine, 80% of the total Hyl is in the form of Hyl, 10% is free and unglycosylated, and the remainder is peptide-bound, which suggests that free Hyl is largely metabolized and not excreted [54]. However, in addition to all structural collagens, both Hyp and Hyl are also found in certain serum proteins, such as the C1q component of complement [55]. This disadvantage, in combination with the effect of age and the circadian rhythm (both have their peak excretion after midnight), make them less specific indices of bone resorption and therefore they have been largely replaced by newer markers.

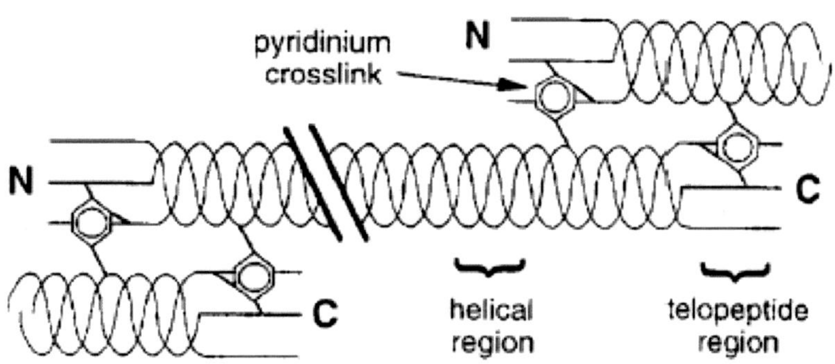


Figure 3. Fibrils of collagen showing the N- and C-terminal ends bonding to helical areas of adjacent fibrils by PYD and DPD.

***Pyridinoline and deoxypyridinoline cross-links of type I collagen:*** In the last decade, collagen cross-links have evolved as promising markers of bone resorption. Pyridinoline (PYD) and deoxypyridinoline (DPD) are formed by the enzymatic action of lysyl oxidase on lysine and Hyl. Newly deposited collagen fibrils in the extracellular matrix are stabilized by cross-links formed by the action of lysyl oxidase on lysine and Hyl residues in telopeptide domains of the collagen molecules. The resulting aldehydes condense with Hyl or lysyl residues on adjacent collagen molecules to form divalent cross-links, which can mature by further condensation with telopeptide aldehydes to the trivalent structures DPD and PYD [44]. PYD and DPD act as mature cross-links in type I collagen of all major connective tissues [56]. These include type I collagen of bone, dentin, tendon, vascular walls, muscle, intestine, etc. Figure 3 depicts the basic crosslinking of collagen fibrils that construct type I collagen, the protein comprising most of the organic matrix of the bone. Each of the fibrils contains aminoterminal and carboxyterminal ends that are termed N-telopeptides (NTX) and

C-telopeptide (CTX), respectively. In type I collagen, these ends are each linked to a helical portion of a nearby molecule by a PYD or DPD crosslink. The pyridinoline cross-links occur essentially at two intermolecular sites in the collagen fibril: two amino-telopeptides are linked to a helical site at or near residue 930 and two carboxy-telopeptides to helical residue 87 [57]. DPD is derived from two hydroxylysines and one lysine residue, while PYD is derived from three hydroxylysine residues. In all tissues, PYD predominates, while DPD is the minor component. The products of collagen degradation by osteoclasts include NTX and CTX fragments of various sizes, still attached to helical portions of a nearby molecule by a pyridinium crosslink, that insert into the circulation [58]. With additional degradation in the liver and kidney the fragments are finally broken down to their constituent amino acids, and the pyridiniums, PYD and DPD. Although it is possible that soft tissues contribute to the normal excretion of DPD and PYD, bone represents the major reservoir of total collagen in the body and turns over faster than most major connective tissues. In contrast to Hyp and Hyl, the measurement of urine DPD and PYD is not influenced by the degradation of newly synthesized collagen fibrils or by dietary collagen intake. The pyridinolines are present in the diet, but unlike Hyp, they are not absorbed [59]. Furthermore, unlike Hyp, the pyridinoline amino acids are fully excreted with no known pathway of metabolic degradation [60].

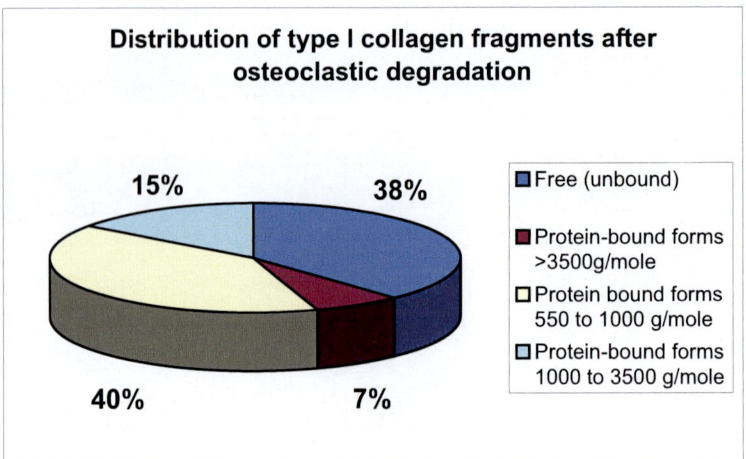


Figure 4. Distribution of type I collagen fragments after osteoclastic degradation

***Amino- and Carboxy-terminal cross-linking telopeptide of type I collagen***: During collagen type I degradation by osteoclasts, N- and C-terminal peptide fragments (NTX and CTX, respectively) are released into the circulation [58]. These fragments represent a spectrum of proteins having different sizes, as shown in Figure 4. The majority of these is relatively small and passes through the glomerulus into the urine. NTX are regarded to be specific for bone tissue breakdown as other tissues comprised of type I collagen, *e.g.* skin, are not actively metabolized by osteoclasts, and, therefore, different types of fragments are formed during breakdown of non-skeletal tissues [61]. An ELISA method has been developed to recognize a discrete pool of NTX isolated from urine [62]. The monoclonal antibody recognizes the $\alpha 2$ chain N-telopeptide fragment. This fragment contains the pyridinium crosslinks, but this assay does not recognize the PYD and DPD per se. This implies bone specificity since the pyridinoline cross-link in bone primarily involves the $\alpha 2$ chain whereas in other tissues the $\alpha 1$ chain predominates [62]. NTX, contains the cross-linked $\alpha 2$ N-telopeptide sequence, QYDGKGVG, which is a product of osteoclastic proteolysis and in which lysine (K) is embodied in a trivalent cross-linkage [63]. Collagen must be broken down to small cross-linked peptides that contain this exact sequence before the antibody can bind to the NTX antigen. This suggests that the NTX peptide is a direct product of osteoclastic proteolysis, does not require further metabolism in the liver or kidney for generation, and is rapidly cleared by the kidney [64].

Other assays have also been developed for the measurement of epitopes associated with the C-terminal telopeptide of type I collagen (α-CTX, β-CTX, ICTP) in serum and urine [65-67]. Due to bone specificity and their unique characteristics NTX, ICTP, and CTX have almost totally replaced the use of older resorption indices in the diagnostic assessment of bone diseases.

***Tartrate resistant acid phosphatase isoform type 5b (TRACP-5b):*** TRACP-5b is a novel marker of bone resorption which has been in use over the last 3-4 years with very encouraging results. TRACP is produced by both osteoclasts and activated macrophages and subsequently is secreted into the circulation [68]. Two forms of TRACP circulate in human serum, macrophage-derived TRACP-5a and osteoclast-derived TRACP 5b [69-71]. The only structural difference between TRACP-5a and 5b is that the former contains sialic acid residue(s) that are not found in TRACP-5b [72]. In human serum, TRACP-5b circulates in a large complex that contains $\alpha_2$-microglobulin and calcium [73]. Osteoclasts secrete TRACP-5b into the blood circulation as a catalytically active enzyme that is inactivated and degraded to fragments in the circulation. Thus, all catalytically active TRACP 5b molecules measured in the serum are freshly liberated from the osteoclasts, providing a sensitive resorptive index [46, 74].

## Formation Markers

***Osteocalcin:*** Osteocalcin is one of the most abundant non-collagenous bone proteins, produced by osteoblasts, odontoblasts, and hypertrophic chondrocytes. Most of the circulating osteocalcin is a product of osteoblast activity and thus considered a marker of bone formation. It is a small protein of 49 amino acids and in most species contains three residues (at 17, 21, and 24) of γ–carboxy glutamic acid, a calcium-binding amino acid [75]. This vitamin K-dependent post-translational modification of newly synthesized proteins results in γ-carboxylation of specific glutamate residues. The reaction is comparable to the activation of vitamin K-dependent blood coagulation factors and is inhibited by warfarin [76]. The human osteoblast produces an 11-kDa molecule consisting of a 23-residue hydrophobic signal peptide, a 26-residue propeptide, and the 49-residue mature protein. The pro-region contains a γ-carboxylation recognition site homologous to corresponding regions in the vitamin K-dependent clotting factors. After the hydrophobic regions cleaved by a signal peptidase, pro-osteocalcin is γ-carboxylated. Subsequently, the propeptide is removed and the mature protein is secreted [44]. In serum, osteocalcin is degraded so that both the intact peptide and fragments coexist in the circulation [77]. Therefore, assays that evaluate both intact osteocalcin and fragments are more accurate for the measurement of serum osteocalcin.

A fraction of newly synthesized osteocalcin is secreted into the circulation, while during bone resorption osteocalcin is also degraded. Thus there is some question whether osteocalcin should be considered an indicator of osteoblast activity or a marker of bone matrix metabolism or turnover [61].

The human osteocalcin gene is located at the distal long arm of chromosome 1 [78]. Various promoter elements contribute to basal expression and osteoblast specificity. The gene is further modulated by vitamin D and glucocorticoid response elements [79, 80]. Although osteocalcin is present in significant amounts in bone, dentin, and calcified cartilage, it has recently also been found in osteosarcomas, prostate, ovarian, lung and brain cancer [81]. Osteocalcin function has not clearly defined yet. However, it is assumed that much of the newly synthesized protein is incorporated into the bone matrix binding calcium. Serum levels of osteocalcin are significantly influenced by gender, age, and renal function [77].

***Bone-specific alkaline phosphatase***: Alkaline phosphatase (ALP) is a ubiquitously expressed, cell-membrane enzyme. ALP belongs to the category of molecules that are localized to cell membranes through a COOH-terminal glycan-phosphatidylinositol anchor, providing a basis for understanding the generation of different isoforms observed in plasma. Isoforms produced by differential cleavage or preservation of the glycan-phosphatidylinositol anchor originate from different tissues, such as liver, bone, intestine, spleen, kidney and placenta [82]. Liver and bone (bALP) isoforms account for almost 95% of the total ALP activity in the serum. Bone ALP is produced by osteoblasts and has been demonstrated in matrix vesicles deposited as "buds" derived from the cells membrane. These deposits seem to play an important role in bone formation [61]. Bone ALP is produced in extremely high amounts during bone formation phase of bone turnover, and is, therefore, an excellent indicator of total bone formation activity [82].

***Type I procollagen propeptides***: Collagen type I, a 300-kDa protein, makes up 90% of the organic bone matrix and is synthesized by osteoblasts in the form of procollagen, having a molecular weight (MW) of 450-kDa. Extracellular processing of procollagen before fiber assembly includes cleavage of the N- and C-terminal extension propeptides, that are termed procollagen type I N- and C-propeptide (PINP, and PICP, respectively), having a MW of 35-kDa and 100-kDa, respectively [61]. PINP is cleared via the scavenger endothelial system in the liver, and PICP via the mannose receptors on liver endothelial cells [83]. Because these peptides are generated in a stoichiometric 1:1 ratio with newly formed collagen molecules, their levels in serum are considered an index of collagen synthesis and thus of bone formation [84]. Serum levels of the PICP have been demonstrated to correlate with histomorphometric measures of bone formation, and hormone replacement or bisphosphonate therapy leads to a reduction in the circulating concentration of this marker. Most recent studies, however, suggest that the PINP has a greater diagnostic validity than PICP [85].

## Markers of Bone remodelling and Myeloma Bone Disease

***Comparison with normal individuals and correlations with the extent of myeloma bone destruction:*** Markers of both resorption and formation have been used in an attempt to better evaluate the extent of bone disease in multiple myeloma and assess clinical correlations. Table 3 summarizes the available data for the use of markers of bone remodelling in MM. Markers of bone resorption are increased in the urine or serum of patients with MM compared to healthy individuals [19, 67, 86-95]. Both PYD and DPD, and NTX in the urine and ICTP in the serum are elevated in patients with MM compared to controls, and correlate with the extent of bone disease [19, 89, 90, 92-95, 96]. Our group has shown that TRACP-5b serum levels also correlate with the extent of bone disease in newly diagnosed myeloma patients [97]. NTX urinary levels have also been found to be increased in myeloma including those patients in plateau phase of myeloma [98], while PYD, DPD and NTX were elevated in myeloma patients before autologous transplantation [99, 100]. A histomorphometric study in bone marrow biopsies of 16 myeloma patients has shown that urinary NTX levels have shown the strongest positive correlation with the dynamic histomorphometric indices of bone resorption, followed by serum ICTP and urine DPD, while urine PYD did not correlate with the histomorphometric findings [101]. Moreover, a comparison between these 4 markers (PYD, DPD, NTX, and ICTP) has revealed that serum ICTP and urine NTX reflected the extent of myeloma bone disease more accurately and could also predict early progression of the bone disease after standard chemotherapy [95]. A further analysis of the same group has confirmed that both ICTP and NTX have predictive value for myeloma bone destruction and disease progression [9]. Furthermore, serum ICTP levels were significantly elevated in myeloma patients with abnormal bone magnetic resonance imaging (MRI) scans compared with myeloma patients with normal MRI findings [102]. In this study by Jakob et al, the sensitivity of ICTP for depiction of MRI abnormalities was 79%, while the positive and

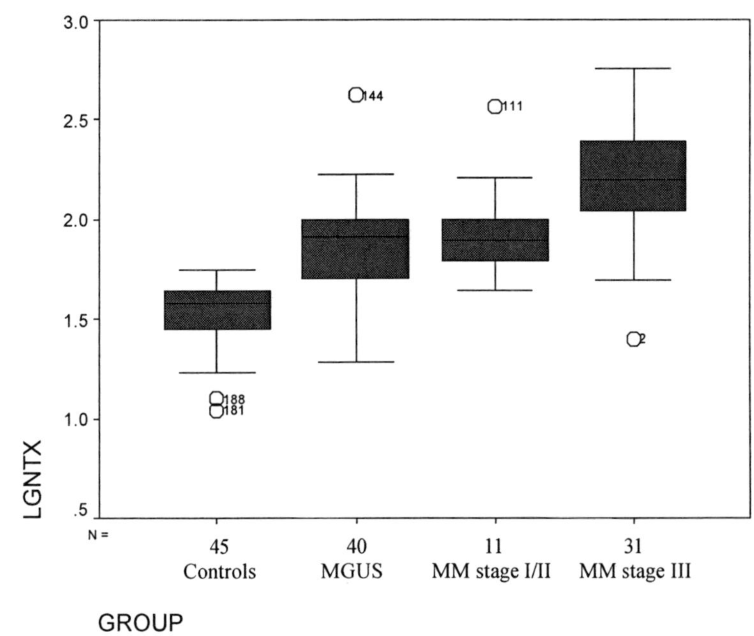


| Parameter | MM (n=42) | MGUS (n=40) | Controls (n=45) | Significance MM vs MGUS | Significance MGUS vs controls |
|---|---|---|---|---|---|
| NTX (nm BCE/mM creatinine) | 132.0 (25-571) | 81.2 (19.1-418.6) | 37.9 (11-56.2) | P<0.001 | P<0.0001 |

Figure 5. NTX urinary levels in MGUS patients, myeloma patients and normal controls (105).

negative predictive values were 85 and 84%, respectively [102]. NTX urinary levels also correlated with the overall score of skeletal involvement as measured by Tc-99m-MIBI scintigraphy, and bone marrow infiltration by plasma cells [103]. These results suggest that serum ICTP and urinary NTX correlate significantly with the extent of myeloma bone disease and we believe that the measurement of these values is feasible in the context of any therapeutic clinical trials.

Markers of bone formation have been used in several studies but the results have been variable [19, 67, 86-92, 94, 104]. In other studies, osteocalcin and bALP were elevated in myeloma patients compared with controls, while in others they were either reduced or within normal limits. In the study of Fonseca et al, which includes the largest number of myeloma patients (313 patients) serum levels of bALP correlated significantly with bone pain, lesions and fractures even if the mean values were not different from control values; osteocalcin levels were lower in myeloma patients than in controls but they showed no correlation with the extent of bone disease [90]. Our data, confirmed that OC levels were decreased in myeloma patients but we found that they were associated with the extent of bone disease, while bALP levels were not [19]. These differences among the different studies may be due to different study population and the different phase of bone turnover in each population. PICP values do not predict the extent of myeloma bone disease [86-90]. As shown in table 3, we believe that markers of bone formation may be of some value but may not necessarily reflect the extent of myeloma bone destruction.

***Correlations with disease activity and survival:*** There are several studies in which markers of bone remodelling have shown strong correlation with the stage of myeloma. Serum levels of ICTP and urinary values of NTX were higher in myeloma stage II/II than stage I disease [87, 90, 94]. Abnormal high DPD urinary levels also correlated with advanced myeloma stage [92, 93]. Our group has also reported in 121 newly diagnosed myeloma patients, that stage of the disease correlated with both TRACP-5b and NTX ($p<0.0001$, and $p=0.014$, respectively), showing a borderline correlation with OC ($p=0.046$) but no correlation with bALP ($p=0.73$) [19]. Figure 5 depicts the differences in NTX urinary levels among myeloma patients at different disease stages, patients with MGUS and normal individuals reported by our group [105]. The association of osteocalcin with stage III disease has also been shown in the study of Woitge et al [104], while two other studies showed no correlation of either osteocalcin or bALP with stage or other clinical parameters [90, 92]. Markers of both formation and resorption also correlated with markers of disease activity, such as $\beta 2$-microglobulin and IL-6, in several studies [19, 90, 92, 101].

However, it is clear that markers of bone resorption and in particular, ICTP correlates with survival in myeloma [87, 89, 90, 93, 106]. Fonseca et al have shown that the median survival was 4.1 years and 3.5 years for patients with low and high ICTP levels, respectively ($p=0.02$) [90]. Furthermore, Jakob et al have shown that ICTP is a prognostic factor for overall survival ($p<0.03$), while urinary NTX showed borderline significance ($p=0.05$) [93]. Turesson et al has shown in an unselected series of 394 myeloma patients that ICTP correlated with survival in the univariate analysis; something that was not confirmed in the multivariate analysis [106]. We had the same results in terms of association of urinary NTX levels with survival; univariate analysis showed a predictive value of NTX, but this was not confirmed by the multivariate analysis [19]. Abildgaard et al, using sequential measurements of both ICTP and NTX showed that both markers predict progression of myeloma [9]. No marker of bone formation has been shown to correlate with survival.

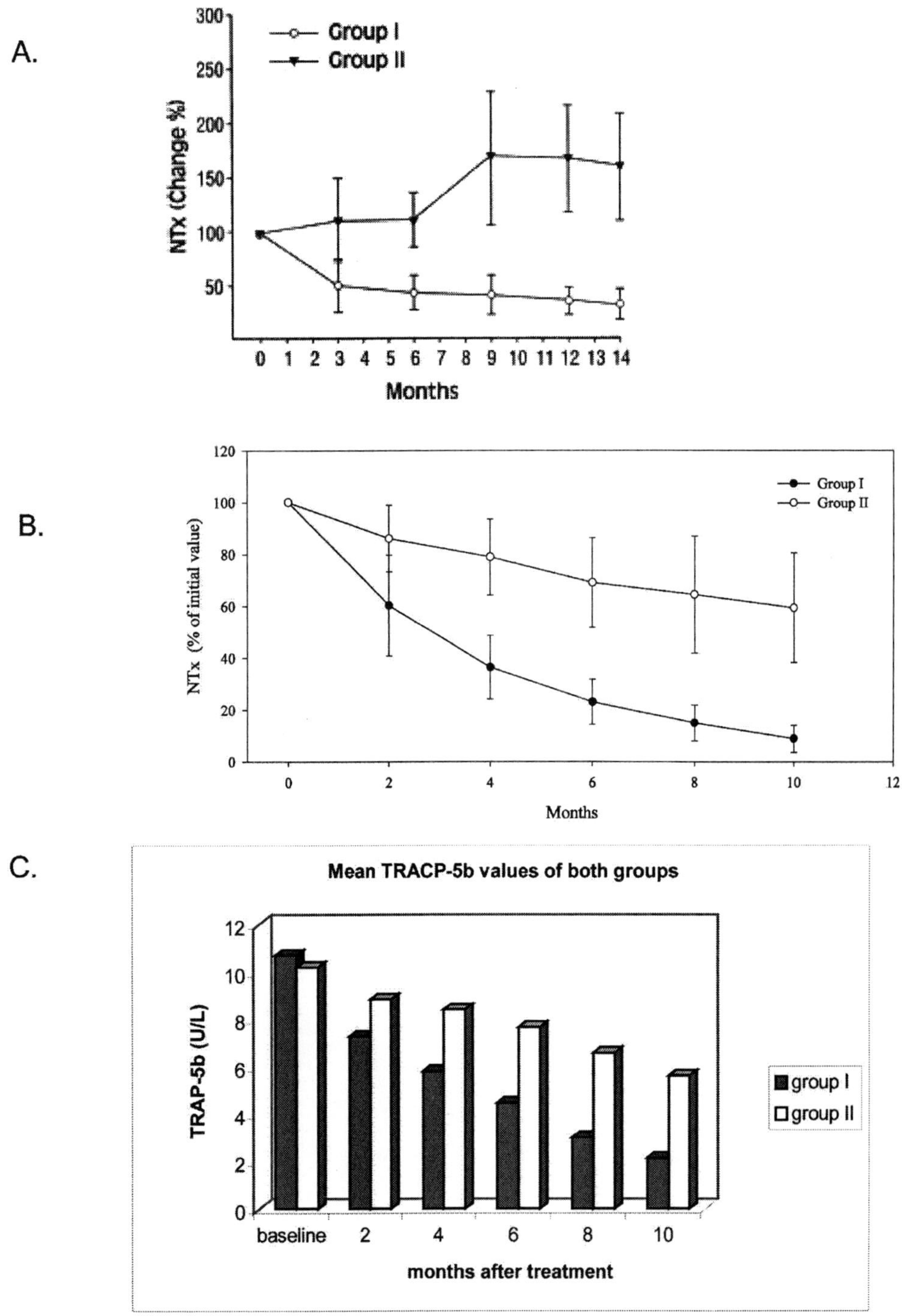


Figure 6. Pamidronate (90 mg per month) in combination with chemotherapy (group I) results in a dramatic decrease of urinary NTX levels compared to controls (group II in A) and patients receiving a combination of ibandronate (4 mg per month) and chemotherapy (group II in B). Pamidronate (group I) was also more effective than ibandronate (group II) in reducing serum TRACP-5b levels in MM patients (C) (91, 109).

***Bone markers for monitoring bisphosphonates or anti-myeloma treatment:*** Biochemical markers of bone turnover have been used in patients with MM in order to monitor bisphosphonate treatment and identify who will benefit the most from bisphosphonate therapy. Both ICTP and NTX have shown a dramatic decrease after clodronate, pamidronate or zoledronic acid administration, in myeloma patients, confirming the strong anti-resorptive activity of these agents that consist part of anti-myeloma therapy in patients with bone lesions [88, 91, 98, 107-109]. Elomaa et al have shown that clodronate administration resulted in a significant decrease of PINP and ICTP in 244 myeloma patients compared to the control group; furthermore high baseline ICTP, PINP and ALP levels indicated a poor prognosis [107]. Our group has shown that pamidronate in combination with chemotherapy reduces urine NTX levels significantly, compared with myeloma patients who receive chemotherapy alone. Figure 6A depicts this difference between the two groups of patients [91]. Furthermore, in addition to the inhibition of osteoclastic activity, pamidronate in combination with interferon-alpha was shown to induce bone formation in patients with myeloma in the plateau phase [98]. In this point it is reasonable to note that bALP and/or OC rises after successful treatment of MM in those patients with bone disease as a sign of repair. Zoledronic acid, which is a potent inhibitor of osteoclastic activity has also shown a reduction in NTX levels at a dose of 4 mg per month in myeloma patients [108], while we reported that pamidronate at a dose of 90 mg could reduce both NTX and TRACP-5b levels more effectively than 4 mg of ibandronate (Figures 6B, and 6C) [109]. In addition, bone remodelling markers seem to be normalized after high dose chemotherapy with autologous stem cell support (ASCT; Figure 7) [99, 100]. However, we believe that bisphosphonate treatment has to be continued post ASCT even if all markers of bone remodelling have been normalized due to the possible antimyeloma effect of bisphosphonates [110].

Abildgaard et al showed that high levels of ICTP and NTX correlated with an increased risk for early progression of bone lesions during standard melphalan-prednisolone treatment in myeloma. Their study suggested that ICTP and NTX are clinically useful for identifying patients with increased risk of early progression of bone disease and therefore of disease progression [9].

A.

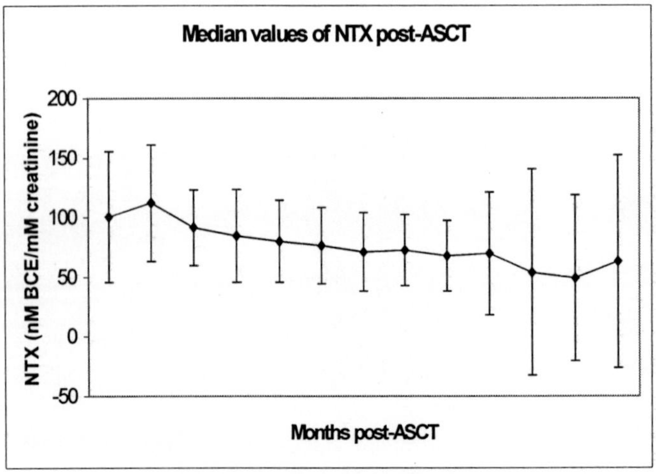


Figure 7. Continued on next page.

B.

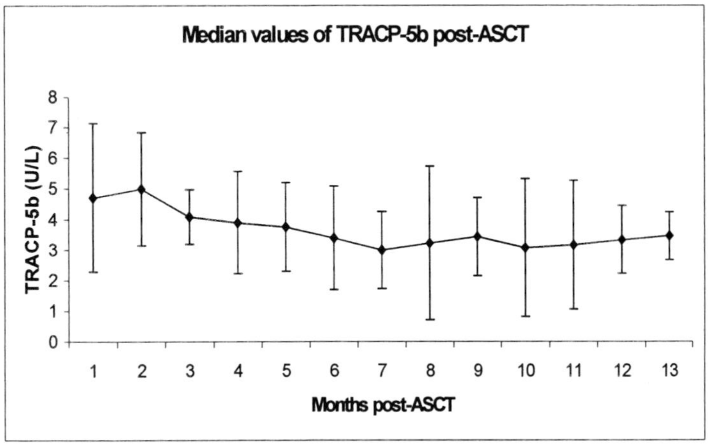


Figure 7. A: Median values (± SD) of NTX post ASCT. B: Median values (± SD) of TRACP-5b post ASCT (100).

Consistent with these findings, an exploratory analysis conducted by Coleman et al showed that NTX levels provide valuable prognostic information in patients with bone metastases from solid tumours or bone lesions from MM who are receiving IV bisphosphonate therapy [111]. Examination of the MM subset (n = 510) of a large randomized trial showed that, compared with patients with solid tumours, MM patients had the lowest baseline NTX levels, and only 1% to 18% of MM patients had high or moderate NTX levels on study. This finding may seem counterintuitive, but likely reflects the fact that antimyeloma chemotherapy and bisphosphonate therapy are very effective at normalizing bone resorption in patients with MM. However, among patients with high NTX levels (≥ 100 nmol/mmol creatinine) during treatment with zoledronic acid, the relative risk for developing a first SRE was 3-fold higher than for patients with low NTX (< 50 nmol/mmol creatinine) during treatment (p=0.008) [111]. Likewise, for patients with moderate on-study NTX levels (50 to 99 nmol/mmol creatinine) versus low levels, the risk of SREs was increased approximately 2-fold (p=0.016). Compared with low bALP levels (< 146 IU/L), high BALP levels (≥ 146 IU/L) were also associated with nearly a 3.3-fold increased risk for all SREs (p<0.001) and a 2.4-fold increased risk for disease progression (p<0.001). Moreover, elevated NTX levels were associated with an increased risk of disease progression in bone and a significantly increased risk of death on study in all patients with bone metastases from solid tumours. These results also support the hypothesis that patients who continue to have high or moderately high levels of bone metabolism during bisphosphonate therapy have an increased risk for skeletal morbidity, more rapid disease progression, and death compared with patients who have normalization of bone metabolism with bisphosphonate therapy.

# Future Developments

## RANKL/Osteoprotegerin

RANKL and OPG play a crucial role in the development of myeloma bone disease (Figure 1). It has been demonstrated that patients with advanced prostate cancer have significantly higher serum OPG levels than patients with early stage disease [112]. In another study, significant differences in OPG serum levels were found between prostate cancer patients with bone metastases compared with healthy controls, patients with non-metastasized cancer, and patients with benign hyperplasia. Even when compared with NTX serum levels, OPG was found to be of higher sensitivity in detecting bone metastases than NTX [113]. However, serum levels of soluble RANKL have no correlation with bone disease in prostate cancer [114].

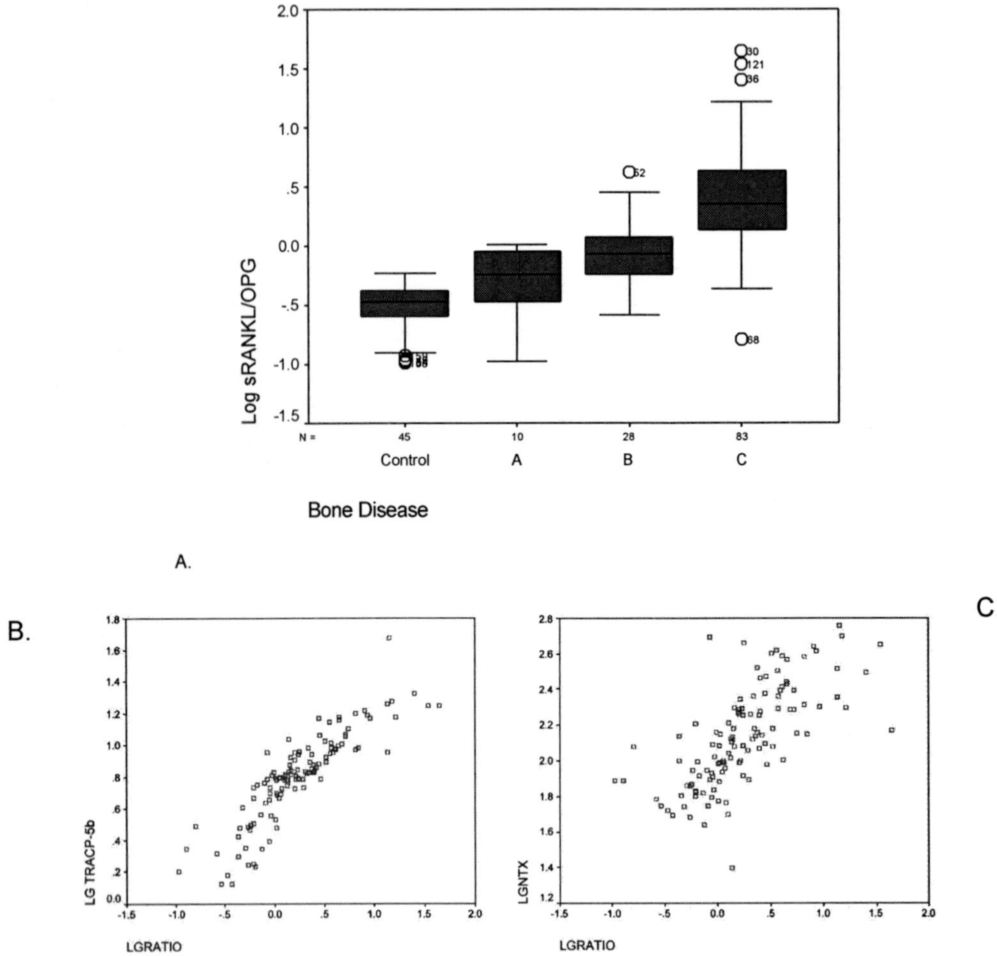


Figure 8.

A. Association between log sRANKL/OPG ratio and extent of bone disease as assessed by radiographic evaluation.

Median values (range) of the sRANKL/OPG ratio for controls and patients were as follows:
Controls: 0.33 (0.10-0.59)
Group A (no lytic lesions and/or osteoporosis): 0.57 (0.10-1.01)
Group B (1-3 lytic lesions): 0.84 (0.26-4.16)
Group C (>3 lytic lesions and/or fractures): 2.25 (0.43-44.04).
Circled numbers referred to patient outliers.

B. Correlation between sRANKL/OPG ratio and TRACP-5b serum levels ($r=0.87$, $p<0.0001$).

C. Correlation between sRANKL/OPG ratio and NTX urinary levels ($r=0.69$, $p<0.0001$) (19).

OPG levels have been found to be reduced in myeloma patients, while the ratio of sRANKL/OPG is increased [17-19]. RANKL/OPG ratio has also reported to be increased in patients with cancer and severe osteolysis [24, 115, 116]. Our group has shown that the ratio of sRANKL/OPG correlates with the extent of bone disease in myeloma, and with markers of bone resorption, such as NTX and TRACP-5b (Figure 8) [19]. The results of a phase I study using a recombinant osteoprotegerin construct in patients with multiple myeloma or breast cancer-related bone metastases were published. A single dose of AMGN-0007, a recombinant osteoprotegerin construct, suppressed bone resorption as indicated by a rapid, sustained, and profound decrease of urinary NTX levels, and the role of OPG as a therapeutic tool in this area will be clarified in future clinical trials [117]. In addition, a single subcutaneous dose of denosumab, a fully human monoclonal antibody to RANKL, given to patients with MM or bone metastases from breast cancer was well tolerated and reduced bone resorption for at least 84 days. The decrease in bone turnover markers was similar in magnitude but more sustained than with IV pamidronate [118].

***Other potential markers reflecting bone destruction in MM*: *Bone sialoprotein*** (BSP) is a phosphorylated 70-80 kDA glycoprotein that accounts for 5-10% of the non-collagenous bone matrix. The protein is a major synthetic product of active osteoclasts and odontoblasts. In bone remodeling BSP is involved in the adhesion of bone resorbing cells to the extracellular bone matrix [119]. BSP levels were associated with skeletal involvement and tumor cell burden and survival in MM patients [47]. The quantification of serum BSP may be a non-invasive method for the diagnosis and follow-up, and may improve the prognostic value of conventional staging in myeloma.

Finally, the novel protein ***Dkk-1***, a *Wnt* pathway inhibitor, has been linked to the function of osteoblasts in myeloma. Immunohistochemical analysis of bone marrow-biopsy specimens showed that myeloma cells contained detectable Dkk-1. Elevated DKK1 levels in bone marrow plasma and peripheral blood from patients with multiple myeloma correlated with the gene-expression patterns of DKK1 and were associated with the presence of focal bone lesions [42]. Our group has recently shown that serum levels of Dkk-1 are increased in MM patients at diagnosis, correlate with disease stage and reduced post-ASCT [120]. Measurement of DKK1 protein in more patients and correlation with markers of bone remodelling will show if the measurement of this protein will provide an accurate reflection of the extent of bone disease in myeloma.

# Conclusion

Biochemical markers of bone resorption are valuable research tools that provide a wealth of information about the pathophysiology of myeloma bone disease and the biologic effects of antiresorptive therapy. Moreover, these markers have been used in several large bisphosphonate trials to monitor response to therapy, and exploratory analyses of these trials have shown that bone resorption markers correlate with clinical outcome. The promising role of bone markers in improving patient outcomes lies in the correlation between bone marker levels and risk for SREs, disease progression, and death. Although some correlation has been established, the only conclusion that can be drawn at present is that patients with elevated bone marker levels at baseline or during treatment with bisphosphonates are at higher risk for negative clinical outcomes relative to patients with normal levels at baseline or patients whose levels normalize with treatment. Elevated bone marker levels clearly have negative prognostic implications, but there is a continuum of risk among all patients with bone lesions because SREs occur even in patients with relatively low bone marker levels.

Biochemical markers of bone metabolism may also have the clinical utility to diagnose bone lesions earlier than is possible with conventional imaging or to identify subgroups of myeloma patients who are not responding to bisphosphonate therapy and are, therefore, at greater risk of skeletal morbidity, disease progression, and death. Consequently, these patients may benefit from alternative treatment approaches. Therefore, although bone markers have clinical utility, they cannot be used as surrogates for other, more robust indicators of clinical outcomes, and they cannot be used to compare treatment regimens or bisphosphonates. Studies are ongoing to determine the optimal use of bone markers to monitor response to antiresorptive therapy and to tailor treatment regimens.

## References

[1] Bataille R, Harousseau JL. Multiple myeloma. *N Engl J Med* 1997;336:1657-64.

[2] Kyle RA, Gertz MA, Witzig TE, et al. Review of 1027 patients with newly diagnosed multiple myeloma. *Mayo Clin Proc* 2003;78:21-33.

[3] Barlogie B, Shaughnessy J, Tricot G, et al. Treatment of multiple myeloma. *Blood* 2004;103:20-32.

[4] Terpos E, Dimopoulos MA. Myeloma bone disease: pathophysiology and management. *Ann Oncol* 2005;16:1223-31.

[5] Terpos E, Rahemtulla A, Dimopoulos MA. Current treatment options for myeloma. *Expert Opin Pharmacother* 2005;6:1127-42.

[6] Terpos E, Politou M, Rahemtulla A. New insights into the pathophysiology and management of bone disease in multiple myeloma. *Br J Haematol* 2003;123:758-69.

[7] Callander NS, Roodman GD. Myeloma bone disease. *Semin Hematol* 2001;38:276-85.

[8] Mileshkin L, Blum R, Seymour JF, et al. A comparison of fluorine-18 fluoro-deoxyglucose PET and technetium-99m sestamibi in assessing patients with multiple myeloma. *Eur J Haematol* 2004;72:32-7.

[9] Abildgaard N, Brixen K, Eriksen EF, et al. Sequential analysis of biochemical markers of bone resorption and bone densitometry in multiple myeloma. *Haematologica* 2004;89:567-77.

[10] Ashcroft AJ, Davies FE, Morgan GJ. Aetiology of bone disease and the role of bisphosphonates in multiple myeloma. *Lancet Oncol* 2003;4:284-92.

[11] Terpos E, Rahemtulla A. Bisphosphonate treatment for multiple myeloma. *Drugs Today* 2004;40:29-40.

[12] Berenson JR, Hillner BE, Kyle RA, et al. American Society of Clinical Oncology clinical practice guidelines: the role of bisphosphonates in multiple myeloma. *J Clin Oncol* 2002;20:3719-36.

[13] Roodman GD. Biology of osteoclast activation in cancer. *J Clin Oncol* 2001;19: 3562-71.

[14] Klein B, Zhang XG, Lu ZY, Bataille R. Interleukin-6 in human multiple myeloma. *Blood* 1995;85:863-72.

[15] Sezer O, Heider U, Zavrski I, et al. RANK ligand and osteoprotegerin in myeloma bone disease. *Blood* 2003;101:2094-8.

[16] Vanderkerken K, Asosingh K, Croucher P, Van Camp B. Multiple myeloma biology: lessons from the 5TMM models. *Immunol Rev* 2003;194:196-206.

[17] Seidel C, Hjertner O, Abildgaard N, et al. Serum osteoprotegerin levels are reduced in patients with multiple myeloma with lytic bone disease. *Blood* 2001;98:2269-71.

[18] Lipton A, Ali SM, Leitzel K, et al. Serum osteoprotegerin levels in healthy controls and cancer patients. *Clin Cancer Res* 2002;8:2306-10.

[19] Terpos E, Szydlo R, Apperley JF, et al. Soluble receptor activator of nuclear factor kappaB ligand-osteoprotegerin ratio predicts survival in multiple myeloma: proposal for a novel prognostic index. *Blood* 2003;102:1064-9.

[20] Standal T, Seidel C, Hjertner O, et al. Osteoprotegerin is bound, internalized, and degraded by multiple myeloma cells. *Blood* 2002;100:3002-7.

[21] Pearse RN, Sordillo EM, Yaccoby S, et al. Multiple myeloma disrupts the TRANCE/ osteoprotegerin cytokine axis to trigger bone destruction and promote tumor progression. *Proc Natl Acad Sci USA* 2001;98:11581-6.

[22] Giuliani N, Bataille R, Mancini C, et al. Myeloma cells induce imbalance in the osteoprotegerin/osteoprotegerin ligand system in the human bone marrow environment. *Blood* 2001;98:3527-33.

[23] Hofbauer LC, Neubauer A, Heufelder AE. Receptor activator of nuclear factor-kappaB ligand and osteoprotegerin: potential implications for the pathogenesis and treatment of malignant bone diseases. *Cancer* 2001;92:460-70.

[24] Grimaud E, Soubigou L, Couillaud S, et al. Receptor activator of nuclear factor kappaB ligand (RANKL)/osteoprotegerin (OPG) ratio is increased in severe osteolysis. *Am J Pathol* 2003;163:2021-31.

[25] Sezer O, Heider U, Jakob C, et al. Immunocytochemistry reveals RANKL expression of myeloma cells. *Blood* 2002;99:4646-7 [letter].

[26] Heider U, Langelotz C, Jakob C, et al. Expression of receptor activator of nuclear factor kappaB ligand on bone marrow plasma cells correlates with osteolytic bone disease in patients with multiple myeloma. *Clin Cancer Res* 2003;9:1436-40.

[27] Farrugia AN, Atkins GJ, To LB, et al. Receptor activator of nuclear factor-kappaB ligand expression by human myeloma cells mediates osteoclast formation in vitro and correlates with bone destruction in vivo. *Cancer Res* 2003;63:5438-45.

[28] Giuliani N, Colla S, Rizzoli V, et al. Do human myeloma cells directly produce the receptor activator of nuclear factor kappaB ligand (RANKL) or induce RANKL in the bone marrow microenvironment? *Cancer Res* 2004;64:772-3 [letter].

[29] Zhang XG, Gu JJ, Lu ZY, et al. Ciliary neurotropic factor, interleukin 11, leukemia inhibitory factor, and oncostatin M are growth factors for human myeloma cell lines using the interleukin 6 signal transducer gp130. *J Exp Med* 1994;179:1337-42.

[30] Lee JW, Chung HY, Ehrlich LA, et al. IL-3 expression by myeloma cells increases both osteoclast formation and growth of myeloma cells. *Blood* 2004;103:2308-15.

[31] Choi SJ, Cruz JC, Craig F, et al. Macrophage inflammatory protein 1-alpha is a potential osteoclast stimulatory factor in multiple myeloma. *Blood* 2000;96:671-5.

[32] Han JH, Choi SJ, Kurihara N, et al. Macrophage inflammatory protein-1alpha is an osteoclastogenic factor in myeloma that is independent of receptor activator of nuclear factor kappaB ligand. *Blood* 2001;97:3349-53.

[33] Abe M, Hiura K, Wilde J, et al. Role for macrophage inflammatory protein (MIP)-1alpha and MIP-1beta in the development of osteolytic lesions in multiple myeloma. *Blood* 2002;100:2195-202.

[34] Hashimoto T, Abe M, Oshima T, et al. Ability of myeloma cells to secrete macrophage inflammatory protein (MIP)-1alpha and MIP-1beta correlates with lytic bone lesions in patients with multiple myeloma. *Br J Haematol* 2004;125:38-41.

[35] Uneda S, Hata H, Matsuno F, et al. Macrophage inflammatory protein-1 alpha is produced by human multiple myeloma (MM) cells and its expression correlates with bone lesions in patients with MM. *Br J Haematol* 2003;120:53-5.

[36] Terpos E, Politou M, Szydlo R, et al. Serum levels of macrophage inflammatory protein-1 alpha (MIP-1alpha) correlate with the extent of bone disease and survival in patients with multiple myeloma. *Br J Haematol* 2003;123:106-9.

[37] Vanderkerken K, De Leenheer E, Shipman C, et al. Recombinant osteoprotegerin decreases tumor burden and increases survival in a murine model of multiple myeloma. *Cancer Res* 2003;63:287-9.

[38] Sordillo EM, Pearse RN. RANK-Fc: a therapeutic antagonist for RANK-L in myeloma. *Cancer* 2003;97 (3 Suppl):802-12.

[39] Oyajobi BO, Franchin G, Williams PJ, et al. Dual effects of macrophage inflammatory protein-1alpha on osteolysis and tumor burden in the murine 5TGM1 model of myeloma bone disease. *Blood* 2003;102:311-9.

[40] Choi SJ, Oba Y, Gazitt Y, et al. Antisense inhibition of macrophage inflammatory protein 1-alpha blocks bone destruction in a model of myeloma bone disease. *J Clin Invest* 2001;108:1833-41.

[41] Silvestris F, Cafforio P, Tucci M, et al. Upregulation of osteoblast apoptosis by malignant plasma cells: a role in myeloma bone disease. *Br J Haematol* 2003;122: 39-52.

[42] Tian E, Zhan F, Walker R, et al. The role of the Wnt-signaling antagonist DKK1 in the development of osteolytic lesions in multiple myeloma. *N Engl J Med* 2003;349: 2483-94.

[43] Oshima T, Abe M, Asano J, et al. Myeloma cells suppress bone formation by secreting a soluble Wnt inhibitor, sFRP-2. *Blood* 2005;106:3160-5.

[44] Calvo MS, Eyre DR, Gundberg CM. Molecular basis and clinical application of biological markers of bone turnover. *Endocrine Rev* 1996;17:333-68.

[45] Hannon RA, Eastell R. Biochemical markers of bone turnover and fracture prediction. *J Br Menopause Soc* 2003;9:10-5.

[46] Hannon RA, Clowes JA, Eagleton AC, et al. Clinical performance of immunoreactive tartrate-resistant acid phosphatase isoform 5b as a marker of bone resorption. *Bone* 2004;34:187-94.

[47] Woitge HW, Pecherstorfer M, Horn E, et al. Serum bone sialoprotein as a marker of tumour burden and neoplastic bone involvement and as a prognostic factor in multiple myeloma. *Br J Cancer* 2001;84:344-51.

[48] Seibel MJ. Biochemical markers of bone metabolism in the assessment of osteoporosis: useful or not? *J Endocrinol Invest* 2003;26:464-71.

[49] Taube T, Beneton MN, McCloskey EV, et al. Abnormal bone remodeling in patients with myelomatosis and normal biochemical indices of bone resorption. *Eur J Haematol* 1992;49:192-8.

[50] Meilman E, Urivetzky MM, Rapoport CM. Urinary hydroxyproline peptides. *J Clin Invest* 1963;42:40-50.
[51] Prockop DJ, Keiser HR, Sjoerdsma A. Gastrointestinal absorption and renal excretion of hydroxyproline peptides. *Lancet* 1962;2:527-8.
[52] Segrest JP. Urinary metabolites of collagen. *Methods Enzymol* 1982;82:398-410.
[53] Prockop DJ, Kivirikko KI. Collagens: molecular biology, diseases, and potentials for therapy. *Annu Rev Biochem* 1995;64:403-34.
[54] Askenasi R, Rao VH, Devos A. Peptide-bound hydroxylysine and large polypeptides related to collagen synthesis. *Eur J Clin Invest* 1976;6:361-3.
[55] Arlaud GJ, Gaboriaud C, Thielens NM, Rossi V. Structural biology of C1. *Biochem Soc Trans* 2002;30 (pt 6):1001-6.
[56] Eyre DR. Bone biomarkers as tools in osteoporosis management. *Spine* 1997;22 (24 Suppl):17S-24S.
[57] Eyre DR, Paz MA, Gallop PM. Cross-linking in collagen and elastin. *Annu Rev Biochem* 1984;53:717-48.
[58] Knott L, Bailey AJ. Collagen cross-links in mineralizing tissues: a review of their chemistry, function, and clinical relevance. *Bone* 1998;22:181-7.
[59] Robins SP. Collagen crosslinks in metabolic bone disease. *Acta Orthop Scand Suppl* 1995;266:171-5.
[60] Garnero P, Delmas PD. New developments in biochemical markers for osteoporosis. *Calcif Tissue Int* 1996;59 (Suppl 1):S2-9.
[61] Christenson RH. Biochemical markers of bone metabolism: an overview. *Clin Biochem* 1997;30:573-93.
[62] Hanson DA, Weis MA, Bollen AM, et al. A specific immunoassay for monitoring human bone resorption: quantitation of type I collagen cross-linked N-telopeptides in urine. *J Bone Miner Res* 1992;7:1251-8.
[63] Eyre DR. The specificity of collagen cross-links as markers of bone and connective tissue degradation. *Acta Orthop Scand Suppl* 1995;266:166-70.
[64] Apone S, Lee MY, Eyre DR. Osteoclasts generate cross-linked collagen N-telopeptides (NTx) but not free pyridinolines when cultured on human bone. *Bone* 1997;21:129-136.
[65] Bonde M, Garnero P, Fledelius C, et al. Measurement of bone degradation products in serum using antibodies reactive with an isomerized form of an 8 amino acid sequence of the C-telopeptide of type I collagen. *J Bone Miner Res* 1997;12:1028-34.
[66] Rosenquist C, Fledelius C, Christgau S, et al. Serum CrossLaps One Step ELISA. First application of monoclonal antibodies for measurement in serum of bone-related degradation products from C-terminal telopeptides of type I collagen. *Clin Chem* 1998;44:2281-9.
[67] Woitge HW, Pecherstorfer M, Li Y, et al. Novel serum markers of bone resorption: clinical assessment and comparison with established urinary indices. *J Bone Miner Res* 1999;14:792-801.
[68] Janckila AJ, Takahashi K, Sun SZ, Yam LT. Tartrate-resistant acid phosphatase isoform 5b as serum marker for osteoclastic activity. *Clin Chem* 2001;47:74-80.
[69] Janckila AJ, Neustadt DH, Nakasato YR, et al. Serum tartrate-resistant acid phosphatase isoforms in rheumatoid arthritis. *Clin Chim Acta* 2002;320:49-58.
[70] Halleen JM, Alatalo SL, Suominen H, et al. Tartrate-resistant acid phosphatase 5b: a novel serum marker of bone resorption. *J Bone Miner Res* 2000;15:1337-45.

[71] Alatalo SL, Halleen JM, Hentunen TA, et al. Rapid screening method for osteoclast differentiation in vitro that measures tartrate-resistant acid phosphatase 5b activity secreted into the culture medium. *Clin Chem* 2000;46:1751-4.

[72] Lam WK, Eastlund DT, Li CY, Yam LT. Biochemical properties of tartrate-resistant acid phosphatase in serum of adults and children. *Clin Chem* 1978;24:1105-8.

[73] Ylipahkala H, Halleen JM, Kaija H, et al. Tartrate-resistant acid phosphatase 5B circulates in human serum in complex with alpha2-macroglobulin and calcium. *Biochem Biophys Res Commun* 2003;308:320-4.

[74] Halleen JM. Tartrate-resistant acid phosphatase 5B is a specific and sensitive marker of bone resorption. *Anticancer Res* 2003;23:1027-9.

[75] Gallop PM, Lian JB, Hauschka PV. Carboxylated calcium-binding proteins and vitamin K. *N Engl J Med* 1980;302:1460-6.

[76] Nelsestuen GL, Shah AM, Harvey SB. Vitamin K-dependent proteins. *Vitam Horm* 2000;58:355-89.

[77] Young MF, Kerr JM, Ibaraki K, et al. Structure, expression, and regulation of the major noncollagenous matrix proteins of bone. *Clin Orthop* 1992;281:275-94.

[78] Puchacz E, Lian JB, Stein GS, et al. Chromosomal localization of the human osteocalcin gene. *Endocrinology* 1989;124:2648-50.

[79] Javed A, Gutierrez S, Montecino M, et al. Multiple Cbfa/AML sites in the rat osteocalcin promoter are required for basal and vitamin D-responsive transcription and contribute to chromatin organization. *Mol Cell Biol* 1999;19:7491-500.

[80] Sierra J, Villagra A, Paredes R, et al. Regulation of the bone-specific osteocalcin gene by p300 requires Runx2/Cbfa1 and the vitamin D3 receptor but not p300 intrinsic histone acetyltransferase activity. *Mol Cell Biol* 2003;23:3339-51.

[81] Koeneman KS, Kao C, Ko SC, et al. Osteocalcin-directed gene therapy for prostate-cancer bone metastasis. *World J Urol* 2000;18:102-10.

[82] Moss DW. Perspectives in alkaline phosphatase research. *Clin Chem* 1992;38:2486-92.

[83] Smedsrod B, Melkko J, Risteli L, Risteli J. Circulating C-terminal propeptide of type I procollagen is cleared mainly via the mannose receptor in liver endothelial cells. *Biochem J* 1990;271:345-50.

[84] Risteli J, Risteli L. Assays of type I procollagen domains and collagen fragments: problems to be solved and future trends. *Scand J Clin Lab Invest Suppl* 1997;227:105-13.

[85] Fohr B, Dunstan CR, Seibel MJ. Clinical review 165: Markers of bone remodeling in metastatic bone disease. *J Clin Endocrinol Metab* 2003;88:5059-75.

[86] Nawawi H, Samson D, Apperley J, Girgis S. Biochemical bone markers in patients with multiple myeloma. *Clin Chim Acta* 1996;253:61-77.

[87] Abildgaard N, Bentzen SM, Nielsen JL, Heickendorff L. Serum markers of bone metabolism in multiple myeloma: prognostic value of the carboxy-terminal telopeptide of type I collagen (ICTP). *Br J Haematol* 1997;96:103-10.

[88] Withold W, Arning M, Schwarz M, et al. Monitoring of multiple myeloma patients by simultaneously measuring marker substances of bone resorption and formation. *Clin Chim Acta* 1998;269:21-30.

[89] Carlson K, Larsson A, Simonsson B, et al. Evaluation of bone disease in multiple myeloma: a comparison between the resorption markers urinary

deoxypyridinoline/creatinine (DPD) and serum ICTP, and an evaluation of the DPD/osteocalcin and ICTP/osteocalcin ratios. *Eur J Haematol* 1999;62:300-6.

[90] Fonseca R, Trendle MC, Leong T, et al. Prognostic value of serum markers of bone metabolism in untreated multiple myeloma patients. Br J Haematol 2000;109:24-9.

[91] Terpos E, Palermos J, Tsionos K, et al. Effect of pamidronate administration on markers of bone turnover and disease activity in multiple myeloma. *Eur J Haematol* 2000;65:331-6.

[92] Corso A, Arcaini L, Mangiacavalli S, et al. Biochemical markers of bone disease in asymptomatic early stage multiple myeloma. A study on their role in identifying high risk patients. *Haematologica* 2001;86:394-8.

[93] Jakob C, Zavrski I, Heider U, et al. Bone resorption parameters [carboxy-terminal telopeptide of type-I collagen (ICTP), amino-terminal collagen type-I telopeptide (NTx), and deoxypyridinoline (Dpd)] in MGUS and multiple myeloma. *Eur J Haematol* 2002;69:37-42.

[94] Alexandrakis MG, Passam FH, Malliaraki N, et al. Evaluation of bone disease in multiple myeloma: a correlation between biochemical markers of bone metabolism and other clinical parameters in untreated multiple myeloma patients. *Clin Chim Acta* 2002;325:51-7.

[95] Abildgaard N, Brixen K, Kristensen JE, et al. Comparison of five biochemical markers of bone resorption in multiple myeloma: elevated pre-treatment levels of S-ICTP and U-Ntx are predictive for early progression of the bone disease during standard chemotherapy. *Br J Haematol* 2003;120:235-42.

[96] Xue Y, Jia W, Zhang H, et al. Urinary cross-linked N-telopeptides of type I collagen and bone metabolic diseases. *Chin Med J* 1999;112:149-52.

[97] Terpos E, de la Fuente J, Szydlo R, et al. Tartrate-resistant acid phosphatase isoform 5b: a novel serum marker for monitoring bone disease in multiple myeloma. *Int J Cancer* 2003;106:455-7.

[98] Terpos E, Palermos J, Viniou N, et al. Pamidronate increases markers of bone formation in patients with multiple myeloma in plateau phase under interferon-alpha treatment. Calcif Tissue Int 2001;68:285-90.

[99] Clark RE, Flory AJ, Ion EM, et al. Biochemical markers of bone turnover following high-dose chemotherapy and autografting in multiple myeloma. *Blood* 2000;96: 2697-702.

[100] Terpos E, Politou M, Szydlo R, et al. Autologous stem cell transplantation normalizes abnormal bone remodeling and sRANKL/osteoprotegerin ratio in patients with multiple myeloma. *Leukemia* 2004;18:1420-6.

[101] Abildgaard N, Glerup H, Rungby J, et al. Biochemical markers of bone metabolism reflect osteoclastic and osteoblastic activity in multiple myeloma. *Eur J Haematol* 2000;64:121-9.

[102] Jakob C, Zavrski I, Heider U, et al. Serum levels of carboxy-terminal telopeptide of type-I collagen are elevated in patients with multiple myeloma showing skeletal manifestations in magnetic resonance imaging but lacking lytic bone lesions in conventional radiography. *Clin Cancer Res* 2003;9:3047-51.

[103] Alexandrakis MG, Kyriakou DS, Passam FH, et al. Urinary N-telopeptide levels in multiple myeloma patients, correlation with Tc-99m-sestaMIBI scintigraphy and other biochemical markers of disease activity. *Hematol Oncol* 2003;21:17-24.

[104] Woitge HW, Horn E, Keck AV, et al. Biochemical markers of bone formation in patients with plasma cell dyscrasias and benign osteoporosis. *Clin Chem* 2001;47: 686-93.

[105] Politou M, Terpos E, Anagnostopoulos A, et al. Role of receptor activator of nuclear factor-kappa B ligand (RANKL), osteoprotegerin and macrophage inflammatory protein-1 alpha (MIP-1α) in monoclonal gammopathy of undetermined significance (MGUS). *Br J Haematol* 2004;126:686-9.

[106] Turesson I, Abildgaard N, Ahlgren T, et al. Prognostic evaluation in multiple myeloma: an analysis of the impact of new prognostic factors. *Br J Haematol* 1999;106:1005-12.

[107] Elomaa I, Risteli L, Laakso M, et al. Monitoring the action of clodronate with type I collagen metabolites in multiple myeloma. *Eur J Cancer* 1996;32A:1166-70.

[108] Berenson JR, Rosen LS, Howell A, et al. Zoledronic acid reduces skeletal-related events in patients with osteolytic metastases. *Cancer* 2001;91:1191-200.

[109] Terpos E, Viniou N, de la Fuente J, et al. Pamidronate is superior to ibandronate in decreasing bone resorption, interleukin-6 and beta 2-microglobulin in multiple myeloma. *Eur J Haematol* 2003;70:34-42.

[110] Gordon S, Helfrich MH, Sati HI, et al. Pamidronate causes apoptosis of plasma cells in vivo in patients with multiple myeloma. *Br J Haematol* 2002;119:475-83.

[111] Coleman RE, Major P, Lipton A, et al. Predictive value of bone resorption and formation markers in cancer patients with bone metastases receiving the bisphosphonate zoledronic acid. *J Clin Oncol* 2005;23:4925-35.

[112] Brown JM, Vessella RL, Kostenuik PJ, et al. Serum osteoprotegerin levels are increased in patients with advanced prostate cancer. *Clin Cancer Res* 2001;7:2977-83.

[113] Jung K, Lein M, von Hosslin K, et al. Osteoprotegerin in serum as a novel marker of bone metastatic spread in prostate cancer. *Clin Chem* 2001;47:2061-3.

[114] Jung K, Stephan C, Semjonow A, et al. Serum osteoprotegerin and receptor activator of nuclear factor-kappa B ligand as indicators of disturbed osteoclastogenesis in patients with prostate cancer. *J Urol* 2003;170:2302-5.

[115] Mountzios G, Dimopoulos MA, Bamias A, et al. Abnormal bone remodeling process is due to an imbalance in the Receptor Activator of Nuclear Factor–κB Ligand (RANKL)/Osteoprotegerin (OPG) axis in patients with solid tumors metastatic to the skeleton. *Acta Oncol* 2006; in press.

[116] Van Poznak C, Cross SS, Saggese M, et al. Expression of osteoprotegerin (OPG), TNF related apoptosis inducing ligand (TRAIL), and receptor activator of nuclear factor kappaB ligand (RANKL) in human breast tumours. *J Clin Pathol* 2006;59:56-63.

[117] Body JJ, Greipp P, Coleman RE, et al. A phase I study of AMGN-0007, a recombinant osteoprotegerin construct, in patients with multiple myeloma or breast carcinoma related bone metastases. *Cancer* 2003;97:887-92.

[118] Body JJ, Facon T, Coleman RE, et al. A study of the biological receptor activator of nuclear factor-kappaB ligand inhibitor, denosumab, in patients with multiple myeloma or bone metastases from breast cancer. *Clin Cancer Res* 2006;12:1221-8.

[119] Nanci A. Content and distribution of noncollagenous matrix proteins in bone and cementum: relationship to speed of formation and collagen packing density. *J Struct Biol* 1999;126:256-69.

[120] Politou MC, Heath DJ, Rahemtulla A, et al. Serum concentrations of Dickkopf-1 protein are increased in patients with multiple myeloma and reduced after autologous stem cell transplantation. *Int J Cancer* 2006;119:1728-31.
[121] Delmas PD. Bone marker nomenclature. *Bone* 2001;28:575-6.

In: Tumor Markers Research Focus
Editor: Deborah H. Chang, pp. 33-46
ISBN: 978-1-60021-544-5


*Chapter II*

# Expression of Hepatoma-Derived Growth Factor in Thoracic Malignancy: Non-Small-Cell Lung Cancer, Malignant Pleural Mesothelioma and Thymoma

***Teruo Iwasaki[1]*, Kunimitsu Kawahara[2], Hideji Nakamura[3] and Katsuhiro Nakagawa[1]***

[1] Department of Respiratory Surgery

[2] Department of Pathology, Osaka Prefectural Hospital Organization, Osaka Prefectural Medical Center for Respiratory and Allergic Diseases, 3-7-1 Habikino, Habikino-City, Osaka 583-8588, Japan

[3]Division of Hepatobiliary and Pancreatic Medicine, Department of Internal Medicine, Hyogo College of Medicine, 1-1 Mukogawa-cho, Nishinomiya, Hyogo 663-8501, Japan

## Abstract

Hepatoma-derived growth factor (HDGF), unrelated to hepatocyte growth factor, is a heparin-binding protein originally purified from human hepatoma HuH-7 cells. Through nuclear targeting in an autocrine or a paracrine manner, HDGF exhibits a mitogenic activity in certain hepatoma cells, fibroblasts and vascular smooth muscle cells (VSMCs), as well as an angiogenic activiy. To date, however, it is unknown if the exogenous mitogenic effect of HDGF is mediated by a cell surface receptor or the protein uptake. Recently, HDGF was found to exert a mitogenic effect on lung epithelial cells *in vitro* and *in vivo*. These findings suggest that HDGF may play a critical role in the development and progression of lung cancer. HDGF expression was analyzed using a rabbit polyclonal antibody raised against the C-terminus of the human HDGF sequence. Weak staining of VSMCs was used as the internal positive control. Then, we investigated the relationship between HDGF expression and clinicopathological variables in 102 patients subjected to complete resection of non-small-cell

* E-mail address: teruteruah@m4.dion.ne.jp; FAX: +81-72-957-8002. Correspondence address: Department of Respiratory Surgery, Osaka Prefectural Hospital Organization, Osaka Prefectural Medical Center for Respiratory and Allergic Diseases, 3-7-1 Habikino, Habikino-City, Osaka 583-8588, Japan.

lung cancer (NSCLC: 70 adenocarcinomas and 32 squamous cell carcinomas). Follow-up of the 102 patients ranged from 4.1 to 150.0 (median 65.8) months; 59 patients (57.8%) died of recurrence of lung cancer during follow-up. HDGF expression was strongly detected in the nucleus of cancer cells; the HDGF-labeling index (LI) was 20—95 (median 64.5)%. There was no significant association between HDGF-expression level and clinicopathological variables. Patients with NSCLC showing a high HDGF-LI (≥65%) had significantly worse overall survival than patients with NSCLC showing a low HDGF-LI. Multivariate analysis showed that pathological stage and HDGF-expression level were significant independent prognostic factors for overall survival, and that HDGF was associated with a higher risk ratio than pathological stage for overall survival (2.572 versus 2.061). Moreover, the Ki-67-LI and the intratumor CD31-positive microvessels density in patients expressing high levels of HDGF were significantly higher than in those expressing low levels of HDGF. We consider HDGF is a useful prognostic marker in patients who have undergone complete resection of NSCLC and may play a critical role in the pathobiology of lung cancer through its mitogenic and angiogenic activities. Moreover, we demonstrated that HDGF expression was higher in malignant pleural mesothelioma cells than in benign mesothelial cells and that many of the thymoma tumor cells highly expressed HDGF but not non-neoplastic lymphocytes. Although the molecular characteristics and biological functions of HDGF warrant further investigation, this factor may be a new tumor marker and a target molecule for the treatment of thoracic malignancy.

# Introduction

Hepatoma-derived growth factor (HDGF), unrelated to hepatocyte growth factor (HGF) produced by non-parenchymal cells, is a secretory heparin-binding protein that was purified from the conditioned medium of human hepatoma HuH-7 cells, and its cDNA was cloned from HuH-7 cells [1, 2]. HDGF represents a new family of growth factors called HDGF-related proteins (HRPs), including HRP1, HRP2, HRP3, HRP4 and p52/p75/lens epithelium-derived growth factor (LEDGF) [3]. These proteins have in common the following characteristics: 1) homology in the N-terminal 100-amino acids [termed homologous to the amino terminus of HDGF (HATH) region], which is the heparin-binding site, 2) bipartite nuclear localization signals responsible for nuclear targeting, and 3) lack of signal peptides [3–6]. HDGF has the PWWP domain within the HATH region and thereby a DNA-binding capacity [7]. Recent studies have shown that HDGF is an exogenous mitogen for HuH-7, Swiss 3T3 fibroblasts [2], endothelial cells [8–10], and vascular smooth muscle cells (VSMCs) [11, 12] and that nuclear targeting of HDGF is essential for its mitogenic activity [12, 13]. HDGF is also a neutrophic factor harbored in the nucleus [14].

As for roles of HDGF in tumor pathobiology, HDGF stimulates *in vitro* proliferation of hepatoma cells such as HuH-7, and antisense oligonucleotides of HDGF can suppress it [15]. HDGF expression is higher in hepatoma cells than in the adjacent non-cancerous tissues [16].

Although HDGF was originally identified in hepatoma cells, HDGF and its mRNA are expressed in various normal adult tissues, including lung tissue [2, 8, 17]. Mori et al. [17] reported that HDGF is also a mitogen for lung epithelial cells *in vitro* and *in vivo*. These findings suggest that HDGF may play a critical role in the development and progression of lung cancer.

Malignant pleural mesothelioma (MPM) is an aggressive tumor arising from the mesothelial surface of the pleura and its incidence is increasing worldwide. Many positive or negative immunohistochemical markers have been used in the diagnosis of MPM, although prognostic factors or molecular targets of clinical use need further investigation [18—21].

Thymomas are neoplasms arising from or exhibiting differentiation towards thymic epithelial cells, regardless of the presence and relative numbers of non-neoplastic lymphocytes [22]. The most relevant prognostic factors in thymomas are tumor stage, WHO histologic type and completeness of resection. In thymomas, tumor markers or molecular targets of clinical relevance remain to be fully clarified.

In the present study, we immunohistochemically investigated the relationship between HDGF expression and clinicopathological variables, as well as the prognostic significance of HDGF in NSCLC patients who underwent complete resection. We show confirmatory data on the basis of a longer follow-up after our previous report [23]. Additionally, we examined the expression of HDGF, as a new potential tumor-marker, in MPM and thymoma.

# Materials and Methods

## Patients and Tumors

**Lung cancer.** Among patients with primary lung carcinoma who were operated on at Osaka Prefectural Medical Center for Respiratory and Allergic Diseases (Osaka, Japan) from 1994 through 1997, one hundred and two patients underwent complete resection for adenocarcinoma (n=70) or squamous cell carcinoma (n=32) without previous chemotherapy or radiotherapy, and adequate paraffin-embedded tissue sections were available. These patients had no other form of malignancy. Tumor specimens were fixed in 10% formaldehyde solution, embedded in paraffin and microscopically examined after hematoxylin and eosin (HE) staining. Histological classification of tumors was based on the World Health Organization (WHO) criteria [22]. Visceral pleural involvement was classified according to the classification established by the Japan Lung Cancer Society [24] as follows: P0, the tumor does not penetrate the elastic layer of the visceral pleura; P1, the tumor penetrates the elastic layer but is not exposed on the pleural surface; P2, the tumor is exposed on the pleural surface but does not involve adjacent anatomic structures; and P3, the tumor involves adjacent anatomic structures. A tumor larger than 3 cm in diameter or a P2 tumor of any size was classified as a T2 tumor. All tumors were staged according to the TNM pathological classification of the American Joint Committee on Cancer (AJCC) and the International Union Against Cancer (UICC) [25]: 40 stage I, 21 stage II, 35 stage III and 6 stage IV (patients with a metastatic nodule in the ipsilateral nonprimary-tumor lobe). The patients (69 men and 33 women) were between 40 and 80 years of age (mean 64 years) and were grouped by age as being either <70 years old or ≥70 years old. Smoking status was 0—232 (median 44.5) pack-year, and patients were divided into 2 groups: those with a <40 pack-year history and those with a ≥40 pack-year history. Survival was calculated from the day of surgery, and follow-up of the 102 patients ranged from 4.1 to 150.0 (median 65.8) months.

**Malignant Pleural Mesothelioma.** Among patients with pathologically confirmed MPM, who were treated at Osaka Prefectural Medical Center for Respiratory and Allergic Diseases from 1977 through 2004, adequate paraffin-embedded tissue sections were available in 29 cases. The patients (23 men and 6 women) were between 30 and 81 years of age (mean 62 years). As treatment for MPM, 6 patients underwent surgery, 18 systemic chemotherapy, 6 irradiation and 5 best supportive care alone. Seven patients were treated with a combination of these modalities. Approaches to biopsy were thoracoscopy in 13 cases, percutaneous needle biopsy in 8 and thoracotomy in 8. Histological classification of tumors was based on the WHO criteria [22]: 18 epithelioid, 7 sarcomatoid and 4 biphasic type mesotheliomas. All tumors were clinically staged according to the TNM classification of the AJCC, the UICC and the International Mesothelioma Interest Group (IMIG) [26, 27]: 7 stage I, 14 stage II, 4 stage III and 4 stage IV cases. Follow-up of the 29 patients ranged from 1.9 to 57.2 (median 16.1) months after the day of pathological diagnosis. For comparison with MPM, 5 cases with a benign lesion such as slight pleuritis or mesothelial hyperplasia with reactive atypia were also examined.

**Thymoma.** Twelve cases of thymoma operated on at Osaka Prefectural Medical Center for Respiratory and Allergic Diseases were examined. Histological classification of thymomas was based on the WHO criteria [22]: 2 cases of type A, 4 cases of type AB and 6 cases of type B thymoma.

## Immunohistochemical Examination

Immunohistochemical staining for HDGF was performed essentially as previously described [9, 15, 17, 28]. The paraffin sections (4 μm thick) were deparaffinized, microwaved in 10 mmol/L citrate buffer (pH 6.0), and then immersed in methanol containing 0.3% hydrogen peroxide. Tissue sections were blocked with normal goat serum, and incubated with 1:5,000 diluted rabbit polyclonal IgG raised against C-terminus (231-240) of the human HDGF sequence for 30 min at room temperature. After washing the sections twice with phosphate-buffered saline, they were incubated with peroxidase-conjugated goat anti-rabbit immunoglobulin (Envision; Dako, Glostrup, Denmark) for 30 min at room temperature. After washing, diaminobenzidine tetrahydrochloride (DAB) solution was applied. The sections were then counterstained with hematoxylin. Specificity of the anti-HDGF antibody (Ab) had been previously demonstrated by Western blot analysis using recombinant human HDGF [17]. Weak staining of VSMCs and endothelial cells of blood vessels was used as the internal positive control [17]. Negative controls were treated in the same way, but anti-HDGF Ab was replaced by non-immune rabbit serum. HDGF was detected mainly in the nucleus of tumor cells more strongly than in that of VSMCs, and weakly in the cytoplasm of some tumor cells. HDGF immunoreactivity was judged positive when HDGF staining in the nucleus of tumor cells was equivalent to or stronger than that in the nucleus of VSMCs. HDGF-labeling index (LI) was defined as the proportion of tumor cells with positive HDGF nuclear reactivity.

Immunohistochemical staining for Ki-67 nuclear antigen was performed using a mouse monoclonal anti-human Ki-67 antigen Ab (MIB-1, DAKO) according to the manufacturer's instructions. Ki-67-LI was defined as the proportion of Ki-67-positive cancer cells. To determine the HDGF- and Ki-67-LI, more than 1,000 lung cancer cells were counted in at least 5 representative areas without necrosis in each section. Intratumor angiogenesis was assessed by counting the microvessels stained for CD31 using a mouse monoclonal anti-human CD31 Ab (JC/70A, DAKO) according to the manufacturer's instructions. Intratumoral microvessels density (MVD) was calculated as the average value of microvessels/$mm^2$ using the criteria previously described elsewhere [29, 30]. After the area of highest vascularization was identified by scanning sections at a low power, individual microvessels counts were determined at ×200 magnification (0.95 $mm^2$ area) in 3 different fields under an Olympus microscope (Tokyo, Japan).

In cases of MPM and benign mesothelial lesions, more than 100 mesothelioma cells and as many mesothelial cells as possible were evaluated, respectively.

### Statistical Analysis

The relationship between HDGF expression and clinicopathological variables was analyzed by the $\chi^2$ test. The significance of differences in HDGF-LI, Ki-67-LI and MVD was tested by Student's *t*-test or Welch's *t*-test as appropriate. The Kaplan-Meier method was used to estimate overall survival as a function of time, and survival difference was analyzed by the log-rank test. Factors potentially related to overall survival were analyzed by the Cox proportional-hazards model. For all statistical analyses, the criterion of significance was defined as $P<0.05$.

## Results

### Lung Cancer

HDGF expression was detected in all lung-cancer sections in various proportions. Many cancer cells exhibited strong HDGF-staining mainly in the nucleus and some cancer cells presented weak staining in the cytoplasm. Representative cases of squamous-cell carcinoma and adenocarcinoma are shown in Figure 1. The median score of HDGF-LI in all cases was 64.5% (20—95%), and therefore we defined 65% as a cut-off value for low (<65%, n=51) and high (≥65%, n=51) expression. Weak staining in the endothelial cells and VSMCs was used as the internal control as mentioned above. HDGF was also detected weakly in 30—40% of the non-cancerous type II pneumocytes and ciliated columnar epithelial cells (data not shown). These findings were consistent with those of a previous report on idiopathic pulmonary fibrosis [17].

The relationship between HDGF expression and clinicopathological variables [age, sex, smoking, tumor size, pathological stage (p-stage), T-factor, N-factor, pleural involvement, vascular involvement, lymphatic involvement, histology and differentiation] in all cases is summarized in Table I. There was no significant relationship between HDGF expression and any clinicopathological variable.

During follow-up, 59 patients (57.8%) died of recurrent lung cancer. Kaplan-Meier overall curves for HDGF expression dichotomized by the median level are shown in Figure 2. Patients with lung cancer expressing high HDGF had a significantly worse overall survival than those with lung cancer expressing low HDGF ($P$=0.0008 by the log-rank test). Among 102 patients, 25 received adjuvant therapy: radiotherapy was given to 6 patients and systemic chemotherapy including cisplatin or a combination of uracil and tegafur (UFT) was given to 19 patients. There was no significant difference in the proportion of patients who received adjuvant therapy between the 2 groups (13/51 in the low-HDGF group and 12/51 in the high-HDGF group).

**Table I. Association between HDGF expression and clinicopathological variables in patients with lung cancer.**

| Variables | high-HDGF | low-HDGF | *P*-value[a] |
|---|---|---|---|
| Age | | | |
| <70 years | 37 (50.0%) | 37 | |
| ▯70 years | 14 (50.0%) | 14 | >0.999 |
| Sex | | | |
| male | 38 (55.1%) | 31 | |
| female | 13 (39.4%) | 20 | 0.204 |
| Smoking | | | |
| <40 pack-year | 28 (54.9%) | 23 | |
| ▯40 pack-year | 23 (45.1%) | 28 | 0.428 |
| Tumor size | | | |
| Š30 mm | 17 (40.5%) | 25 | |
| >30 mm | 34 (59.5%) | 26 | 0.159 |
| p-Stage[b] | | | |
| Stage I + II | 30 (49.2%) | 31 | |
| Stage III + IV | 21 (51.2%) | 20 | >0.999 |
| pT-factor[b] | | | |
| T1 + T2 | 42 (49.4%) | 43 | |
| T3 + T4 | 9 (52.9%) | 8 | >0.999 |
| pN-factor[b] | | | |
| N0 | 25 (51.0%) | 24 | |
| N1 + N2 | 26 (49.0%) | 27 | >0.999 |
| Pleural involvement[c] | | | |
| P0 + P1 | 40 (49.4%) | 41 | |
| P2 + P3 | 11 (50.6%) | 10 | >0.999 |
| Vascular involvement | | | |
| v (–) | 19 (48.7%) | 20 | |
| v (+) | 32 (50.8%) | 31 | >0.999 |
| Lymphatic involvement | | | |
| ly (–) | 16 (50.0%) | 16 | |
| ly (+) | 35 (50.0%) | 35 | >0.999 |
| Histology[d] | | | |
| Ad | 38 (54.3%) | 32 | |
| Sq | 13 (40.6%) | 19 | 0.286 |
| Differentiation | | | |
| well | 25 (45.5%) | 30 | |
| moderate/poor | 26 (55.3%) | 21 | 0.427 |

[a]$\chi^2$-test. [b]According to the AJCC/UICC TNM pathological classification. p-Stage=pathological stage; pT=pathological tumor; pN=pathological lymph node. [c]According to the general rules for clinical and pathological records of lung cancer established by the Japan Lung Cancer Society. [d]Ad=adenocarcinoma; Sq=squamous cell carcinoma.

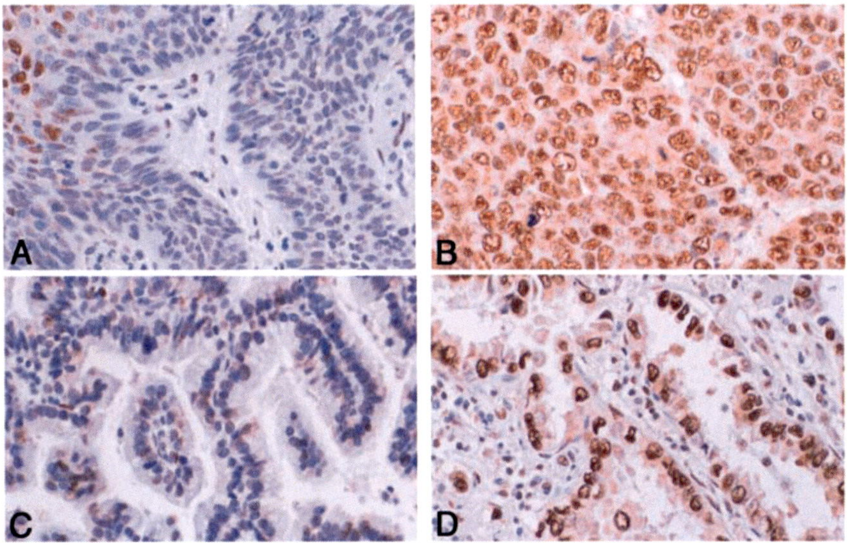


Figure 1. Representative photomicrographs of immunohistochemically stained HDGF in squamous cell carcinoma (A and B) and adenocarcinoma (C and D) cases. HDGF is expressed weakly in the nucleus of <65% of tumor cells in A and C (defined as low HDGF-expression). To the contrary, HDGF staining was more intense in the nucleus and weak in the cytoplasm of ≥65% of tumor cells in B and D (defined as high HDGF-expression). Original magnification: ×100.

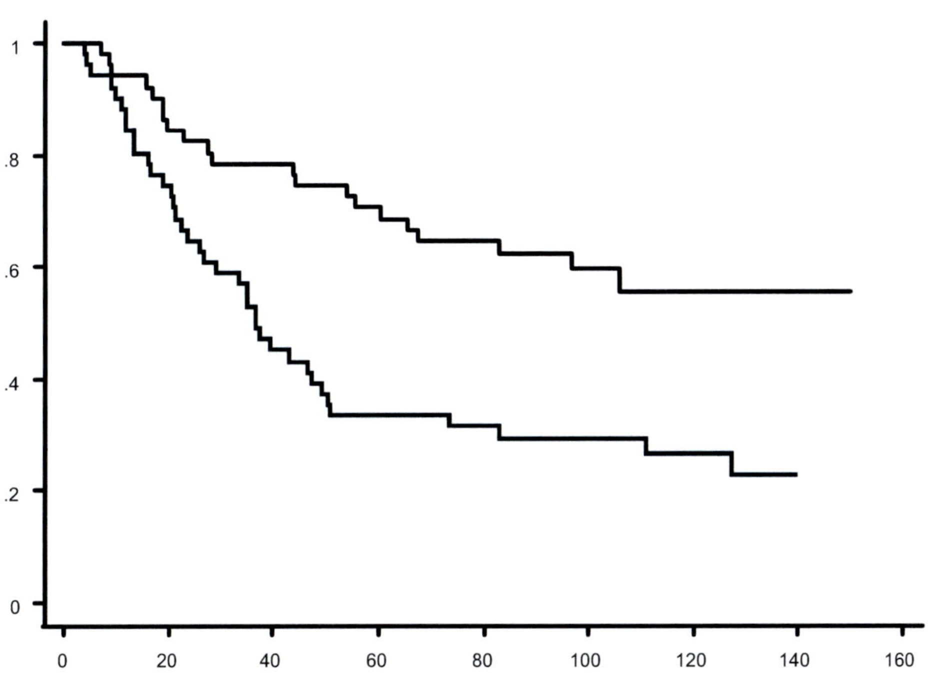


Figure 2. Kaplan-Meier analysis of the overall survival of NSCLC patients showing low (a solid line) and high (a dotted line) HDGF-expression. *P*=0.0008 by the log-rank test.

By univariate analysis of correlations between prognosis and potential prognostic factors (HDGF expression, adjuvant therapy and the 12 clinicopathological variables shown in Table I), lymphatic involvement, vascular involvement, N-factor, sex, p-stage and HDGF were found to be significant prognostic factors ($P<0.05$) for overall survival. Adjuvant therapy was not a significant factor for overall survival in this study. These 6 significant variables were entered into the Cox proportional-hazards model and multivariate analysis was performed (Table II). HDGF-expression level and p-stage were significant independent prognostic factors for overall survival, and moreover HDGF was associated with higher risk-ratios than p-stage for overall survival (2.572 *versus* 2.061).

**Table II. Multivariate analysis of prognostic factors in patients with lung cancer**

| Variables | Unfav./Fav.[a] | Risk ratio (95% CI[b]) | *P*-value |
|---|---|---|---|
| Lymphatic involvement | ly (+)/ly (–) | 0.899 (0.417—1.938) | 0.7866 |
| Vascular involvement | v (+)/v (–) | 1.186 (0.606—2.320) | 0.6178 |
| pN-factor[c] | N1+N2/N0 | 1.685 (0.843—3.367) | 0.1400 |
| Sex | male/female | 1.878 (0.987—3.572) | 0.0547 |
| p-Stage[c] | III+IV/I+II | 2.061 (1.149—3.698) | 0.0153 |
| HDGF | high/low | 2.572 (1.484—4.458) | 0.0008 |

[a]unfavorable vs. favorable characteristics.
[b]CI=confidence interval.
[c]According to the AJCC/UICC TNM pathological classification.
pN=pathological lymph node;
p-Stage=pathological stage.

The role of HDGF in the biological behavior of NSCLC remains to be fully elucidated. HDGF was very recently reported to be not only a mitogenic factor for lung epithelial cells but also an angiogenic factor [8, 11, 12, 17]. We, therefore, examined the relationship between HDGF-expression level and Ki-67-LI or MVD in serial sections. Ki-67-LI values for low and high HDGF-expressing cases were 19.3 ± 14.3% and 34.1 ± 17.7%, respectively (mean ± SD, $P<0.00005$ by Student's *t*-test). MVD values for low and high HDGF-expressing cases were 49.8 ± 23.6 and 68.5 ± 20.7 vessels/mm$^2$, respectively (mean ± SD, $P<0.00005$ by Student's *t*-test). These findings suggested that HDGF may promote the proliferation of tumor cells and intratumor angiogenesis in lung cancer.

## Malignant Pleural Mesothelioma

HDGF expression was detected in all MPM sections in various proportions. Many MPM cells irrespective of the histologic type exhibited stronger HDGF-staining, mainly in the nucleus, than benign mesothelial cells. Representative cases of a benign mesothelial lesion and MPM are shown in Figure 3. The HDGF-LI was 58.9±25.9% (mean±SD) in MPM and

23.2±10.0% in benign mesothelial cells, and this difference was significant by Welch's *t*-test ($P<0.001$).

During follow-up, 25 patients (86.2%) died of disease progression, and the median survival time was 16.4 (95%CI: 15.1—17.6) months; which was consistent with previous reports [18, 19]. The univariate and multivariate analysis of correlations between prognosis and potential prognostic factors [HDGF expression (HDGF-LI≥65% vs. <65%), sex, affected side (left vs. right), age (≥65 vs. 65>), Eastern Cooperative Oncology Group (ECOG) performance status (PS) (0 or 1 vs. ≥2), clinical stage (c-stage) (I+II vs. III+IV) and histologic type (epithelioid vs. sarcomatoid or biphasic)] revealed that only histologic type was a significant independent prognostic factor for overall survival. Patients with sarcomatoid or biphasic type MPM had a worse prognosis after diagnosis than those with epithelioid type MPM [$P$=0.0294, hazard ratio 2.663 (95%CI: 1.103—6.429)]. HDGF expression was not a significant factor for overall survival in this small-size population.

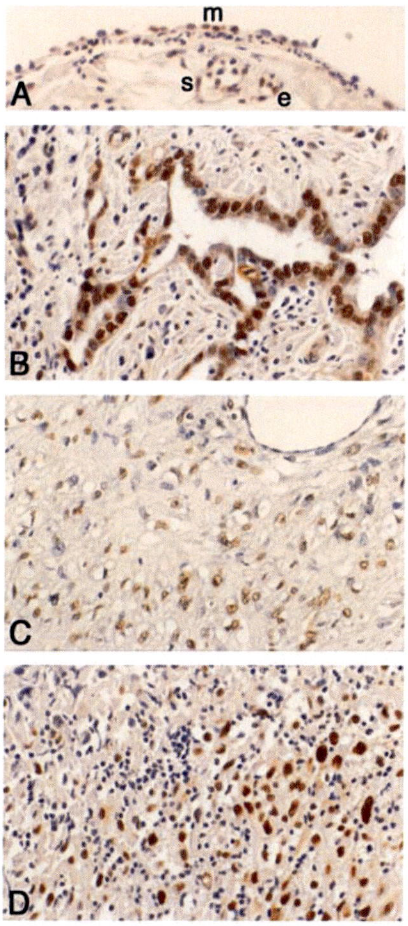


Figure 3. Representative photomicrographs of immunohistochemically stained HDGF in a benign mesothelial lesion (A), epithelioid (B) and sarcomatoid (C and D) type malignant pleural mesothelioma. A: Some of benign mesothelial cells (m), and smooth muscle cells (s) and endothelial cells (e) of blood vessels are positive for HDGF. To the contrary, MPM tumor-cells are more frequently positive for HDGF (B—D). Original magnification: ×100.

### Thymoma

HDGF was strongly expressed mainly in the nucleus of many thymoma cells but not in non-neoplastic lymphocytes. Representative cases of type A and type B3 thymoma are shown in Figure 4.

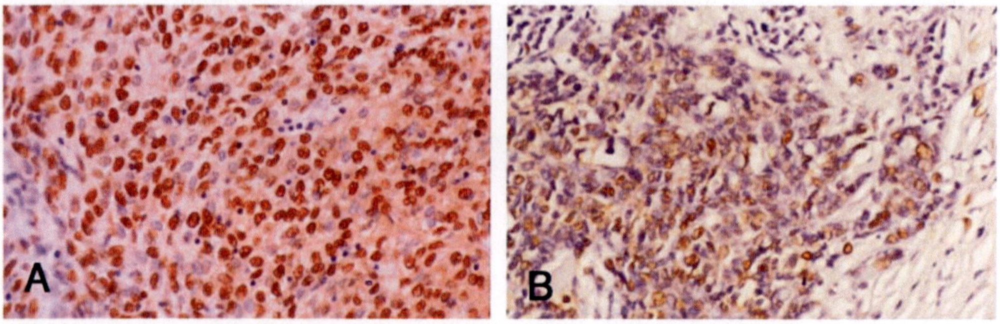


Figure 4. Representative photomicrographs of immunohistochemical staining of HDGF in type A (A) and type B3 (B) thymoma. Original magnification: ×100.

## Discussion

We demonstrated that HDGF is mainly expressed in the nucleus of NSCLC cells and that high expression of HDGF is a significant independent factor for worse overall survival of patients with completely resected NSCLC. We also showed that HDGF-expression was associated with both a high Ki-67-LI and a high intratumor MVD. Ren et al. [31] reported that HDGF was a poor prognostic indicator in patients with stage I NSCLC. To the contrary, we demonstrated that HDGF-expression is a prognostic factor independent of and more powerful than the p-stage of NSCLC by multivariate analysis in stage I—IV patients.

Exogenous HDGF promotes *in vitro* DNA synthesis and cell proliferation in rat and human lung epithelial cells. Endogenous HDGF overexpressed via transient gene transfer translocates into the nucleus and promotes the proliferation of human lung epithelial A549 cells. Using short interfering RNA (siRNA) technique, Mori et al. [17] confirmed that endogenously produced HDGF has a mitogenic effect on A549 cells. Collectively, HDGF probably stimulates the proliferation of lung epithelial cells, at least partially, in an autocrine manner. These findings support our result that high expression of HDGF correlates with a high Ki-67-LI in NSCLC cells.

Recent studies demonstrate the existence of 2 different pathways through which HDGF exerts its mitogenic activity: 1) one pathway depends on the C-terminal non-HATH region responsible for intranuclear localization, and 2) the other depends on the HATH81—100 region and binding of HDGF to a putative cell surface receptor [32]. Further exploration of this mechanism will contribute to the precise understanding of the biological functions of HDGF.

HDGF induced tumorigenesis of NIH3T3 cells in nude mice via direct angiogenic activity and induction of VEGF [9]. Moreover, HDGF is a highly expressed vascular endothelial cell protein *in vivo* and is a potent endothelial mitogen and regulator of endothelial cell migration that acts through mechanisms distinct from those of VEGF [8]. Since we could not observe a remarkable enhancement of HDGF expression in endothelial cells or VSMCs in NSCLC sections (data not shown), overproduction of HDGF by cancer cells might induce a high intratumor MVD possibly in a paracrine manner.

HDGF shows homology to high mobility group-1 (HMG-1), a DNA binding protein [33], but lacks the characteristics of an HMG-1 protein, especially of the HMG box responsible for DNA bindings [2]. HMG-1 enhances the activity of several transcription factors, including the glucocorticoid receptor, as well as the activity of RAG recombinase [33, 34]. No molecules controlled by HDGF in the nucleus or subsequent functions of HDGF have been identified. However, several HDGF-associated proteins were identified using mass spectrometric analysis and computer-assisted sequence searching: heterogeneous nuclear ribonucleoproteins (hnRNPs) K and I, and the sarcoma oncoprotein TLS/Fus [35]. These proteins have RNA-binding ability and are commonly overexpressed in colon cancers. A very recent study using siRNA demonstrated that HDGF is involved in anchorage-independent growth, cell invasion and formation of the neovasculature in NSCLC [36]. Therefore, HDGF may display other tumorigenic and aggressive behaviors besides tumor-cell proliferation or angiogenesis.

With regard to other malignancies, melanoma cells express HDGF more strongly than benign nevoid cells [37]. A recent study using differential display revealed that HDGF expression was associated with radiosensitivity in esophageal cancer [38]. Expression profiling of gastric adenocarcinoma using cDNA array revealed that HDGF was one of overexpressed genes in gastric cancer as compared with normal gastric mucosa [39], and thereafter its prognostic significance was shown in patients with completely resected gastric cancer [40]. HDGF expression was a poor prognostic indicator even for hepatocellular carcinoma [41]. Thus, HDGF probably plays a critical role in the development and progression of various malignancies.

In the present study, we demonstrated for the first time that HDGF was highly expressed in MPM and thymoma tumor-cells. HDGF expression was not a significant prognostic factor in MPM patients in this study, where only 6 out of 29 patients (21%) underwent surgery. Only patients with early-stage MPM suitable for extrapleural pneumonectomy followed by adjuvant therapy can expect a good prognosis. Further investigation should be done in a larger number of patients with early-stage MPM.

## Conclusion

Based on the above findings, we consider HDGF is a useful marker of poor prognosis in patients who have undergone complete resection of NSCLC, and high HDGF-expression might be a potential indicator of the need for adjuvant therapy. Besides NSCLC, MPM and thymoma tumor-cells highly express HDGF. Although further investigations need to be done on the molecular characteristics and biological functions of HDGF, this factor may become a target molecule for the treatment of thoracic malignancy.

# References


[1] Nakamura H., Kambe H., Egawa T., Kimura Y., Ito H., Hayashi E., Yamamoto H., Sato J. & Kishimoto S. (1989). Partial purification and characterization of human hepatoma-derived growth factor. *Clin Chim Acta,* 183, 273—284.

[2] Nakamura H., Izumoto Y., Kambe H., Kuroda T., Mori T., Kawamura K., Yamamoto H. & Kishimoto T. (1994). Molecular cloning of complementary DNA for a novel human hepatoma-derived growth factor. *J Biol Chem,* 269, 25143—25149.

[3] Dietz F., Franken S., Yoshida K., Nakamura H., Kappler J. & Gieselmann V. (2002). The family of hepatoma-derived growth factor proteins: characterization of a new member HRP-4 and classification of its subfamilies. *Biochem J,* 366, 491—500.

[4] Everett A.D. & Bushweller J. (2003). Hepatoma derived growth factor is a nuclear targeted mitogen. *Curr Drug Targets,* 4, 367—371.

[5] Izumoto Y., Kuroda T., Harada H., Kishimoto T. & Nakamura H. (1997). Hepatoma-derived growth factor belongs to a gene family in mice showing significant homology in the amino terminus. *Biochem Biophys Res Commun,* 238, 26—32.

[6] Sue S., Chen J., Lee S., Wu W. & Huang T. (2004). Solution structure and heparin interaction of human hepatoma-derived growth factor. *J Mol Biol,* 343, 1365—1377.

[7] Lukasik S.M., Cierpicki T., Borloz M., Grembecka J., Everett A. & Bushweller J.H. (2006). High resolution structure of the HDGF PWWP domain: a potential DNA binding domain. *Protein Sci,* 15, 314—323.

[8] Everett A.D., Narron J.V., Stoops T., Nakamura H. & Tucker A. (2004). Hepatoma-derived growth factor is a pulmonary endothelial cell-expressed angiogenic factor. *Am J Physiol Lung Cell Mol Physiol,* 286, L1194—L1201.

[9] Okuda Y., Nakamura H., Yoshida K., Enomoto H. Uyama H., Hirotani T., Funamoto M., Ito H., Everett A.D., Hada T. & Kawase I. (2003). Hepatoma-derived growth factor induces tumorigenesis *in vivo* through both direct angiogenic activity and induction of vascular endothelial growth factor. *Cancer Sci,* 94, 1034—1041.

[10] Oliver J.A. & Al-Awqati Q. (1998). An endothelial growth factor involved in rat renal development. *J Clin Invest,* 102, 1208—1219.

[11] Everett A.D., Lobe D.R., Matsumura M.E., Nakamura H. & McNamara C.A. (2000). Hepatoma-derived growth factor stimulates smooth muscle cell growth and is expressed in vascular development. *J Clin Invest,* 105, 567—575.

[12] Everett A.D., Stoops T. & McNamara C.A. (2001). Nuclear targeting is required for hepatoma-derived growth factor-stimulated mitogenesis in vascular smooth muscle cells. *J Biol Chem,* 276, 37564—37568.

[13] Kishima Y., Yamamoto H., Izumoto Y., Yoshida K., Enomoto H., Yamamoto M., Kuroda T., Ito H., Yoshizaki K. & Nakamura H. (2002). Hepatoma-derived growth factor stimulates cell growth after translocation to the nucleus by nuclear localization signals. *J Biol Chem,* 277, 10315—10322.

[14] Zhou Z., Yamamoto Y., Sugai F., Yoshida K., Kishima Y., Sumi H., Nakamura H. & Sakoda S. (2004). Hepatoma-derived growth factor is a neutrophic factor harbored in the nucleus. *J Biol Chem,* 279, 27320—27326.

[15] Kishima Y., Yoshida K., Enomoto H., Yamamoto M., Kuroda T., Okuda Y., Uyama H. & Nakamura H. (2002). Antisense oligonucleotides of hepatoma-derived growth factor

(HDGF) suppress the proliferation of hepatoma cells. *Hepato-Gastroenterology,* 49, 1639—1644.

[16] Yoshida K., Nakamura H., Okuda Y., Enomoto H., Kishima Y., Uyama H., Ito H., Hirasawa T., Inagaki S. & Kawase I. (2003). Expression of hepatoma-derived growth factor in hepatocarcinogenesis. *J Gastroenterol Hepatol,* 18, 1293—1301.

[17] Mori M., Morishita H., Nakamura H., Matsuoka H., Yoshida K., Kishima Y., Zhou Z., Kida H., Funakoshi T., Goya S., Yoshida M., Kumagai T., Tachibana I., Yamamoto Y., Kawase I. & Hayashi S. (2004). Hepatoma-derived growth factor is involved in lung remodeling by stimulating epithelial growth. *Am J Respir Cell Mol Biol,* 30, 459—469.

[18] Robinson B.W.S. Musk A.W. & Lake R.A. (2005). Malignant mesothelioma. *Lancet,* 366, 397—408.

[19] Sterman D.H. & Albelda S.M. (2005). Advances in the diagnosis, evaluation, and management of malignant pleural mesothelioma. *Respirology,* 10, 266—283.

[20] Steele J.P.C., Klabatsa A., Fennell D.A., Palläska A., Sheaff M.T., Evans M.T., Shamash J. & Rudd R. M. (2005). Prognostic factors in mesothelioma. *Lung Cancer,* 49*S*1, S49—S52.

[21] Kumar P. & Kratzke R.A. (2005). Molecular prognostic markers in malignant mesothelioma. *Lung Cancer,* 49S1, S53—S60.

[22] Travis W.D., Brambilla E., Müller-Hermelink H.K. & Harris C.C. (2004). *WHO Classification: Tumours of the lung, pleura, thymus and heart.* Lyon, France: IARC Press.

[23] Iwasaki T., Nakagawa K., Nakamura H., Takada Y., Matsui K. & Kawahara K. (2005). Hepatoma-derived growth factor as a prognostic marker in completely resected non-small-cell lung cancer. *Oncol Rep,* 13, 1075—1080.

[24] The Japan Lung Cancer Society. (2003). *General rule for clinical and pathological record of lung cancer (6th edition).* [in Japanese]. Tokyo, Japan: Kanehara.

[25] Mountain C.F. (1997). Revisions in the International System for Staging Lung Cancer. *Chest,* 111, 1710—1717.

[26] Greene F.L., Page D.L., Fleming I.D., Fritz A.G., Balch C.M., Haller D.G. & Morrow M. (2002). *AJCC Cancer Staging Manual (6th Edition).* New York, NY: Springer.

[27] The International Mesothelioma Interest Group. (1995). A proposed new international TNM staging system for malignant pleural mesothelioma. *Chest,* 108, 1122—1128.

[28] Enomoto H., Yoshida K., Kishima Y., Kinoshita T., Yamamoto M., Everett A.D., Miyajima A. & Nakamura H. (2002). Hepatoma-derived growth factor is highly expressed in developing liver and promotes fetal hepatocyte proliferation. *Hepatology,* 36, 1519—1527.

[29] Bosari S., Lee A.K.C., DeLellis R.A., Wiley B.D., Heatley G.J. & Silverman M.L. (1992). Microvessel quantitation and prognosis in invasive breast carcinoma. *Hum Pathol,* 23, 755—761.

[30] Weidner N. (1995). Intratumor microvessel density as a prognostic factor in cancer. *Am J Pathol,* 147, 9—19.

[31] Ren H., Tang X., Lee J.J., Feng L., Everett A.D., Hong W.K., Khuri F.R. & Mao L. (2004). Expression of hepatoma-derived growth factor is a strong prognostic predictor for patients with early-stage non-small-cell lung cancer. *J Clin Oncol,* 22, 3230—3237.

[32] Abouzied M.M., El-tahir H.M., Prenner L., Häberlein H., Gieselmann V. & Franken S. (2005). Hepatoma-derived growth factor. Significance of amino acid residues 81—100 in cell surface interaction and proliferative activity. *J Biol Chem,* 280, 10945—10954.

[33] Bianchi M.E. & Beltrame M. (2000). Upwardly mobile proteins: the role of HMG proteins in chromatin structure, gene expression and neoplasia. *EMBO Rep,* 1,109—119.

[34] Bustin M. (1999). Regulation of DNA-dependent activities by the functional motifs of the high-mobility-group chromosomal proteins. *Mol Cel Biol,* 19, 5237—5246.

[35] Lepourcelet M., Tou L., Cai L., Sawada J., Lazar A.J.F., Glickman J.N., Williamson J.A., Everett A.D., Redston M., Fox E.A., Nakatani Y. & Shivdasani R.A. (2005). Insights into developmental mechanisms and cancers in the mammalian intestine derived from serial analysis of gene expression and study of the hepatoma-derived growth factor (HDGF). *Development,* 132, 415—427.

[36] Zhang J., Ren H., Yuan P., Lang W., Zhang L. & Mao L. (2006). Down-regulation of hepatoma-derived growth factor inhibits anchorage-independent growth and invasion of non-small cell lung cancer cells. *Cancer Res,* 66, 18—23.

[37] Bernard K., Litman E., Fitzpatrick J.L., Shellman Y.G., Argast G., Polvinen K., Everett A.D., Fukasawa K., Norris D.A., Ahn N.G. & Resing K.A. (2003). Functional Proteomic analysis of melanoma progression. *Cancer Res,* 63, 6716—6725.

[38] Matsuyama A., Inoue H., Shibuta K., Tanaka Y., Barnard G.F., Sugimachi K. & Mori M. (2001). Hepatoma-derived growth factor is associated with reduced sensitivity to irradiation in esophageal cancer. *Cancer Res,* 61, 5714—5717.

[39] El-Rifai W., Frierson H.F., Jr, Harper J.C., Powell S.M. & Knuutila S. (2001). Expression profiling of gastric adenocarcinoma using cDNA array. *Int J Cancer,* 92, 832—838.

[40] Yamamoto S., Tomita Y., Hoshida Y., Takiguchi S., Fujiwara Y., Yasuda T., Doki Y., Yoshida K., Aozasa K., Nakamura H. & Monden M. (2006). Expression of hepatoma-derived growth factor is correlated with lymph node metastasis and prognosis of gastric carcinoma. *Clin Cancer Res,* 12, 117—122.

[41] Yoshida K., Tomita Y., Okuda Y., Yamamoto S., Enomoto H., Uyama H., Ito H., Hoshida Y., Aozasa K., Nagano H., Sakon M., Kawase I., Monden M. & Nakamura H. (2006). Hepatoma–derived growth factor is a novel prognostic factor for hepatocellular carcinoma. *Ann Surg Oncol,* 13, 159—167.

In: Tumor Markers Research Focus
Editor: Deborah H. Chang, pp. 47-61
ISBN: 978-1-60021-544-5


*Chapter III*

# Minichromosome Maintenance (MCM) Proteins as Tumor Markers: The Detection of MCM Proteins as Markers of Aberrant S-Phase Entry in Cervical Neoplasia

***Douglas P. Malinowski****
Research, TriPath Oncology

## Abstract

The Minichromosome Maintenance (MCM) Proteins constitute a family of 6 related proteins that participate in the initiation of DNA replication during the cell cycle. These proteins are essential components of proliferating eukaryotic cells. Although the MCM proteins are detected in normal proliferating cells, they are not detected in differentiated cells or cells that have exited the cell cycle. In cancer, the high proliferation state of these cells is associated with an increased expression of MCM proteins that can be detected in both the malignant precursor lesions and carcinomas. In cervical neoplasia, the detection of the MCM proteins is commonly observed in squamous cell carcinoma, adenocarcinoma and cervical intraepithelial neoplasia (i.e., precancerous lesions). The specific detection of MCM proteins in cervical neoplasia has been described in both cervical histology specimens and cervical cytology specimens. In cervical neoplasia, this increased expression of the MCM genes has been described at both the mRNA level and the protein level. Recent investigations have suggested that a semi-quantitative difference in MCM protein expression in cervical disease is associated with more advanced cervical dysplasia. In addition to the detection of proliferating cells, the use of MCM over-expression can be used to distinguish between mild dysplasia and moderate/severe dysplasia. During the pathogenesis of cervical neoplasia, the over-expression of the MCM genes appears to be a direct consequence of oncogenic HPV alteration of the cell cycle and specific activation of the E2F-1 transcription factor. This constitutive activation of

* E-mail address: dmalinowski@tripathimaging.com; Contact information: Douglas P. Malinowski, Ph.D., TriPath Oncology, 4025 Stirrup Creek Drive – Suite 400, Durham, North Carolina 27703, Office Telephone: (919) 206-7102

E2F-1, independent of cell cycle regulation, leads to aberrant entry of the infected cells into the S-phase of the cell cycle. Increased expression of many S-phase genes occurs in response to this effect of high risk HPV on aberrant S-phase entry, but the MCM proteins appear most useful in terms of stable and reproducible detection within these abnormal cells. Continued research into the MCM proteins is anticipated to further define the clinical utility of the MCM proteins for improved detection and diagnosis of high-grade cervical disease.

## Introduction

In eukaryotic cells, the replication of DNA and the duplication of chromosomes prior to cellular division is a complex process that is controlled through the regulatory processes of the cell cycle. The cell cycle is characterized by four discrete phases which collectively control and maintain the accuracy and integrity of DNA replication and subsequent cell division. The G1 phase is the gap phase that precedes the replication of DNA. In the G1 phase, the cell integrates various signals from its environment which ultimately determines the fate of the cell – whether the cell proceeds with replication, exits the cell cycle and enters quiescence, proceeds to terminal differentiation or enters into apoptosis and cell death. The next phase of the cell cycle is the S-phase, or Synthesis phase, where the cell replicates its genome. This is followed by another gap phase, the G2 phase. Finally, chromosomal separation and cell division occurs during the M phase, or mitotic phase. This stepwise progression through each phase of the cell cycle is controlled through a coordinated series of discrete biochemical events that insure DNA replication and chromosomal separation occurs error-free prior to cell division. This process leads to progeny cells with a complete and accurate set of chromosomes (and the accompanying integrity of the genome sequence) and thus insures that each daughter cell has the exact copy of genetic material originally present in the cell prior to division. A number of key enzymes are responsible for progression through the cell cycle and include the cyclins, cyclin-dependent kinases (CDK), CDK inhibitors and a variety of cell cycle checkpoint kinases [1]. Initiation of DNA replication during the S-phase of the cell cycle involves a separate set of key proteins which form the origin of replication (ORC) complex and that are responsible for the assembly and function of the DNA replication complex and subsequent DNA replication. The assembly of the pre-replication complex involves a series of proteins including CDC6, cdt-1 and the minichromosome maintenance (MCM) proteins [2, 3].

## MCM Proteins and the Control of DNA Replication

The minichromosome maintenance (MCM) proteins represent a family of highly conserved proteins present in all eukaryotic cells. Normally the MCM proteins are only expressed within proliferating cells and are not observed in quiescent cells that have exited the cell cycle or have terminally differentiated. The MCM protein family consists of 6 distinct protein members, MCM2-7, which form a hexamer and participate in both the formation of the pre-replication complex and function as a helicase to unwind DNA during replication [2]. The MCM proteins participate in the early stages of eukaryotic DNA replication through the regulated assembly of the pre-replication complex onto DNA during the G1 phase of the cell cycle. In this process, the origin of replication complex (ORC) interacts with CDC6 and cdt-1 to recruit additional proteins into the pre-replication complex including the MCM hexamer. This multi-protein pre-replication complex is responsible for the initiation of DNA replication during the S-phase of the cell cycle. This assembled pre-replication complex permits the initiation of DNA replication. Furthermore, the MCM hexamer binds to the chromatin and the ORC only once per cell-cycle (in the G1 phase) and thereby insures that DNA replication proceeds only once in the cell cycle. As such, these MCM proteins are referred to as "licensing factors' since their participation in the appropriate assembly of the pre-replication complex is a pre-requisite to permit (or license) DNA replication [4-8]. The subunit assembly of the MCM proteins into the hexamer has been postulated to function as a helicase to unwind the replicating DNA ahead of the replication fork [9]. Recently it has been postulated that the MCM hexamer functions mechanistically as a rotary pump to unwind double stranded DNA in advance of the replication fork [10].

# MCM Proteins in Human Cancer

Given the central role of the MCM proteins in DNA replication, it is not surprising that these proteins would be associated with the proliferative state of cancer. Detection of the MCM proteins has been reported in a number of human cancers including cancers of the uterine cervix, skin, esophagus, bladder, colon and lung. In many of these normal tissue types, MCM detection is restricted to the proliferating cells of these tissue with no detection observed in the differentiated cells present within these tissues. In contrast, as neoplastic transformation occurs, many of the differentiated cells re-enter the cell cycle and these newly proliferating cells can be detected based upon MCM expression. MCM expression throughout the neoplastic tissue correlates with the degree of dysplasia and can be detected in both squamous epithelial carcinomas (cervix, skin, esophagus) and glandular carcinoma (breast, colon) tissues. In addition, the degree of MCM expression has been reported to correlate with the grade of carcinoma. These data are summarized in Table 1 [11, 12].

**Table 1. Tissue Distribution of MCM Labeling and Grade of Human Neoplasia**

| Tissue | Grade | MCM Staining | % Positive Nuclei in Tissue |
|---|---|---|---|
| Skin | Normal | MCM5 | 17% restricted to basal layer |
| | Well differentiated squamous cell carcinoma (SCC) | MCM5 | 69% |
| | Moderately differentiated SCC | MCM5 | 78% |
| | Poorly differentiated SCC | MCM5 | 80% |
| Cervix | Normal | MCM5 | 14% restricted to basal layer |
| | CIN1 | MCM5 | 52% |
| | CIN3 | MCM5 | 98% |
| | SCC | MCM5 | 95% |

**Table 1. (Continued)**

| Tissue | Grade | MCM Staining | % Positive Nuclei in Tissue |
|---|---|---|---|
| Bladder | Normal | MCM5 | 20% |
| | Well differentiated transitional cell carcinoma (TCC) | MCM5 | 38% |
| | Moderately differentiated TCC | MCM5 | 70% |
| | Poorly differentiated TCC | MCM5 | 76% |
| Esophagus | Normal | MCM5 | 17% |
| | SCC | MCM5 | 97% |
| Lung | Normal | MCM5 | 15% (alveolar pneumocytes) |
| | SCC | MCM5 | 94% |
| Colon | Normal | MCM5 | 43% |
| | Adenoma | MCM5 | 91% |
| | Carcinoma | MCM5 | 84% |

Summary complied from data published in [11].

## Clinical Utility of MCM Detection in Cancer

Continued studies on MCM detection in cancer have reported on various aspects of the clinical utility of these proteins. MCM2 and MCM5 detection in muscle-invasive bladder cancer has been reported as a prognostic factor in histopathology assessment of bladder carcinoma as well as the detection of recurrent bladder cancer in urine specimens [13,14]. MCM2 detection in breast cancer has been reported as a prognostic factor in predicting disease recurrence and shown to correlate with poorly differentiated breast carcinomas [15,16]. Prognostic utility has also been reported in endometrial [17] and esophageal cancer [18]. Diagnostic utility in the detection of esophageal cancer [19, 20] and oral squamous cell carcinoma [21, 22] has also been reported. These results are summarized in Table 2.

**Table 2. Clinical Utility Observations on MCM Detection in Human Carcinoma**

| Cancer | Cancer-Type | MCM Marker | Clinical Observation | Reference |
|---|---|---|---|---|
| Urothelial Bladder Cancer | Muscle-invasive bladder cancer | MCM2 and MCM5 | MCM detection correlated with proliferation index<br>MCM detection correlated with grade of cancer and poor disease-free survival | 13 |
| | Primary and recurrent bladder cancer | MCM5 | Detection of MCM5 in urine sediment predictive of bladder cancer | 14 |

**Table 2. (Continued)**

| Cancer | Cancer-Type | MCM Marker | Clinical Observation | Reference |
|---|---|---|---|---|
| Breast Cancer | Invasive breast carcinoma | MCM2 | MCM2 labeling correlated with tumor size, mitotic index, histology grade and Nottingham Prognostic Index. MCM2 labeling correlated with overall survival, disease-free survival. MCM2 reported to be a prognostic factor in predicting clinical outcome | 15 |
| | | | MCM2 labeling correlated with Nottingham Prognostic Index | 16 |
| Endometrial Cancer | | MCM7 | MCM7 labeling correlated with proliferation status MCM7 labeling correlated with histologic grade MCM7 labeling index increased in poorly differentiated relative to well differentiated carcinoma Independent prognostic utility demonstrated by multivariate analysis | 17 |
| Esophageal Cancer | Esophageal squamous cell carcinoma | MCM2 | MCM2 labeling correlated with tumor status, lymph node status, metastatic status, histologic grade, pathologic grade and poor prognosis | 18 |
| | | MCM5 | MCM5 detection in gastric aspirates correlated with esophageal cancer | 20 |
| Oral Cancer | Oral Squamous Cell Carcinoma | MCM2 | Detection of MCM2 expression in greater than 10% of the cancer cells correlated with poor disease-free survival | 21 |
| | | MCM2 and MCM5 | Detection of oral SCC using MCM proteins in oral cytology specimens | 22 |

# MCM Proteins and Cervical Neoplasia

As mentioned above, the MCM proteins can be detected in cervical neoplasia including cervical carcinoma and the malignant precursors of dysplasia. The development of cervical carcinoma is preceded by the malignant precursors of moderate-severe dysplasia, which constitute Cervical Intraepithelial Neoplasia 2, 3 (CIN2, 3) in histology specimens and High-Grade Squamous Intraepithelial Lesion (HSIL) in cytology specimens. Mild dysplasia, which can harbor underlying CIN2/3 cervical disease, is referred to as CIN1 in histology and Low-Grade Squamous Intraepithelial Lesion (LSIL) in cytology. Suspicious appearing cells detected in cervical specimens can be categorized as either Atypical Squamous Cells – cannot rule out HSIL (ASC-H) or Atypical Squamous Cells of Uncertain Significance (ASC-US). Likewise, underlying CIN2/3 disease can still be present within the LSIL (CIN1), ASC-H and ASC-US specimens. Many atypical cells described as ASC-US and LSIL simply reflect morphological alterations associated with HPV infections and do not reflect neoplastic transformation.

MCM5 was the first member of the MCM family that was described as a potential biomarker in cervical neoplasia [23]. Subsequently, the proteins for MCM2, MCM3 and MCM7 were also shown to be promising biomarkers in the detection of cervical neoplasia. This detection was consistent with re-entry of the differentiated keratinocytes into the proliferative phase of the cell cycle [11, 24, 25]. Independent analysis of the gene expression profile of cervical carcinoma in comparison to normal cervical epithelium has also identified increased expression of MCM6 and MCM4 mRNA in cervical carcinoma [26]. Likewise, transcriptional profiling of HPV infected keratinocytes in organotypic raft cultures has also identified over-expression of MCM genes in response to the HPV infection of these cultured keratinocytes [27].

# Characteristics of MCM Expression in Cervical Neoplasia

As previously mentioned, MCM expression can be detected in the proliferative component of the stratified epithelium, namely the parabasal layer of the cervical epithelium. The cells within the stratified epithelium of normal cervical tissue do not express MCM proteins given the fact that these cells are differentiated and have exited the cell cycle. In cervical dysplasia (CIN1-3), the cells within the stratified epithelium undergo re-entry into the cell cycle and these cells re-express the MCM proteins. This expression pattern mirrors the degree of dysplasia. For example, CIN1 lesions which constitute the lower one-third of the cervical epithelium next to the parabasal layer demonstrate expression of MCM5. CIN2 lesions which constitute the lower two-thirds of the epithelial layer demonstrate MCM5 expression. CIN3 lesions which constitute the entire cervical epithelium have been shown to express MCM5 [11].

Examples of MCM5 and MCM2 staining in CIN3 lesions and in HSIL cervical cytology specimens are shown in Figures 1 and 2. As noted in these examples, expression of the various MCM proteins is restricted to the nucleus of proliferating cells. This nuclear localization is consistently observed in cells within the proliferating parabasal layer cells, CIN1-3 and cervical carcinoma specimens.

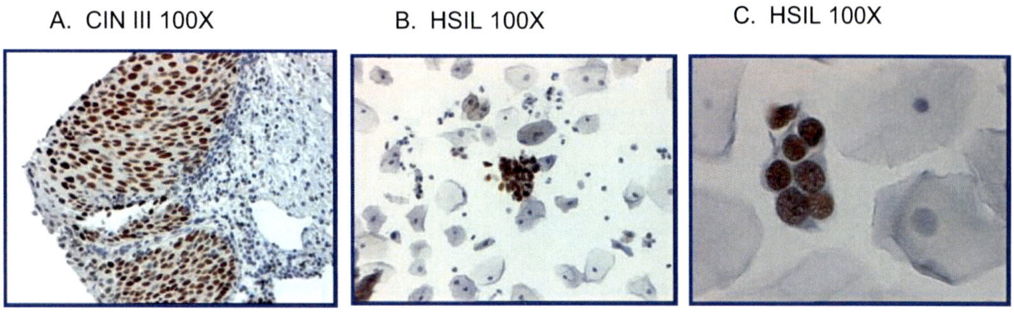


Figure 1. Detection of MCM5 in Cervical Neoplasia. A. The staining of MCM5 in cervical intraepithelial neoplasia – grade 3 (CIN3). The detection of MCM5 is restricted to the nucleus of the proliferating dysplastic cells. B and C. The staining of MCM5 in HSIL cervical cytology specimens. The MCM5 expression is localized to the nucleus without obscuring cytoplasm.

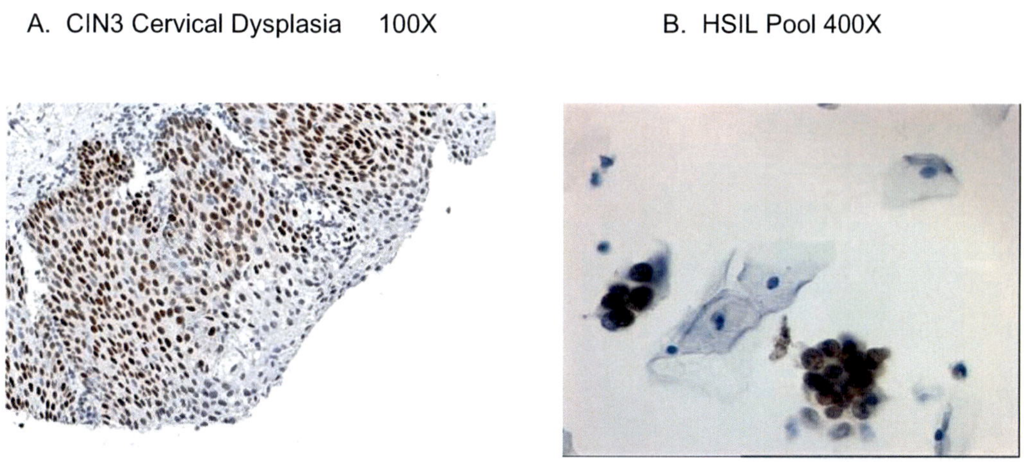


Figure 2. Detection of MCM2 in Cervical Neoplasia. A. The staining of MCM2 in cervical intraepithelial neoplasia – grade 3 (CIN3). The detection of MCM2 is restricted to the nucleus of the proliferating dysplastic cells. B and C. The staining of MCM2 in HSIL cervical cytology specimens. The MCM2 expression is localized to the nucleus without obscuring cytoplasm.

## Analysis of MCM mRNA and Protein Expression in Cervical Neoplasia

Transcriptional profiling of cervical carcinoma using DNA microarrays demonstrated an increase in MCM6 mRNA expression levels in HSIL, cervical squamous cell carcinoma and cervical adenocarcinoma relative to LSIL and normal cervical tissue [26]. This observation has been extended to MCM5 which has demonstrated increase in MCM5 mRNA using PCR analysis [28]. Likewise, characterization of MCM2, MCM6 and MCM7 expression in cervical neoplasia has been reported and shown to be elevated at both the mRNA and the protein levels for moderate-severe dysplasia and carcinoma [29, 30]. As shown in Figure 3, TaqMan analysis comparing the mRNA expression levels of MCM2 in matched cervical carcinoma and the corresponding adjacent normal cervical epithelium tissue demonstrates an over-expression of this gene in cervical carcinoma (Figure 3)

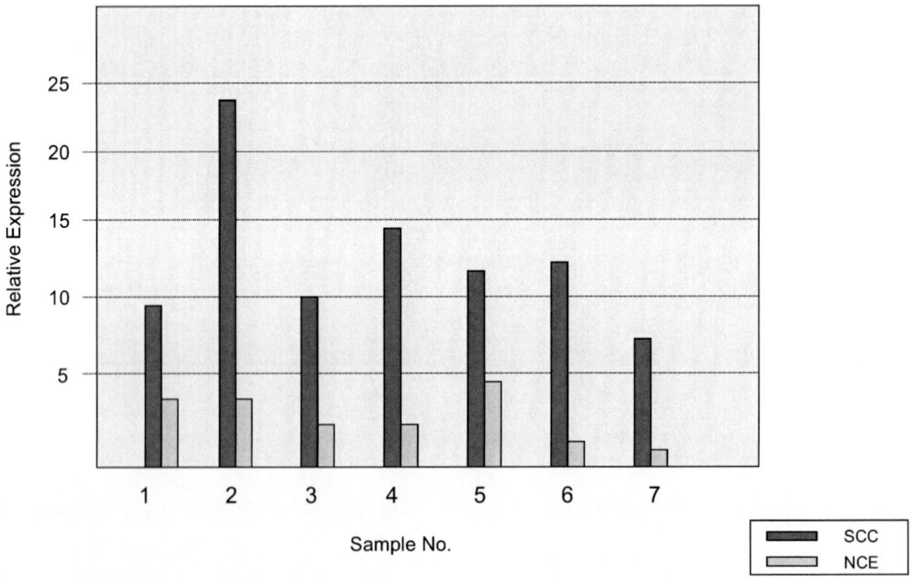


Figure 3. TaqMan analysis of MCM2 expression in cervical carcinoma. Matched cervical biopsy specimens of squamous cell cervical carcinoma (SCC) and the adjacent normal cervical epithelium (NCE) were analyzed for MCM2 mRNA using TaqMan analysis. MCM2 mRNA expression levels were determined relative to rRNA levels in these samples.

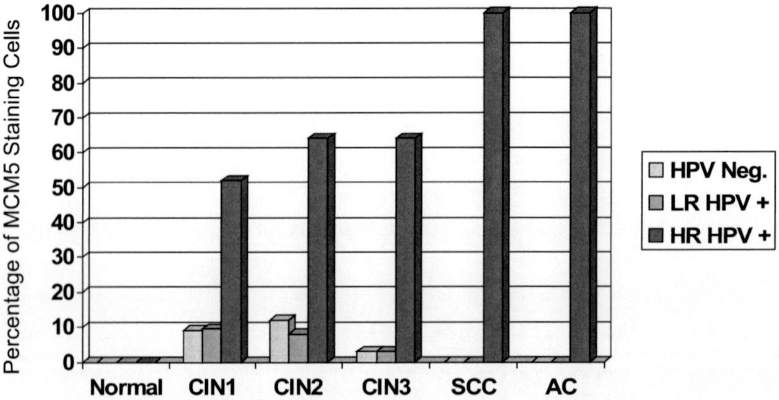


Figure 4. Detection of MCM5 in Various Stages of Cervical Neoplasia. The percentage of MCM5 expressing cells increases with stage of CIN with the highest levels detected in CIN3 and cervical carcinoma. MCM5 expression is closely associated with the presence of oncogenic types of HPV present in the cervical neoplasia specimens.

Investigations using immortalized cervical cancer cell lines have indicated a quantitative increase in the expression levels of MCM3 and MCM4 proteins relative to normal proliferating cells. Furthermore, these cell lines displayed MCM3 and MCM4 expression beyond the S-phase of the cell cycle [31].

Furthermore, in cervical neoplasia, the number of cells that express MCM5 has been reported to increase in relation to the stage of cervical dysplasia and is associated with the presence of high-risk HPV viral subtypes in these dysplastic lesions as shown in Figure 4 [32].

The detection of MCM proteins in cervical cytology specimens has been reported as adjunctive information to aid in the detection of cervical abnormalities. The detection of MCM5 in cervical liquid-based cytology specimens demonstrated a good correlation with the presence of cellular abnormalities as defined as LSIL or higher malignancy [28]. These results and the calculated diagnostic performance of MCM5 from this study are summarized in Table 3.

**Table 3. MCM5 Detection of Cervical Dysplasia in Cytology Specimens**

| Cytology Category | True Positives (TP) | False Positives (FP) | True Negatives (TN) | False Negative (FN) |
|---|---|---|---|---|
| Normal (NIL) | 0 | 4 | 26 | 0 |
| LSIL | 9 | 0 | 0 | 0 |
| HSIL | 16 | 0 | 0 | 0 |
| Adenocarcinoma | 3 | 0 | 0 | 0 |

Positive specimen defined as LSIL or higher

Sensitivity = TP/(TP+FN)
Specificity = TN/(TN+FP)
Positive Predictive Value (PPV) = TP/(TP+FP)
Negative Predictive Value (NPV) = TN/(TN+FN)

**Detection of LSIL+**

| | |
|---|---|
| **Sensitivity** | 100% |
| **Specificity** | 86.7% |
| **PPV** | 87.5% |
| **NPV** | 100% |

Performance characteristics calculated from data represented in [23]

## MCM Markers and the Proliferation Signature of Cervical Cancer

The application of DNA microarray transcriptional profiling of primary cervical carcinoma lesions, cultured primary cervical carcinoma cell lines and HPV infected cell line model systems has yielded information related to both the over-expression and the reduction of gene expression associated with HPV-induced cervical neoplasia [27,30,31]. Among these different experimental approaches, a common set of genes with increased gene expression activity has consistently been detected. These genes are related to the control and regulation of cellular proliferation (including cell cycle regulation, signal transduction, DNA replication, and cellular proliferation). As such, this set of activated genes can be considered a proliferation signature within HPV induced cervical neoplasia. Among this proliferation signature are genes associated with DNA replication including PCNA, CDC6, members of the MCM family of DNA licensing factors (MCM2-7) and Topoisomerase II alpha (TOP2A) [26,27,33-36]. Similar proliferative signatures have been identified in both HPV infected raft keratinocytes and primary cervical carcinoma [27, 33]. A series of genetically engineered cell lines with defined sequential alterations in key oncogenes (c-myc; telomerase) and tumor suppressors (p53) have identified a proliferation signature that correlates with the transformation of cells from hyperplastic to dysplastic and finally experimental neoplasia [36]. The relationship between activation of the proliferation signature and the effects of HPV oncoproteins E6 and E7 on cell cycle regulation can be summarized in Figure 5.

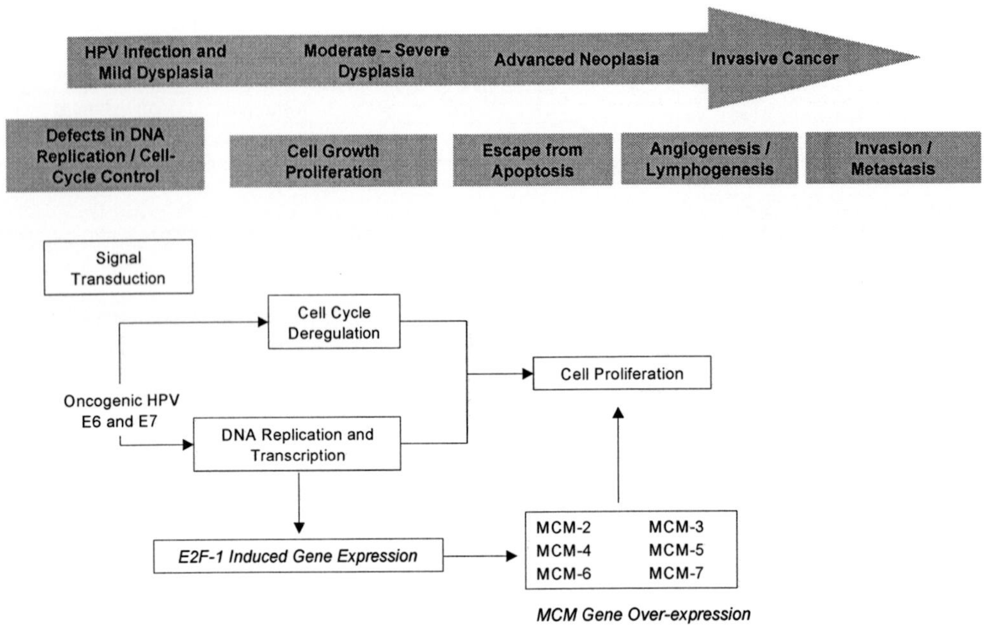


Figure 5. Molecular pathways of MCM gene expression in cervical neoplasia. The effects of oncogenic HPV viral subtypes on cell cycle de-regulation include activation of the E2F-1 transcription factor and entry into the S-phase of the cell cycle independent of cell cycle regulatory control. This constitutive activation of E2F-1 results in aberrant S-phase entry and activation of MCM gene expression at both the mRNA and the protein levels.

Activation of proliferation within keratinocytes includes HPV activation of the E2F1 transcription pathway leading to over-expression of genes related to entry into the S-phase of the cell cycle and DNA replication [37, 38]. The MCM gene family is known to be under the control of the E2F-1 transcription factor. As a result of HPV E7 disruption of the Rb tumor suppressor pathway, the constitutive activation of the E2F-1 transcription factor results in constitutive transcription of S-phase genes and permits the aberrant entry of the transfected cells into the S-phase of the cell cycle within control via cell cycle regulation [37, 39, 40]. The aberrant over-expression of the S-phase genes, including MCM2-7 and TOP2A, appears similar to the same set of genes implicated in the proliferation signature of tumorigenic cell lines mentioned above [36]. This aberrant expression of the S-phase genes also appears to be a characteristic of cervical neoplasia with potential diagnostic applications [39, 40] (Figures 6 and7).

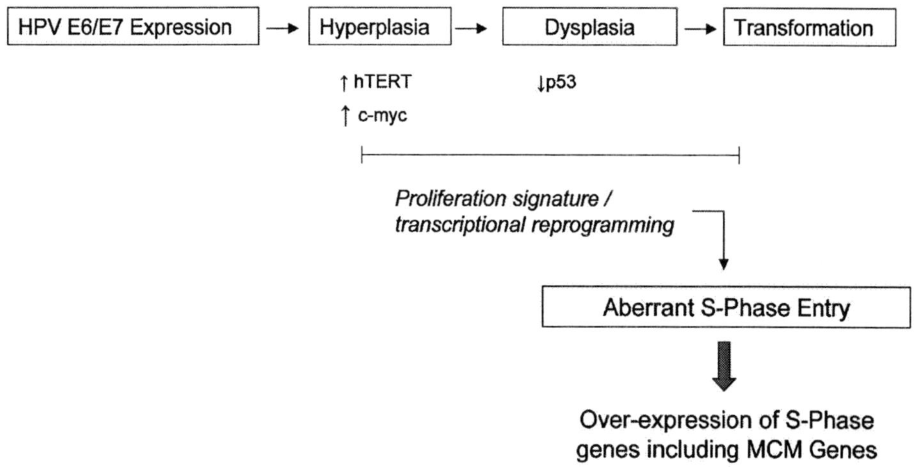


Figure 6. Molecular pathogenesis of cervical neoplasia. The persistent infection of cervical keratinocytes with oncogenic subtypes of HPV ultimately results changes in key tumor suppressors Rb and p53 and activation of the proliferation proteins c-myc and telomerase. The combined action of key tumor suppressor inactivation and aberrant S-phase entry through E2F-1 transcriptional activation contributes to the development of neoplastic transformation in the infected cervical keratinocytes.

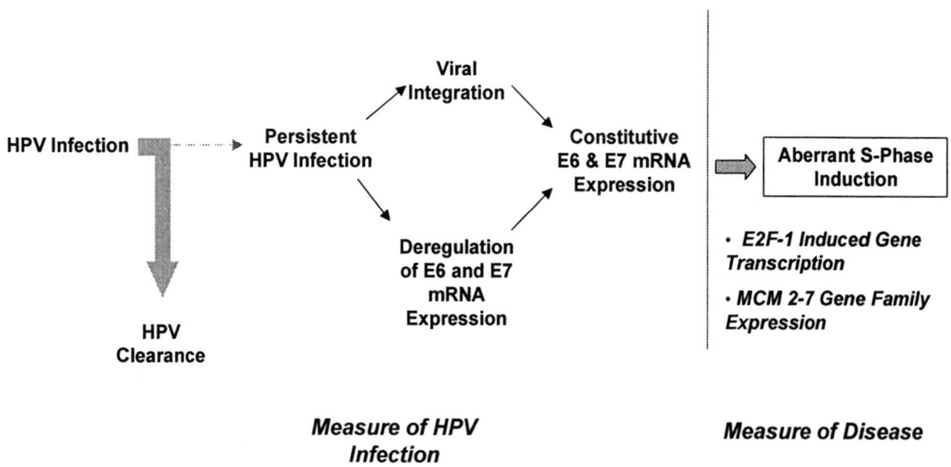


Figure 7. MCM expression in HPV induced cervical neoplasia. The presence of HPV DNA in cervical specimens is a measure of transient HPV infections. The majority of these viral infections are normally cleared within 12 months. HPV DNA testing is thus a measure of risk for future cervical disease development. The detection of the E6 and E7 transcripts is associated with a higher incidence of cervical disease and appears to be a useful measurement of active viral replication and a higher likelihood of disease development within 12-24 months. Finally the detection of MCM proteins is representative of aberrant S-phase induction and appears to be is a characteristic of neoplastic transformation and a measure of current cervical disease.

## Future Directions on MCM Biomarkers and Clinical Utility

The application of the MCM markers has been shown to detect atypical cervical cells which display with a high likelihood of CIN2+ disease upon biopsy [29,30,41,42]. The detection of these cells is consistent with aberrant S-phase entry. Furthermore, the MCM markers appear to represent a feature of neoplastic transformation within cervical cells [40-42]. As noted previously, the expression level of the MCM proteins appears to increase in advanced lesions suggesting that this quantitative difference in MCM protein expression can be used to distinguish between mild and moderate-severe dysplasia [41,42]. Additional clinical studies are required to validate the utility of the MCM detection to improve the detection of cervical neoplasia in both the detection of CIN2+ disease within the atypical cervical cytology specimen and in a primary screening application. The clinical data published to date suggests that these markers are suitable for use in the detection of cervical dysplasia with the ability to detect all stages of cervical dysplasia in both histology and cytology samples. As such, these markers would appear useful to help resolve suspicious lesions and cells where the morphology is inadequate to permit a clear diagnosis of cervical dysplasia versus more benign squamous metaplasia or reactive repair processes within the uterine-cervix. Furthermore, the apparent quantitative differences in the expression of the MCM genes suggest that these markers can be used to distinguish between moderate-severe dysplasia or cervical carcinoma and mild dysplasia or normal proliferating cervical cells. Examples of the biomarkers that display this specific over-expression in high-grade cervical disease (CIN2+) are MCM2, MCM6, MCM7 and TOP2A. It is anticipated that future investigations into these markers will permit the development of specific molecular diagnostic tests to detect high-grade cervical disease within suspicious ASCUS and ASC-H cases or within indeterminate SIL cases.

## Acknowledgements

The author would like to acknowledge Timothy J. Fischer for the MCM images and Hewei Li for assistance with the TaqMan analysis.

### Conflict of Interest Statement

The author is an employee of TriPath Oncology which develops, manufactures and sells diagnostic products for molecular oncology applications. TriPath Oncology has developed several molecular diagnostic products related to MCM detection in cervical neoplasia.

## References

[1] Morgan, David O. *The Cell Cycle: Principles of Control* (2006). New Science Press, Ltd. ISBN 0878935088

[2] Diffley JF, Labib K. The chromosome replication cycle. *J Cell Sci.* 2002;115:869-72.

[3] Diffley JF. Regulation of early events in chromosome replication. *Curr Biol.* 2004;14:R778-86.

[4] Labib K, Kearsey SE, Diffley JF. MCM2-7 proteins are essential components of prereplicative complexes that accumulate cooperatively in the nucleus during G1-phase and are required to establish, but not maintain, the S-phase checkpoint. *Mol Biol Cell.* 2001;12:3658-67.

[5] Prasanth SG, Mendez J, Prasanth KV, Stillman B. Dynamics of pre-replication complex proteins during the cell division cycle. *Phil Trans R Soc. London B*(2004) 359; 7-16.

[6] Forsburg SL. Eukaryotic MCM proteins: beyond replication initiation. *Microbiol Mol Biol Rev.* 2004;68:109-31.

[7] Lei M, Tye BK. Initiating DNA synthesis: from recruiting to activating the MCM complex. *J Cell Sci.* 2001;114:1447-54.

[8] Tye BK. MCM proteins in DNA replication. *Annu Rev Biochem.* 1999; 68:649-86

[9] Tye BK, Sawyer S. The hexameric eukaryotic MCM helicase: building symmetry from nonidentical parts. *J Biol Chem.* 2000;275: 34833-6.

[10] Laskey RA, Madine MA. A rotary pumping model for helicase function of MCM proteins at a distance from replication forks. *EMBO Rep.* 2003; 4:26-30.

[11] Freeman A, Morris LS, Mills AD, Stoeber K, Laskey RA, Williams GH, Coleman N. Minichromosome maintenance proteins as biological markers of dysplasia and malignancy. *Clin Cancer Res.*, 1999; 5: 2121-2132.

[12] Laskey R. The Croonian Lecture 2001 hunting the antisocial cancer cell: MCM proteins and their exploitation. *Philos Trans R Soc Lond B Biol Sci.* 2005; 360:1119-32.

[13] Korkolopoulou P, Givalos N, Saetta A, Goudopoulou A, Gakiopoulou H, Thymara I, Thomas-Tsagli E, Patsouris E. Minichromosome maintenance proteins 2 and 5 expression in muscle-invasive urothelial cancer: a multivariate survival study including proliferation markers and cell cycle regulators. *Hum Pathol.* 2005; 36:899-907.

[14] Stoeber K, Swinn R, Prevost AT, de Clive-Lowe P, Halsall I, Dilworth SM, Marr J, Turner WH, Bullock N, Doble A, Hales CN, Williams GH. Diagnosis of genito-urinary tract cancer by detection of minichromosome maintenance 5 protein in urine sediments. *J Natl Cancer Inst.* 2002; 94:1071-9.

[15] Gonzalez MA, Pinder SE, Callagy G, Vowler SL, Morris LS, Bird K, Bell JA, Laskey RA, Coleman N. Minichromosome maintenance protein 2 is a strong independent prognostic marker in breast cancer. *J Clin Oncol.* 2003; 21:4306-13.

[16] Shetty A, Loddo M, Fanshawe T, Prevost AT, Sainsbury R, Williams GH, Stoeber K. DNA replication licensing and cell cycle kinetics of normal and neoplastic breast. *Br J Cancer.* 2005; 93:1295-300.

[17] Li SS, Xue WC, Khoo US, Ngan HY, Chan KY, Tam IY, Chiu PM, Ip PP, Tam KF, Cheung AN.Replicative MCM7 protein as a proliferation marker in endometrial carcinoma: a tissue microarray and clinicopathological analysis. *Histopathology.* 2005; 46:307-13.

[18] Kato H, Miyazaki T, Fukai Y, Nakajima M, Sohda M, Takita J, Masuda N, Fukuchi M, Manda R, Ojima H, Tsukada K, Asao T, Kuwano H. A new proliferation marker, minichromosome maintenance protein 2, is associated with tumor aggressiveness in esophageal squamous cell carcinoma. *J Surg Oncol.* 2003; 84:24-30.

[19] Going JJ, Keith WN, Neilson L, Stoeber K, Stuart RC, Williams GH. Aberrant expression of minichromosome maintenance proteins 2 and 5, and Ki-67 in dysplastic squamous oesophageal epithelium and Barrett's mucosa. *Gut*. 2002; 50:373-7.

[20] Williams GH, Swinn R, Prevost AT, De Clive-Lowe P, Halsall I, Going JJ, Hales CN, Stoeber K, Middleton SJ. Diagnosis of oesophageal cancer by detection of minichromosome maintenance 5 protein in gastric aspirates. *Br J Cancer*. 2004; 91: 714-9.

[21] Szelachowska J, Dziegiel P, Jelen-Krzeszewska J, Jelen M, Matkowski R, Pomiecko A, Spytkowska B, Jagas M, Gisterek I, Kornafel J. Mcm-2 protein expression predicts prognosis better than Ki-67 antigen in oral cavity squamocellular carcinoma. *Anticancer Res*. 2006; 26:2473-8.

[22] Scott IS, Odell E, Chatrath P, Morris LS, Davies RJ, Vowler SL, Laskey RA, Coleman N. A minimally invasive immunocytochemical approach to early detection of oral squamous cell carcinoma and dysplasia. *Br J Cancer*. 2006; 94:1170-5.

[23] Williams GH, Romanowski P, Morris L, Madine M, Mills AD, Stoeber K, Marr J, Laskey RA, Coleman N. Improved cervical smear assessment using antibodies against proteins that regulate DNA replication. *Proc Natl Acad Sci USA*., 1998; 95: 14932-14937.

[24] Ha SA, Shin SM, Namkoong H, Lee H, Cho GW, Hur SY, Kim TE, Kim JW. Cancer-associated expression of minichromosome maintenance 3 gene in several human cancers and its involvement in tumorigenesis. *Clin Cancer Res*. 2004; 10:8386-95.

[25] Brake T, Connor JP, Petereit DG, Lambert PF. Comparative analysis of cervical cancer in women and in a human papillomavirus-transgenic mouse model: identification of minichromosome maintenance 7 protein as an informative biomarker of human cervical cancer. *Cancer Res*., 2003; 63: 8173-8180.

[26] Chen Y, Miller C, Mosher R, Zhao X, Deeds J, Morrissey M, Bryant B, Yang D, Meyer R, Cronin F, Gostout BS, Smith-McCune K, Schlegel R. Identification of cervical cancer markers by cDNA and tissue microarrays. *Cancer Res*., 2003; 63: 1927-1935.

[27] Garner-Hamrick PA, Fostel JM, Chien WM, Banerjee NS, Chow LT, Broker TR, Fisher C. Global effects of human papillomavirus type 18 E6/E7 in an organotypic keratinocyte culture system. *J Virol*., 2004; 78: 9041-9050.

[28] Murphy N, Ring M, Heffron CC, Martin CM, McGuinness E, Sheils O, O'Leary JJ. Quantitation of CDC6 and MCM5 mRNA in cervical intraepithelial neoplasia and invasive squamous cell carcinoma of the cervix. *Mod Pathol*., 2005; 18; 844-849.

[29] Malinowski DP, Parker MR, Sampson SJ, Hessling JJ, Prpic DK, Hall LB, Wingate SD, Taylor AJ, Fischer TJ. Development of a Molecular Diagnostic Assay to Detect Moderate-Severe Dysplasia and Cervical Neoplasia. *Acta Cytologica*., 2004; 48: 696.

[30] Sampson SJ, Parker MR, Hessling JJ, Wingate S, Prpic D, Hall L, Taylor AJ. Data comparison of three molecular markers (MCM7, p16 and integrin beta 6) for the detection of cervical dysplasia in SurePathTM cytology specimens. *Acta Cytologica*., 2004; 48: 658.

[31] Ishimi Y, Okayasu I, Kato C, Kwon HJ, Kimura H, Yamada K, Song SY. Enhanced expression of Mcm proteins in cancer cells derived from uterine cervix. *Eur J Biochem*. 2003; 270:1089-101.

[32] Murphy N, Ring M, Heffron CC, King B, Killalea AG, Hughes C, Martin CM, McGuinness E, Sheils O, O'Leary JJ. $p16^{INK4a}$, CDC6 and MCM5: predictive biomarkers in cervical preinvasive neoplasia and cervical cancer. *J Clin Pathol.* 2005; 58: 525-534.

[33] Rosty C, Sheffer M, Tsafrir D, Stransky N, Tsafrir I, Peter M, de Cremoux P, de La Rochefordiere A, Salmon R, Dorval T, Thiery JP, Couturier J, Radvanyi F, Domany E, Sastre-Garau X. Identification of a proliferation gene cluster associated with HPV E6/E7 expression level and viral DNA load in invasive cervical carcinoma. *Oncogene.* 2005; 24:7094-7104.

[34] Santin AD, Zhan F, Bignotti E, Siegel ER, Cane S, Bellone S, Palmieri M, Anfossi S, Thomas M, Burnett A, Kay HH, Roman JJ, O'Brien TJ, Tian E, Cannon MJ, Shaughnessy J Jr, Pecorelli S. Gene expression profiles of primary HPV16- and HPV18-infected early stage cervical cancers and normal cervical epithelium: identification of novel candidate molecular markers for cervical cancer diagnosis and therapy. *Virology.*, 2005; 331: 269-291.

[35] Ruutu M, Peitsaro P, Johansson B, Syrjanen S.et.al. Transcriptional Profiling of a Human Papillomavirus 33-Positive Squamous Epithelial Cell Line Which Acquired a Selective Growth Advantage After Viral Infection. *Int. J. Cancer.*, 2002; 100: 318-322.

[36] Milyavsky M, Tabach Y, Shats I, Erez N, Cohen Y, Tang X, Kalis M, Kogan I, Buganim Y, Goldfinger N, Ginsberg D, Harris CC, Domany E, Rotter V. Transcriptional programs following genetic alterations in p53, INK4A, and H-Ras genes along defined stages of malignant transformation. *Cancer Res.*, 2005; 65: 4530-4543.

[37] Clarke B, Chetty R. Cell cycle aberrations in the pathogenesis of squamous cell carcinoma of the uterine cervix. *Gynecol Oncol.* 2001; 82:238-46.

[38] Cho NH, Kim YT, Kim JW. Alteration of cell cycle in cervical tumor associated with human papillomavirus: cyclin-dependent kinase inhibitors. *Yonsei Med J.*, 2002; 43: 722-728.

[39] Malinowski DP. Molecular diagnostic assays for cervical neoplasia: emerging markers for the detection of high-grade cervical disease. *BioTechniques.*, 2005; 38: S17-S23.

[40] Malinowski DP. The Use of Biomarkers to Detect Cervical Neoplasia and to Diagnose High-Grade Cervical Disease. *Frontiers of Drug Design and Discovery.* Vol.2_(2006) Chapter3; pp. 35-54 (G. Caldwell, B. Springer, A. Rahman and M. D'Andrea, editors); Bentham Science Publishers.

[41] Malinowski DP, Avissar PL, Li H, Hall LB, Parker MS, Taylor AJ, Fischer TJ. Aberrant S-Phase induction in high-grade cervical disease: specific over-expression of minichromosome maintenance protein-2 (MCM2) as a diagnostic marker for moderate-severe dysplasia and cervical carcinoma. *Journal of Cytopathology*, 2005; 16: 19.

[42] Malinowski DP, Avissar PL, Li H, Hall LB, Parker MS, Taylor AJ, Fischer TJ. Aberrant S-phase induction as a molecular parameter for the detection of CIN2+ disease in cervical histology and cytology specimens. *Cancer Cytopathology*, 2005; 105: 356.

In: Tumor Markers Research Focus
Editor: Deborah H. Chang, pp. 63-79
ISBN: 978-1-60021-544-5


*Chapter IV*

# Advances in Tumour Biomarker Discovery for Screening Gynaecological Malignancy: CA125 and Beyond

***Kothandaraman Narasimhan and Mahesh Choolani****
Obstetrics and Gynaecology Department, National University Hospital, Singapore,
5 Lower Kent Ridge Crescent Road, 119704

## Abstract

Tumour markers are either sent into the blood, urine or tissues by the tumour itself, or by the body in response to the tumour. With the advent of sophisticated technologies more sensitive tumour markers have been reported in the last few years. One of the major cancers being investigated for serum tumour markers is for gynaecological cancers, especially cancer of the ovary. In this report we will focus on the new developments after the discovery of cancer antigen-125. Broadly the approaches leading to tumour marker discovery could be classified into three (1) biomarker discovery using proteomic approaches (2) using genomic approaches and (3) more recently using metabolomics approaches. And there is another entirely different approach using mass spectrometry based pattern profiling for cancer diagnosis. Using proteomics approach more than 30 serum markers have been evaluated alone and in combination with CA-125 by different investigators. Some of the promising markers include: HE4, mesothelin, M-CSF, osteopontin, kallikrein(s), soluble EGF receptor, serum amyloid A1, bikunin, leptin, prolactin, osteopontin, and insulin-like growth factor-II. Serum secretory leukocyte protease inhibitor levels as well as creatine kinase B are some other promising serum markers identified for ovarian cancer. Currently the focus is on the development of multiplex platforms for simultaneous assay of several markers with small volumes of serum. A more recent advance is to use immune system as a biosensor where serum immunoglobulins from cancer patients could be used as bait for detecting cancer specific antigens. This global

* E-mail address: obgmac@nus.edu.sg, Phone: +65-67724279, Fax: +65-67794753 Correspondence address: Diagnostic Biomarker Discovery Laboratory, Obstetrics and Gynaecology Department, National University Hospital, 5 Lower Kent Ridge Road, Singapore 119074

approach to antigenic profiling, epitomics, has applications to cancer diagnostics. Molecular genetic markers for ovarian cancer include BRCA-1, BRCA-2, Ras oncogenes, C-erb2 proto-oncogene, p53 suppressor gene and Bcl-2 oncogene. Using rigorous genomic approaches, whole transcriptome have been investigated for biomarker discovery. Interrogation of the entire transcriptome in human cancers and normal tissues, coupled with refined methods for sequence motif searching, and biological methods for enrichment are likely to yield many more tumour marker candidates. The other novel approaches developed from the above platform technologies include use of (1) anti-tumor antibodies which have the potential as cancer biomarkers were the anti-tumor response tends to be confined to individuals with ovarian cancer (2) another approach is to use a multianalyte cytokine panel profiling technology for simultaneous measurement of concentrations of 24 cytokines (cytokines/chemokines, growth, and angiogenic factors) in combination with CA-125. Using mass spectrometry approaches, pattern based recognition has reported higher sensitivity and specificity. The same technology has helped in the identification of 3 biomarkers (a) apolipoprotein A1 (down-regulated in cancer); (b) a truncated form of transthyretin (down-regulated); and (c) a cleavage fragment of inter-alpha-trypsin inhibitor heavy chain H4 (up-regulated). The other promising technology is to use metabolites as markers for cancer. One of the first markers identified using metabolites, lysophophatidic acid, happens to be a marker for ovarian cancer. Recently a new potential marker, Carcinoma cell-specific Mig7, have been identified for circulating and migrating cancer cells. This would form the next generation of imaging techniques which would play key role in the noninvasive screening for early detection of cancer.

In 2005, more than 22,000 American women were diagnosed with ovarian cancer and 16,000 women died from the disease (American Cancer Society Statistics, 2005). The five-year relative survival rate for stage III and IV ovarian cancer is 31%, and the five-year relative survival rate for stage I is 95%. From an Asian perspective taking Singapore as an ideal centre due to its multiracial ethnic population, 1028 new cases of ovarian cancer were reported for a period from 1998 – 2002 (Singapore Cancer Registry, 2002). About half of these women would die from the cancer within two years. In most cases, early detection offers a high cure rate while 75% of patients suffering from ovarian cancer are detected at an advanced stage. Ultimately early diagnosis could significantly lower the fatality rate.

## Difficulties Associated with Detection of Ovarian Cancer

A key challenge in cancer control and prevention is detection of the disease at an early stage itself, which could result in effective intervention and therapies to contribute to reduction in mortality and morbidity. Ovarian cancer is difficult to diagnose because the symptoms are vague and there are currently no reliable means of detecting the disease. Unfortunately, early diagnosis is difficult because of the physically inaccessible location of the ovaries, the lack of specific symptoms in early disease, and the limited understanding of ovarian oncogenesis. Screening tests for ovarian cancer need high sensitivity and specificity to be useful because of the low prevalence of undiagnosed ovarian cancer. Because currently available screening tests do not achieve high levels of sensitivity and specificity, screening is not recommended for the general population. The theoretical advantage of screening is much higher for women at high risk (such as those with a strong family history of ovarian cancer and those with BRCA 1 or BRCA 2 mutations). However, even for women at high risk, no prospective studies have shown benefits of screening. The public health challenge is that 90% of ovarian cancer occurs in women who are not in an identifiable high-risk group, and most women are diagnosed with advanced-stage disease. Currently available tests using cancer antigen 125 (CA125), transvaginal ultrasound, or a combination of both lacks the sensitivity and specificity to be useful in screening the general population.

## Ovarian Cancer Tumour Markers

At a specific time, biomarkers serve as molecular signposts of the physiologic state of a cell. These signposts are the result of genes, their products (proteins) and other organic chemicals made by the cell. Biomarkers could prove to be vital for the identification of early cancer and subjects at risk of developing cancer as a normal cell progresses through the complex process of transformation to a cancerous state. A variety of biomarkers have been developed to monitor growth of ovarian cancer and to detect disease at an early phase. CA125 also known as MUC16 has served as a useful serum tumor marker for (1) screening ovarian cancer, (2) monitoring response to chemotherapy, (3) detecting disease recurrence, (4) distinguishing malignant from benign pelvic masses, and (5) potentially improving clinical trial design. Several studies now document that CA125 can serve as a surrogate marker for response in phase II trials. Serial measurement of CA125 might also provide a useful marker for monitoring stabilization of disease with cytostatic targeted therapeutic agents. The greatest potential for serum markers may be in detecting ovarian cancer at an early stage.

## A Brief History on the Discovery and Application of CA125

CA125 was discovered as human tumor marker by Dr. Robert C. Bast, Jr. in 1983 (Bast et al., 1983). History for the discovery of CA125 dates backs to the early 70's associated with the attempts to obtain monoclonal reagents for serotherapy of patients with ovarian cancer. It was observed in animal model studies that the intraperitoneal injection of a heteroantiserum developed in rabbits against a partially purified tumor- associated antigen could inhibit the intraperitoneal growth of syngeneic murine ovarian cancer transplants (Order et al., 1973 & 74). With the advent of the monoclonal antibody technology by Kohler and Milstein in 1975 (Kohler et al., 1975), attempts were made to develop antibodies reactive with ovarian cancer that might be administered in combination with *Corynebacterium parvum* (Knapp et al., 1977). Mice were repeatedly injected with a human ovarian cancer cell line and hybridomas were prepared from immune spleen cells and the P3NS-1 plasmacytoma. From these hybridomas, clones were isolated based on the production of antibodies that bound to the ovarian cancer cell line used for immunization. One the clone ($125^{th}$ clone) produced an IgG1 antibody of the desired specificity and was designated OC (ovarian cancer) 125.

Using immunohistochemical analysis, the OC 125 antibody was found to bind antigen expressed by approximately 80% of epithelial ovarian cancers, as well as by other gynecologic, breast, lung, and colon carcinomas; this antigen was designated CA (cancer antigen) 125 (Bast et al., 1981). Mucinous ovarian cystadenocarcinomas were less frequently positive than serous and endometrioid tumors. In addition, OC 125 was found to reach with amnion and coelomic epithelium in embryos, as well as with a fraction of secretory endometria in adults.

Progress toward the characterization of CA125 began in the middle of 1980s. CA125 determinants were found to be associated with a family of high molecular weight glycoproteins, that differed from classical mucins by means of carbohydrate conversion (less than 50%) and the presence of both N- and O-linked carbohydrate residues (Davis et al., 1986). The smallest subunit retaining reactivity with OC 125 exhibited a mass of approximately 220 kD. It has been shown by many studies that CA125 is not a specific marker for ovarian cancer. It has been found elevated in sera obtained from patients with gynecological adenocarcinomas, as well as lymphomas, malignant mesotheliomas, immature teratomas, and carcinomas of the pancreas, colon, breast and lung. Elevations were also observed with benign conditions including severe endometriosis, adenomyosis, uterine fibroids, ovarian cysts, salpingitis, peritonitis, pleuritis, pericarditis, alcoholic hepatitis, and the first trimester of normal pregnancy. Although many of these conditions might complicate use of CA125 for screening a general population, they can be readily excluded when monitoring patients with known ovarian cancer. The CA125 assay was originally developed to monitor the course of patients with epithelial ovarian cancer. Most of the time chemotherapy which is highly cytotoxic is often administered for many months without a clear knowledge of whether the disease is responding to treatment. If a cutoff of 35 U/ml is chosen, which excludes 95% of apparently healthy individuals, more than 80% of patients with clinically evident ovarian cancer will have elevated CA125 levels (Bast et al., 1983). In patients with early stage disease and in those mucinous tumors, a smaller percentage exhibit elevated antigen levels.

It has been shown that a persistently rising level of CA125 has been associated with progressive growth of ovarian cancer in more than 90% of instances studied (Jacobs and Bast, 1989). Decreasing levels of CA125 have correlated with decreases in the volume of disease sufficiently often that CA125 has been proposed as an appropriate surrogate for measurable disease in conducting phase II trials of new drugs in patients with ovarian cancer (Rustin et al., 1996). CA125 can, however, return to less than 35 U/mL prior to "reassessment" of those ovarian cancer cases, and most often small volumes of disease can still be found in approximately half of patients. Consequently, CA125 is not optimally sensitive as a marker for residual disease, but, if elevated, can predict the persistence of disease with greater than 95% accuracy (Jacobs and Bast, 1989). This correlation prompted approval of the CA125 assay by the United States Food and Drug Administration.

## Tissue Expression of CA125 versus Serum CA125 Levels

A novel approach using ten potential markers for ovarian cancer was shown by Rosen et al., (2005) were tissue expression of CA125 was compared to serum CA125 levels. From 296 ovarian cancers, 65 (22%) were found to have weak or absent CA125 expression on immunoperoxidase staining. Using immunoperoxidase staining of tissue arrays, expression of 10 potential serum tumor markers in the 65 epithelial ovarian cancers with little or no CA125 expression and in ovarian cystadenomas, tumors of low malignant potential, normal ovaries, and 16 other normal tissues was reported in this study by Rosen et al., (2005). Low or absent expression of CA125 in surgical specimens of epithelial ovarian cancer was associated with low levels of serum CA125 in pre-operative serum specimens. In ovarian cancers that lacked CA125, all specimens (100%) expressed human kallikrein 10 (HK10), human kallikrein 6 (HK6), osteopontin (OPN), and claudin 3. A smaller fraction of CA125-deficient ovarian cancers expressed DF3 (95%), vascular endothelial growth factor (VEGF) (81%), MUC1 (62%), mesothelin (MES) (34%), HE4 (32%), and CA19-9 (29%). At the level of tissue expression, each of 10 potential serum markers could be detected in 29-100% of ovarian cancers that had low or absent expression of CA125.

### Screening Studies for Ovarian Cancer

One of the most comprehensive studies involving ovarian cancer marker CA125 was reported in UK in 2005 (Bast et al., 2005). It is a well followed practice that most of the time a rising CA125 can be used to generate transvaginal sonography (TVS) in a small fraction of patients. With this general observation the group led by Bast has developed an algorithm that calculates the risk of ovarian cancer based on serial CA125 values and refers patients at highest risk for TVS. Use of the algorithm is currently being evaluated in a trial with 200,000 women in the UK that will test critically the ability of a two-stage screening strategy to improve survival in ovarian cancer. However approximately 20% of ovarian cancers have little or no expression of CA125, additional serum markers will be required to detect all patients in an initial phase of screening.

## The Advent of New Technology Post CA125: Role of Multiplex Panel of Markers

Approximately more than 30 serum markers have been evaluated alone or in combination with CA125 by different investigators (Bast et al., 2005). Some of the most promising include: HE4, mesothelin, M-CSF, osteopontin, kallikrein(s), and soluble EGF receptor. Numerous other markers such as NB 70K, IAP, PLAP, CA 15-3 and TAG 72, are actually in the clinical evaluation phase, for the most part in association with CA125. Several groups are placing markers on multiplex platforms to permit simultaneous assay of multiple markers with very small volumes of serum. With increasing complexity and large amount of data generated, mathematical techniques are being developed to analyze combinations of marker levels to improve sensitivity and specificity (Bast et al., 2005). Several approaches were followed to identify these potential markers. Most of the current approaches follow a similar trend were both genomic and proteomic techniques are used to identify candidate markers for potential screening on a larger cohort. In one such study, protein microarray based assay was carried out using 169 proteins in serum from 28 healthy women, 18 women newly diagnosed with EOC, and 40 women with recurrent disease (Mor et al., 2005). Evaluation of those proteins which showed significant differences in expression between controls and cancer patients by ELISA assays yielded four candidates. These four proteins were later evaluated in a blind cross-validation study by using 106 healthy females and 100 patients with EOC (24 stage I/II and 76 stage III/IV). As in most of other studies it was found that no single protein could completely distinguish the cancer group from the healthy controls. However, the combination of the four analytes exhibited a sensitivity of 95%, positive predictive value (PPV) 95%, specificity 95%, and negative predictive value (NPV) 94%, which could be considered a considerable improvement of current methodology.

The greatest potential for serum markers may be in detecting ovarian cancer at an early stage. Another marker widely found acceptable is osteopontin (OPN). OPN is a putative plasma biomarker that was recently identified using high-throughput cDNA microarray technology (Brakora et al., 2004). OPN has been shown to be clinically useful adjunct to CA125 in detecting recurrent ovarian cancer (Schorge et al., 2004). OPN levels tend to decline after treatment was initiated, but decreasing CA125 measurements were more consistently observed. Although inferior to CA125 in predicting clinical response to therapy, OPN rose earlier in 90% of the patients developing recurrent disease (median lead time, 3 months) (Schorge et al., 2004).

## Role of Complementary Serum Markers with CA125 for Ovarian Cancer Screening

Since the existing markers lack both sensitivity and specificity, multiple serum markers have been proposed and followed for screening women for detecting early stage epithelial ovarian cancer. The use of serum tumor markers for the early detection of ovarian cancer has been limited because of their low sensitivity and low positive predictive value. CA125 levels are elevated in only about one half of women with Stage I ovarian cancer, thus researchers have focused on using the serial measurement of complementary markers to improve the sensitivity, specificity, and positive predictive value of this approach for screening. CA125, CA15-3, C19-9, CA54-61, CA72-4, CEA, HMFG2, IL-6, IL-10, LSA, M-CSF, NB70K, OVX1, PLAP, TAG72, TNF, TPA, and UGTF have been studied alone and in combination (Berek et al., 1995). It has been found that by using a serial analysis of a second-generation CA125 to measure the intercept (initial level) and slope (change of levels over time) could be used to discriminate malignant cases from benign and normal cases. Studies has shown that the serial measurement of the new, more sensitive CA125 has a high sensitivity (83%), specificity (99.7%), and positive predictive value (16%) for the early detection of ovarian cancer. It has been found that OVX1 used in combination with CA125 provides the best complementarity. Serial measurements of the two markers have sensitivities in the range of that for transvaginal ultrasonography. The serial measurement of complementary serum markers can improve the use of marker screening for epithelial ovarian cancer. With the use of several different methods of analysis, it has been shown that this approach improves the sensitivity, specificity, and positive predictive value of serum markers CA125 and OVX1.

Thus a procedure that measures complementary serum markers over time can be used as a primary screening technique followed by transvaginal ultrasonography. This could provide a cost-effective means of early detection and could significantly decrease the probability of surgical intervention for false-positive test results. In another study a panel of three tumor markers (CA125, M-CSF and OVX1) (Woolas et al., 1993) when used could successfully identify early-stage ovarian cancer with extremely high sensitivity and moderate specificity, by studying 204 apparently healthy women, 46 patients with stage I ovarian cancer of different histologies and 237 patients with benign pelvic masses. At least one of the serum markers was elevated in 98% of patients with stage I ovarian cancer and at the same time

CA125 levels were found to be elevated in 67%. By the same criteria, 11% of healthy individuals and 51% of patients with benign pelvic masses had at least one elevated marker value. Thus, the sensitivity of the combination of assays for the three serum markers was significantly greater than the sensitivity of the CA125 assay and specificity was found to be moderate.

Use of protein microarray helps in studying hundreds of target proteins at a single time. A more recent study (Mor et al., 2005) was reported using protein microarray approach to determine the levels of 169 candidate proteins in serum from 28 healthy women, 18 women newly diagnosed with EOC, and 40 women with recurrent disease. Four candidate proteins (1) leptin, (2) prolactin, (3) osteopontin, and (4) insulin-like growth factor-II, was used for this purpose. The study could discriminate between disease-free and EOC patients, including patients diagnosed with stage I and II disease, with high efficiency (95%). Evaluation of proteins that showed significant differences in expression between controls and cancer patients by ELISA assays yielded the four analytes. These four proteins then were evaluated in a blind cross-validation study by using an additional 106 healthy females and 100 patients with EOC (24 stage I/II and 76 stage III/IV). As in previous studies (Woolas et al., 1993) no single protein could completely distinguish the cancer group from the healthy controls. However, the combination of the four analytes exhibited the following: sensitivity 95%, positive predictive value (PPV) 95%, specificity 95%, and negative predictive value (NPV) 94%, a considerable improvement.

## Serum Markers for Distinguishing Subclasses with in Ovarian Cancers

Some studies have focussed on categorising subclasses within the ovarian cancer (An et al., 2006). Studies showed distinct properties for ovarian mucinous tumors from other ovarian epithelial tumours. It was found that LMP mucinous tumours showing histologically aggressive features belong to mucinous carcinoma based on proteomic analysis. The following five proteins were found to be upregulated in the LMP mucinous tumors, (1) NM23, annexin-1, (2) protein phosphatase-1, (3) ferritin light chain, (4) proteasome alpha-6, and (5) NAGK (N-acetyl glucosamine kinase) (An et al., 2006).

## Kallikreins as Serum Markers for Ovarian Cancer

Kallikreins are a family of secreted serine proteases, encoded by 15 genes which all localize in tandem on chromosome 19q13.4. Several members of this family have been previously associated with ovarian cancer. Kallikreins 6 (KLK6) and 10 (KLK10) are elevated in tumour cells, serum and ascites fluid of ovarian cancer patients and correlate with disease prognosis (Oikonomopoulou et al., 2006). Kallikrein expression by ovarian cancer cells is not specific enough for detecting disseminated disease. Kallikrein expression may have some value for differentiating ovarian cancer from other types of cancer or from non-malignant diseases that lead to ascites accumulation. Other kallikreins that have been related to ovarian cancer include KLK4, 5, 7, 8, 9, 11, 13, 14 and 15 (Yousef and Diamandis, 2003;

Bast et al., 2005). These markers were used to monitor dissemination of ovarian cancer cells in blood and ascites fluid of ovarian cancer patients. Screening for disseminated cancer cells in blood from 24 ovarian cancer patients, with RT-PCR for KLK6 mRNA, resulted in 75% positivity; however, this was not different from the positivity of normal controls. By utilizing KLK10 as a marker, the positivity of patients was 40% versus 20% of controls. Screening of ascites fluid of ovarian cancer patients revealed 90% positivity for KLK6 and KLK10 mRNA compared with 33% for other cancer types. Significant correlations were identified among mRNA of KLK4, 5, 6, 7, 8, 9, 10, 11, 13, 14 and 15 in cancer cells isolated from ascites fluid.

Human kallikrein 8 has been used as an independent marker of favourable prognosis in ovarian cancer (Borgono et al., 2006). Human kallikrein 8 (hK8/neuropsin/ovasin; encoded by KLK8) is a steroid hormone-regulated secreted serine protease differentially expressed in ovarian carcinoma. KLK8 mRNA levels are associated with a favourable patient prognosis and hK8 protein levels are elevated in the sera of 62% ovarian cancer patients, suggesting that KLK8/hK8 is a prospective biomarker. Using ELISA, hK8 was quantified in 136 ovarian tumor extracts and correlated with clinicopathologic variables and outcome [progression-free survival (PFS); overall survival (OS)] over a median follow-up period of 42 months. hK8 levels in ovarian tumor cytosols ranged from 0 to 478 ng/mg total protein, with a median of 30 ng/mg. The optimal cutoff value of 25.8 ng/mg total protein was reported based on the ability of hK8 values to predict the PFS of the study population and to categorize tumors as hK8 positive or negative (Borgono et al., 2006). Women with hK8-positive tumors most often had lower-grade tumors (G1), no residual tumor after surgery, and optimal debulking success. Studies showed that patients with hK8-positive tumors had a significantly longer PFS and OS than hK8-negative patients. Further detailed studies confirmed a reduced risk of relapse and death in women with hK8-positive tumours.

Using cDNA database mining strategies and real-time quantitative reverse transcription-PCR, B7-H4 was identified as a novel membrane-bound protein and a candidate serum and tissue biomarker for ovarian cancer (Simon et al., 2006). Studies using this strategy showed that B7-H4 was found to be overexpressed in ovarian and breast cancer tissues when compared with normal tissues. The gene encodes a protein of 282 amino acids with a signal sequence, an immunoglobulin domain, and a −COOH-terminal hydrophobic transmembrane domain. Immunohistochemistry experiments showed plasma membrane staining in serous ovarian and breast cancer, confirming the tissue specificity and cell surface localization for B7-H4. Using a sensitive dual monoclonal antibody sandwich ELISA method the levels of B7-H4 protein tested on more than >2,500 serum samples, ascites fluids, and tissue lysates showed high levels of B7-H4 protein were detected in ovarian cancer tissue lysates when compared with normal tissues. B7-H4 showed an elevated level in serum samples from ovarian cancer patients when compared with healthy controls or women with benign gynecologic diseases. The median B7-H4 concentration in endometrioid and serous histotypes was found to be higher than in mucinous histotypes, consistent with results of immunohistochemical staining. In early-stage patients, the sensitivity at 97% specificity increased from 52% for CA125 alone to 65% when used in combination with B7-H4.

## Interleukins

Cytokines produced by leucocytes and acting mainly on other white blood cells are called interleukins. Some studies have shown the role of cytokines as a new group of tumor markers for ovarian cancer. Similar to protein markers studies have shown the use of a panel of multiple cytokines, which individually may not show strong correlation with the disease, might provide higher diagnostic power (Gorelik et al., 2005). To evaluate the diagnostic utility of cytokine panel, a novel multianalyte (panel of markers) termed as LabMAP profiling technology was designed that allows simultaneous measurement of multiple markers was reported recently by Gorelik et al., (2005). Concentrations of 24 cytokines (cytokines/chemokines, growth, and angiogenic factors) in combination with cancer antigen-125 (CA-125) were measured in sera of 44 patients with early-stage ovarian cancer, 45 healthy women, and 37 patients with benign pelvic tumors. Six markers, interleukin (IL)-6, IL-8, epidermal growth factor (EGF), vascular endothelial growth factor (VEGF), monocyte chemoattractant protein-1 (MCP-1), and CA-125, showed significant differences in serum concentrations between ovarian cancer and control groups. Out of this group, IL-6, IL-8, VEGF, EGF, and CA-125, were used in a classification tree analysis that resulted in 84% sensitivity at 95% specificity. The receiver operator characteristic curve created using the combination of markers produced sensitivities between 90% and 100% in the area of 80% to 90% specificity, whereas the receiver operator characteristic curve for CA125 alone resulted in sensitivities of 70% to 80%. The classification tree analysis for discrimination of benign condition from ovarian cancer used CA125, granulocyte colony-stimulating factor (G-CSF), IL-6, EGF, and VEGF resulting in 86.5% sensitivity and 93.0% specificity. The study showed that simultaneous testing of a panel of serum cytokines and CA-125 using LabMAP technology may present a promising approach for ovarian cancer detection.

In another study (Le Page et al., 2006), three markers (IL-18, FGF-2, and CA125) showed similar sensitivity in scoring for ovarian cancer (35/45 patients) compared to that of CA125 alone (37/45) and significantly improved the specificity of detection (20/25 patients) compared to each marker individually (15/25 for CA125; 18/25 FGF-2; 16/25 for IL-18).

## Biomarker Discovery Using Genomics Approaches

The main challenge in cancer control and prevention is to detect the cancer early. The identification and definition of the molecular profiles of cancer will require the development and dissemination of high-throughput molecular analysis technologies, as well as elucidation of all of the molecular species embedded in the genome of cancer and normal cells. This could then enable effective interventions and therapies contributing to reduction in mortality and morbidity. Cancer is not a single disease but more often due to an accumulation of several events, genetic and epigenetic, arising from a single cell over a long time interval. A high priority in the cancer field is to identify these events. Most often this can be achieved by characterizing cancer-associated genes and their protein products. Ongoing research in the field of genomics could be broadly classified into genetic and proteomic approaches to identify molecular signatures such as protein profiles, microsatellite instability, hypermethylation, and single nucleotide polymorphisms. Identifying the molecular alterations that distinguish any particular cancer cell from a normal cell will ultimately help to define the nature and predict the pathologic behaviour of that cancer cell. Understanding the profile of molecular changes in any particular cancer will be extremely useful as it will become possible to correlate the resulting phenotype of that cancer with molecular events.

Genetic abnormalities occur in all cancers and genes that safe guard the integrity of the cell are those which are most studied to be associated with cancer. The most characterised genes associated ovarian and breast cancers are the tumour suppressor genes BRCA1 and BRCA2. BRCA-related pathways are critical because they serve to safeguard genetic content. Germline mutations in the tumor suppressor genes BRCA1 and BRCA2 predispose women to breast and ovarian cancer. Female carriers of BRCA1 or BRCA2 gene mutations have very high lifetime risks for breast and ovarian cancers. Although protecting genetic information is a general function, BRCA-related pathways seem largely specific to preventing breast and ovarian cancer. Although mutations target breast and ovary, a broader spectrum of cancers also occur with statistically significant elevated frequencies. Risks for "all cancers except breast or ovary" are elevated, with some population subgroups differing with regard to how frequently elevated risks were found at individual sites (Friedenson et al., 2005). Additional sites at risk (risk range from 20% to 60%) included stomach, pancreas, prostate, and colon. Studies from several groups suggest applying an increased level of clinical alertness to those with defects in BRCA-related pathways.

A novel approach by merging genomic and proteomic approaches Huddleston (2005) identified creatine kinase B (CKB) is elevated in pre-operative sera from ovarian cancer patients compared to patients with benign pelvic masses and normal controls. cDNA microarray system and RNA derived from pooled ovarian cancer cell lines and normal ovary surface epithelial cells (HOSE) were used to identify differentially expressed genes. Microarray technology revealed that CKB gene expression had a cancer to HOSE ratio of 18. RNA levels of CKB, measured by real-time PCR, were elevated a by 36 fold in cancer cell lines compared with HOSE cells and 22.75 fold in microdissected ovarian cancer epithelial cells compared with normal ovarian epithelial cells. CKB activity was measured in pre-operative serum samples obtained from 45 ovarian cancer patients, 49 patients with a benign pelvic mass, as well as 37 normal controls showed the CKB enzyme activity in cancer cases as 24.7 U/L units (+/- 5.1) compared to 9.6 U/L (+/- 1.6) for benign mass cases and to 8.5 U/L (1.7) for normal controls.

In another recent report (Adib et al., 2004) using microarray approach identified mammaglobin-2 (MGB2) which found to be highly expressed and specific to ovarian cancer. MGB2, in combination with other putative markers identified here, could have the potential for screening.

## Pattern Based Diagnosis for Ovarian Cancer Diagnosis

Considerable interest and controversy has been generated by initial results utilizing surface-enhanced laser desorption/ionization (SELDI) in ovarian cancer (Diamandis, 2003 & 2004). There are challenging issues related to the design of studies to evaluate SELDI and other proteomic technology, as well as the reproducibility, sensitivity, and specificity of this new technology. Large serum banks such as that assembled in UKCTOCS at UK, which contain preclinical samples from patients who later developed ovarian cancer and other disorders, provide a unique resource for carefully designed studies of proteomic technology. There is a sound basis for optimism that further developments in serum proteomic analysis will provide powerful methods for screening in ovarian cancer and many other diseases. Studies using protein profiling mainly rely on the use of serum samples from diseased and healthy controls for identifying patterns or fingerprints associated with the disease. The pioneering study using this technology was reported for diagnosing ovarian cancer by Petricoin's group in 2002 (Petricoin et al., 2002). Later this technology has been used for mostly all different types of human cancers (Wiesner , 2004; Bons, 2005; Engwegen, 2006). Mostly all the studies have reported more that 90% accuracy in diagnosing the disease condition. However due the technical limitations as well as no general guidelines on sample preparation and storage this technology is still in its nascent stages but still hold immense promise towards development as a promising technology for cancer screening. The major advantages of this technology are being high-throughput and require very little quantity for the whole analysis. And the results could be achieved in 2-3 hours following preparation of serum samples.

Attempts have been made to characterise the so called unique proteins identified in the protein spectra. Most of the biomarkers either identified or still under characterisation belong to the low molecular mass range, between 0-20 kDa. These markers have been postulated to be fragments from high abundance proteins. The proteins or peptides could have originated through degradation or through protein cleavage by endo-proteinases floating in serum. These proteases could also arise during sample perpetration or during the thawing process.

One of the biggest challenges is to characterise the identity of the unique peaks/features present in the protein profile/spectrum as identified using profiling approaches. Very few reports are available in this regard. Recently by Kozak's group, (2005) reported the identification of three ovarian cancer biomarker panels comprised of SELDI-TOF-MS peaks representing 14 differentially expressed serum proteins for the diagnosis of ovarian cancer. Using another highly sensitive technique called micro-LC-MS/MS, they identified five m/z peaks as transthyretin (TTR 13.9 kDa, TTR fragment 12.9 kDa), beta-hemoglobin (Hb, 15.9 kDa), apolipoprotein AI (ApoAI, 28 kDa) and transferrin (TF, 79 kDa). Western and/or ELISA methods confirmed the differential expression of TTR, Hb, and TF, and multivariate analyses resulted in improving the detection of early stage ovarian tumors as compared to cancer antigen CA125 alone.

## Scepticism Associated with Low Molecular Weight Biomarkers

One of the major concerns associated with these markers is that they are mostly associated with the high abundance proteins in serum. And most of the time they appear in association with some form of inflammatory response which could render them non-specific to a particular type of disease. A truncated form of Transthyretin (TTR) has recently been described to be part of a set of biomarkers for the diagnosis of ovarian cancer (Kozak et al., 2005). TTR was also known to be a traditional biomarker for nutritional and inflammatory status exists in different molecular variants however their functions are not yet clear. A recent study (Gericke et al., 2005) has investigated the source of differences in microheterogeneity between ascitic fluid and plasma of women affected with ovarian cancer and to evaluate the tumor site as the possible source of TTR. The results show that the severity of the cancer associated catabolism as well as the inflammation status affect serum TTR and RBP levels. Neither TTR nor its truncated form originates from tumor tissue and its occurrence in ascites may well reflect the filtration from blood into ascitic fluid.

## Tumour Antigens

To gain a comprehensive understanding of the physiology and pathophysiology of cancer an approach that harmoniously integrates the various 'omic' platforms are key to unravelling the complexity of biomarker/tumour antigen discovery (Miles et al., 2006). Altered proteins or changes in gene expression in malignant cells may lead to the expression of tumour antigens recognised by host immune system. Current research in this filed focuses on the use of molecular technologies to study the global genomic-wide analysis of changes in DNA (genotyping), RNA expression (transcriptomics) and protein expression (proteomics) that have enabled the acceleration for the new biomarker/tumour antigen discovery. A recent study by Chatterjee et al., (2006) have reported the use of a combination of high-throughput selection and array-based serologic detection of many antigens indicative of the presence of cancer, thereby using the immune system as a biosensor. This high-throughput selection involved biopanning of an ovarian cancer phage display library using serum immunoglobulins from an ovarian cancer patient as bait. Protein macroarrays containing 480 of these selected antigen clones revealed 65 clones that interacted with immunoglobulins in sera from 32 ovarian cancer patients but not with sera from 25 healthy women or 14 patients having other benign or malignant gynecologic diseases. Sequence analysis data of these 65 clones revealed 62 different antigens. Among the markers identified some known antigens, including RCAS1, signal recognition protein-19, AHNAK-related sequence, nuclear autoantogenic sperm protein, Nijmegen breakage syndrome 1 (Nibrin), ribosomal protein L4, Homo sapiens KIAA0419 gene product, eukaryotic initiation factor 5A, and casein kinase II, as well as many previously uncharacterized antigenic gene products. Using these 65 antigens on protein microarrays, neural networks were trained on two-colour fluorescent detection of serum IgG binding. The results showed an average sensitivity and specificity of 55% and 98%, respectively. In addition, the top 6 of the most specific clones resulted in an average sensitivity and specificity of 32% and 94%, respectively. This global approach to antigenic profiling, epitomics, has applications to cancer and autoimmune diseases for diagnostic and therapeutic studies. Further work with larger panels of antigens should provide a comprehensive set of markers with sufficient sensitivity and specificity suitable for clinical testing in high-risk populations.

## Anti-tumor Antibodies have Potential as Cancer Biomarkers

Another novel approach is the use of anti-tumor antibodies which has the potential to be used as cancer biomarkers (Luborsky et al., 2005). There is limited information on the prevalence of anti-tumor antibodies among ovarian cancer patients. Although most anti-tumor antibodies react with antigens common to both tumor and normal tissue, the anti-tumor response tends to be confined to individuals with ovarian cancer, similar to other cancers. Antibodies to HOXA7, a differentiation antigen, have the highest reported prevalence in ovarian cancer (67%). Antibodies to other ubiquitous antigens including NY-ESO-1, Ep-CAM (epithelial cell adhesion molecule), HSP-90 (heat shock protein 90), and mutated p53 have been identified in ovarian cancer. Anti-tumor antibody specificity reflects the heterogeneity of antigen expression in tumors. Tests based on panels of a combination of anti-tumor antibodies may be more predictive for ovarian cancer, as no single specificity accounts for ovarian tumors. In addition to characterization of anti-tumor antibodies as diagnostic markers, study of anti-tumor antibodies is likely to provide insights into mechanisms of tumor development. There is evidence of antibodies to tumor antigens and of activated T cells, suggesting immune recognition of tumor antigens occurred. Nonetheless, as tumors are not 'rejected', it is likely that there are alterations in the immune system. The basis for tumor growth in the face of immune activity remains to be determined.

## Metabolites as Markers for Ovarian Cancer

Lysophosphatidic acid (LPA) has been shown to stimulate proliferation of ovarian cancer cells and is present in the ascitic fluid of patients with ovarian cancer. Plasma LPA levels may represent a potential biomarker for ovarian cancer and other gynaecologic cancers. However, these findings are preliminary and require confirmation in larger studies (Xu et al., 1998). Patients in the ovarian cancer group had significantly higher plasma LPA levels compared with the healthy control group. Elevated plasma LPA levels were detected in 9 of 10 patients with stage I ovarian cancer, 24 of 24 patients with stage II, III, and IV ovarian cancer, and 14 of 14 patients with recurrent ovarian cancer. Elevated plasma LPA levels were detected in 5 of 48 controls and 4 of 17 patients with benign gynecologic diseases and in no women with breast cancer or leukemia. In comparison, among a subset of patients with ovarian cancer, 28 of 47 had elevated CA125 levels, including 2 of 9 patients with stage I disease. In another study LPA and other lysophospholipids (LPL) were found to be useful markers for diagnosis and/or prognosis of ovarian cancer in a controlled setting (Sutphen et al., 2004). Blinded LPL analysis, including 23 individual LPL species, was performed on case patients with epithelial ovarian cancer (n = 117) and healthy control subjects (n = 27). The combination of 16:0-LPA and 20:4-LPA yielded the best discrimination between preoperative case samples and control samples, with 93.1% correct classification, 91.1% sensitivity, and 96.3% specificity.

## Imaging Cancer Cells: Potential Applications in Cancer Diagnosis

The more recent advance and highly promising technique in detecting ovarian cancer is using imaging techniques. CAT (computed tomography) Scan, PET (positron emission tomography) Scan, Mammogram, MRI (magnetic resonance imaging), Nuclear medicine scan and bone scan and Ultrasonography or Ultrasound. Transvaginal ultrasonography is the most efficient, accurate, and least expensive of the imaging modalities (transabdominal ultrasonography, computed tomography, magnetic resonance imaging, radioimmunoscintigraphy) for this purpose. Doppler flow imaging and morphology index values improve the accuracy of transvaginal ultrasonography.

However newer technologies are set to replace the existing technologies in the near future. The detection of cell-bound proteins that are produced due to aberrant gene expression in malignant tumours can provide important diagnostic information influencing patient management. Affibody molecules represent a new class of affinity molecules that can provide small sized, high affinity cancer-specific ligands, which may be well suited for tumor imaging (Orlova et al., 2006). The use of small radiolabeled targeting proteins would enable high-contrast radionuclide imaging of cancers expressing such antigens if adequate binding affinity and specificity could be provided. HER2-specific 6 kDa Affibody molecule at a concentration of 22 pmol/L affinity that can be used for the visualization of HER2 expression in tumours in vivo using gamma camera. When radioiodinated, the affinity-matured Affibody molecule showed clear, high-contrast visualization of HER2-expressing xenografts in mice as early as 6 hours post-injection. The tumor uptake at 4 hours post-injection was improved 4-fold (due to increased affinity) with 9% of the injected dose per gram of tissue in the tumor (Orlova et al., 2006).

Another protein which could aid in the detection of migrating cancer cell is the Carcinoma cell-specific Mig-7 (Phillips et al., 2005). Mig-7 is highly specific localization to cancer cells in contrast to an absence in normal cells. By immunohistochemistry and by RT-PCR, Mig-7 mRNA was detected in lymph nodes from 7 out of 9 (77.8%) endometrial carcinoma xenograft in mice but not from any of the 5 negative control animals. The preliminary data from this group indicate that Mig-7 (Phillips et al., 2005) may be a potential early marker of migrating and circulating carcinoma cells.

## Summary

A wide gap currently exists between the ability to discover potential biomarkers and the ability to assess the real value of these proteins for ovarian cancer screening. The challenge in biomarker validation is the inherent variability in biomarker levels. This variability stems from the diversity across the human population and the considerable molecular heterogeneity between individual ovarian tumors. Another challenge for a promising biomarker is the low prevalence of these tumours in the general population meaning that the assay specificity must be very high. Otherwise, the number of false positives will be much greater than the number of true positives. Due to these challenges associated with biomarker validation, it becomes a necessity to analyse many thousands of samples in order to obtain a clear picture of the utility of a screening protocol using a promising serum tumour marker. Currently the most cost effective and easy to use technology is using Enzyme-linked immunosorbent assay (ELISA) technology. Other promising technologies such as protein microarray, multiple panels of biomarkers and assays using mass spectrometry will soon replace the existing technologies in the near future.

## Reference


[1] Adib, TR; Henderson, S; Perrett, C. et al., Predicting biomarkers for ovarian cancer using gene-expression microarrays. *Br J Cancer*. 2004, 90, 686-92.

[2] American Cancer Society Statistics, 2005. http://www.cancer.org/docroot/STT/stt_0.asp

[3] An, HJ; Kim, DS; Park, YK. Et al., Comparative proteomics of ovarian epithelial tumors. *J Proteome Res*. 2006; 5, 1082-90.

[4] Bast, RC Jr; Badgwell, D; Lu, Z et al., CA125 and beyond. *Int J Gynecol Cancer*. 2005,15 Suppl, 3, 274-81.

[5] Bast, RC Jr; Feeney, M; Lazarus, H. et al. Reactivity of a monoclonal antibody with human ovarian carcinoma. *Journal of Clinical Investigation,* 1981, 68, 1331-1337.

[6] Bast, RC Jr; Klug, TL; St. John, E; et al. A radioimmunoassay using a monoclonal antibody to monitor the course of epithelial ovarian cancer. *New England Journal of Medicine*, 1983, 309, 883-887.

[7] Berek, J.S. & Bast, R.C. Jr. Ovarian cancer screening. The use of serial complementary tumor markers to improve sensitivity and specificity for early detection. *Cancer*. 1995, 76, 2092-6.

[8] Bons, JA ; Wodzig, WK ; van Dieijen-Visser MP. Protein profiling as a diagnostic tool in clinical chemistry: a review. *Clin Chem Lab Med*. 2005, 43, 1281-90.

[9] Borgono, CA; Kishi, T; Scorilas, A. et al., Human kallikrein 8 protein is a favorable prognostic marker in ovarian cancer. *Clin Cancer Res*. 2006, 12, 1487-93.

[10] Brakora, KA; Lee, H; Yusuf, R et al., Utility of osteopontin as a biomarker in recurrent epithelial ovarian cancer. *Gynecol Oncol*. 2004, 93, 361-5.

[11] Chatterjee, M; Mohapatra, S; Ionan, A. et al., Diagnostic markers of ovarian cancer by high-throughput antigen cloning and detection on arrays. *Cancer Res*. 2006, 66,1181-90.

[12] Davis, HM ; Zurawski, VR Jr ; Bast, RC Jr . et al., Characterization of the CA 125 antigen associated with human epithelial ovarian carcinomas. *Cancer Research,* 1986, 46, 6143-6148.

[13] Diamandis, EP. Analysis of serum proteomic patterns for early cancer diagnosis: drawing attention to potential problems. *J Natl Cancer Inst*. 2004, 96, 353-6.

[14] Diamandis, EP. Point: Proteomic patterns in biological fluids: do they represent the future of cancer diagnostics? *Clin Chem*. 2003, 49, 1272-5.

[15] Engwegen, JY; Gast, MC; Schellens, JH; Beijnen, JH. Clinical proteomics: searching for better tumour markers with SELDI-TOF mass spectrometry. *Trends Pharmacol Sci*. 2006, 27, 251-9.

[16] Friedenson, B. BRCA1 and BRCA2 pathways and the risk of cancers other than breast or ovarian. *MedGenMed*. 2005, 7, 60.

[17] Gericke, B; Raila, J; Sehouli, J. et al., Microheterogeneity of transthyretin in serum and ascitic fluid of ovarian cancer patients. *BMC Cancer*. 2005, 5, 133.

[18] Gorelik, E; Landsittel, DP; Marrangoni, AM. Et al., Multiplexed immunobead-based cytokine profiling for early detection of ovarian cancer. *Cancer Epidemiol Biomarkers Prev*. 2005, 14, 981-7.

[19] Huddleston, HG; Wong, KK; Welch, WR. E et al., Clinical applications of microarray technology: creatine kinase B is an up-regulated gene in epithelial ovarian cancer and shows promise as a serum marker. *Gynecol Oncol*. 2005, 96, 77-83.

[20] Jacobs, I; Bast, RC Jr; The CA125 tumour-associated antigen: A review of the literature. *Human Reproduction*, 1989, 4, 1-12.

[21] Knapp, R.C. & Berkowitz, R.S. Corynebacterium parvum as an immunotherapeutic agent in an ovarian cancer model. A*merican Journal of Obstetrics & Gynecology,* 1977; 128: 782-786.

[22] Kohler, G. & Milstein, C; Continuous cultures of fused cells secreting antibody of predefined specificity. *Nature,* 1975, 257: 495-497.

[23] Kozak, KR; Su, F; Whitelegge, JP. et al., Characterization of serum biomarkers for detection of early stage ovarian cancer. *Proteomics*. 2005, 5, 4589-96.

[24] Le Page, C ; Ouellet, V ; Madore, J. et al., From gene profiling to diagnostic markers: IL-18 and FGF-2 complement CA125 as serum-based markers in epithelial ovarian cancer. *Int J Cancer*. 2006, 118, 1750-8.

[25] Luborsky, JL; Barua, A; Shatavi, SV. Et al., Anti-tumor antibodies in ovarian cancer. *Am J Reprod Immunol*. 2005, 54, 55-62.

[26] Miles, AK; Matharoo-Ball, B; Li, G. et al., The identification of human tumour antigens: current status and future developments. Cancer Immunol Immunother. 2006, 55, 996-1003.

[27] Mor, G; Visintin, I; Lai, Y et al, Serum protein markers for early detection of ovarian cancer. *Proc Natl Acad Sci U S A*, 2005, 102, 7677-82.

[28] Oikonomopoulou, K; Scorilas, A; Michael, IP. et al., Kallikreins as markers of disseminated tumour cells in ovarian cancer-- a pilot study. *Tumour Biol*. 2006, 27, 104-14.

[29] Order, SE; Donahue, VC; Knapp, RC; Immunotherapy of ovarian carcinoma: *An experimental model. Cancer* 1973, *32,* 573-579.

[30] Order, SE; Kirkman, R; Knapp, RC; Serologic immunotherapy: Results and probable mechanisms of action. *Cancer,* 1974, 34, 175-183.

[31] Orlova, A; Magnusson, M; Eriksson, TL et al., Tumor imaging using a picomolar affinity HER2 binding affibody molecule.*Cancer Res*. 2006, 66, 4339-48.

[32] Petricoin, EF III; Ardekani, AM, Hitt, BA. et al., Use of proteomic patterns in serum to identify ovarian cancer. *Lancet,* 2002, 359, 572-577.

[33] Phillips, T.M. & Lindsey, J.S. Carcinoma cell-specific Mig-7: a new potential marker for circulating and migrating cancer cells. *Oncol Rep.* 2005, 13, 37-44.

[34] Rosen, DG; Wang, L; Atkinson, JN. Et al., Potential markers that complement expression of CA125 in epithelial ovarian cancer. Gynecol Oncol. 2005, 99, 267-77.

[35] Rustin, G.J; Nelstrop, A.E; McClean, P; et al. Defining response of ovarian carcinoma to initial chemotherapy according to serum CA 125. *Journal of Clinical Oncology,* 1996, 14, 1545-51.

[36] Schorge, JO; Drake, RD; Lee, H al., Osteopontin as an adjunct to CA125 in detecting recurrent ovarian cancer. *Clin Cancer Res.* 2004, 10, 3474-8.

[37] Seow, A; Koh, WP; Chia, KS; Shi, LM; Lee, HP; Shanmugaratnam, K. Trends in cancer Incidence in Singapore 1968-2002. *Singapore Cancer Registry Report No. 6.*

[38] Simon, I; Zhuo, S; Corral, L. Et al., B7-h4 is a novel membrane-bound protein and a candidate serum and tissue biomarker for ovarian cancer. *Cancer Res*. 2006, 66, 1570-5.

[39] Sutphen, R; Xu, Y; Wilbanks, GD. et al., Lysophospholipids are potential biomarkers of ovarian cancer. *Cancer Epidemiol Biomarkers Prev*. 2004;13:1185-91.

[40] Wiesner A. Detection of tumor markers with ProteinChip technology. *Curr Pharm Biotechnol.* 2004, 5, 45-67.

[41] Woolas, RP; Xu, FJ; Jacobs, IJ. Et al., Elevation of multiple serum markers in patients with stage I ovarian cancer. *J Natl Cancer Inst.* 1993, 85, 1748-51.

[42] Xu, Y; Shen, Z; Wiper, DW et al., Lysophosphatidic acid as a potential biomarker for ovarian and other gynecologic cancers. *JAMA.* 1998 26, 280, 719-23.

[43] Yousef, G.M. & Diamandis, E.P. Tissue kallikreins: new players in normal and abnormal cell growth? *Thromb Haemost.* 2003, 90, 7-16.

In: Tumor Markers Research Focus
Editor: Deborah H. Chang, pp. 81-91
ISBN: 978-1-60021-544-5


*Chapter IV A*

# Tumor Markers in Ovarian Neoplasia

***Beatriz M. Tavares-Murta*[1], *Rosekeila S. Nomelini*[2] *and Eddie Fernando C. Murta*[2]**
[1]Department of Biological Sciences
[2]Research Institute of Oncology (IPON)/Discipline of Gynecology and Obstetrics, Federal University of Triângulo Mineiro, Uberaba-MG, Brazil

## Abstract

Ovarian cancer is characterized by a lack of clinical symptoms, presentation in advanced stages and poor survival. Despite major research development leading to an increased comprehension of the pathophysiology of this disease, advances in successful therapeutics have lagged. It is the most frequent cause of death by gynecological cancer. To date, new strategies have been considered in order to improve the early diagnosis of the disease by means of image techniques, tumor marker assays, proteomics and gene-expression microarrays. Tumor markers will be discussed in this review as an alternative to the early diagnosis, follow-up of patients already undergone treatment and in the differentiation between benign and malignant ovarian masses, with intent to optimize and amplify the benefits of treatment. CA 125 is the most frequent tumor marker for ovarian tumors, but due to the difficulties in the differentiation between benign and malignant tumors, it has been associated to other biomarkers such as CA 15.3, CA 19.9 and CA 72.4 to improve the accuracy of the method in the screening of ovarian cancer. Besides, serial measurements of CA 15.3, CA 19.9 and CA 72.4 constitute an alternative to patients with negative CA 125. In mucinous tumors, measurements of CA 72.4 are recommended in the differentiation between benign and malignant tumors, although the positivity rate of CA 72.4 has been found to be significantly lower than CA 125 in patients with borderline tumor. The tumor markers ß-human chorionic gonadotropin and alpha-fetoprotein are useful in the diagnosis and follow-up in women with ovarian tumor of germinal origin. The serum levels of inhibin and estrogen can be increased in tumors of the sex cord and from stromal origin. However, it will also be emphasized that the detection of tumor markers in diseases other than cancer, reflecting its heterogeneity, has turned difficult its use as an isolated method, being necessary new discoveries to optimize its use in ovarian tumors. Despite the new advances, the diagnosis of ovarian cancer is late and the treatment in advanced stages is still based on surgery of cytoreduction and chemotherapy. Combination of transvaginal ultrasound, Doppler and quantification of serum tumor markers is a good strategy for the diagnosis of ovarian neoplasia.

# Introduction

Tumor markers are substances related to the presence or the progression of a tumor. The ideal tumor marker should present the following characteristics: (1) detectable only when malignancy is present, (2) specific for the histological type, (3) specific for the area of malignancy, (4) correlates with the quantity of the malignant tissue present and (5) quickly respond to changes in the size of the tumor [1].

Oncologists have always demonstrated great interest in tumor markers. These substances can represent specific tumor types, but they can also be present in even non-neoplastic diseases. Some examples of tissue-specific biomarkers are α-fetoprotein (AFP) and ß-human chorionic gonadotropin (ß-hCG) for ovarian tumors of germinative origin, while others, such as cancer antigen 125 (CA 125), CA 15.3 and carcinoembryonic antigen (CEA) are less specific, since their elevated levels can be associated to a subtype of tumor but they can also be found in cancer of different origins such as breast, ovary and colon [2].

CA 125 is a high-molecular-mass glycoprotein found in the epithelium of the embryonic colon. This antigen has been identified by a monoclonal antibody OC 125 by use of radioimmunoassay [3]. A very recent study analyzing results obtained from different automated assays showed acceptable performance characteristics and the methods generally compared well [4]. CA 125 is a typical example of biomarker that can be increased in benign and malignant ovarian tumors but also in non-neoplastic diseases. It can be identified in serous, endometrioid, clear-cells and in undifferentiated ovarian tumors. Besides, systemic levels of CA 125 can be augmented in any type of peritoneal irritation, in the first trimester of pregnancy, pelvic infections, leiomyomas and endometriosis [5,6]. In this condition, a comparison of the levels of CA 125, CA 15.3 and CA 19.9 in the peritoneal fluid of patients with and without endometriosis found that only CA 125 levels were higher in women with endometriosis [7].

CA 125 can also be related to the severity of the chronic congestive heart failure showing significant changes in response to the clinical treatment. This marker presents significant elevations in patients from classes III and IV compared to classes I and II, stratified according to the severity of the disease (New York Heart Association). In a smaller number of cases, increased levels of CA 15.3, CA 19.9 and CEA could also be detected in patients with chronic heart failure [8,9].

One great clinical utility of the determination of tumor marker levels is during the follow-up of patients submitted to treatment, in order to evaluate the evolution of the disease by monitoring response to treatment, as can be detected for ß-hCG in gestational trophoblastic disease Also, tumor markers are useful to early detect recurrent disease, since during follow-up increased levels of tumor markers can be observed even months before the clinical demonstration of the recurrence of the disease [2].

## Tumor Markers and the Ovarian Cancer

Epithelial ovarian cancer is the fourth cause of death related to cancer in women in the United States, and the main cause of death by gynecological cancer. It is characterized by lack of symptoms, diagnosis at advanced stages and poor survival [10]. In patients with early diagnosis, at I or II stages, survival in 5 years is about 60 to 90%, depending on the level of differentiation of the tumor [11,12]. In patients with advanced disease, which constitutes approximately 80% cases, initially 80 to 90% will respond to chemotherapy, but less than 10-15% will stay in permanent remission [13]. Despite advances in treatment that have improved the survival rate in 5 years, reaching 45% survival, the global survival has not improved yet [11,14].

One important cause of detection of ovarian cancer mainly at advanced stages is due to the anatomical localization of the ovaries, not easy to access by physical examination, associated to the fact that clinical signs and symptoms at initial stages of the disease do not exist or are unspecific. Early ovarian cancer-associated symptoms are mostly non-gynecological complaints, suggesting a visceral disturbance, which do not point immediately to a pelvic origin. Abdominal bloating and pain predominate with recent onset and multiple symptomatic episodes, but gastrointestinal and urinary symptoms and fatigue may be part of the symptom complex [15].

Screening tests available do not reach high levels of sensitivity and specificity. Thus, screening is not recommended to the general population, and it is also questioned the real value of the screening in patients with high risk for the disease; for example positive BRCA1 and BRCA2. Since ovarian cancer is not very frequent, a low index of false positives would result in a great number of women being incorrectly classified as having ovarian cancer [16].

In addition, the differentiation between benign and malignant adnexal masses is difficult by using the available diagnostic methods. Bimanual pelvic examination is too limited in detecting and evaluating small ovarian alterations. A prospective study comprising 373 women found that the majority of ovarian masses with the largest diameter ≤5 cm were not detected at gynecological examination [17]. These findings reinforce the importance of transvaginal ultrasound in the diagnosis of adnexal masses, although as an isolated method it presents low sensitivity for detecting ovarian neoplasia [17,18]. In this context, tumor marker assay can be added to improve the accuracy of the diagnostic methods.

The tumor marker assay is a non-invasive test of easy appliance by physicians. When combined to Doppler an increased sensitivity and sensibility could be demonstrated in the detection of ovarian neoplasias and, mainly, cancer [17]. This strategy could avoid unnecessary surgical procedures of functional cysts resulting in adherences, chronic pelvic pain and infertility, guiding the surgeon to a more specific treatment [18].

Many tumor markers used in ovarian cancer are also used in breast cancer. But in the malignant breast neoplasia the early diagnosis and the differentiation between benign and malignant alterations are turned easier by other efficient methods such as mammography. In the case of the ovarian masses, the differentiation between benign and malignant is still a challenge. That is why one has tried to detect new tumor markers with intent to improve diagnosis, avoid unnecessary surgical interventions and facilitating the diagnosis of the recurrent disease.

## Tumor Markers in the Screening of Ovarian Cancer

The relative rareness of ovarian cancer, which has a prevalence in the general population of 17 cases per 100 000 women, makes it difficult to devise a diagnosis screening method for pre-clinical disease [16].

CA 125 is the most frequent biomarker used for ovarian cancer. It has been considered useful for monitoring disease progression, response to surgical treatment or chemotherapy and in the early detection of recurrent disease during the follow-up [19,20]. Although the levels of CA 125 are elevated in the serum of the majority of ovarian carcinoma patients, unfortunately as an isolated tumor marker it does not present a very satisfactory accuracy in the screening of the ovarian cancer. This is because CA 125 shows high rates of false-positive results, poor sensibility and specificity, that would result in increased cost and patient anxiety [21].

Serum levels of CA 125 present a positive predictive value lower than 10% and addition of the ultrasound to CA 125 in the screening increases the positive predictive value to approximately 20% [22]. By the combined information with CA 125II (containing antibody M11 in addition to OC-125), CA 72.4 and macrophage colony stimulating factor (M-CSF) for early stage ovarian cancer, an increase in the preoperative sensitivity was obtained from 45% with CA125II alone to 70%, keeping 98% specificity in patients with diagnosis of active disease [23].

The association of CA 125 to CA 15.3, CA 19.9 and CA 72.4 can improve the management of the pelvic masses, with appliance in the screening of the ovarian cancer [24]. Unfortunately, despite all advances, these biomarkers still fail to detect ovarian cancer at initial stages.

## Tumor Markers as a Factor of Differentiation between Benign and Malignant Tumors

The associated use of transvaginal ultrasonography and tumor marker assay have increased the diagnosis of pelvic masses. However, these non-invasive methods frequently do not distinguish a benign condition from a malignant one, since they can present similar morphological characteristics. The association with Color Doppler and tumor markers may improve the accuracy of the method. Gene expression array, proteomics, and mathematical models are new approaches, but proper prospective studies are necessary for validation [18].

While the role of CA 125 in the screening of malignancy is a matter of controversy, its serum levels can be useful in differentiating between benign and malignant ovarian tumors, mainly in the post-menopause [25]. CA 125 can help to eliminate false-positive results in the ultrasound evaluation of solid masses in the discrimination between benign and malignant tumors. So, combining transvaginal ultrasound and CA 125, an accurate prediction can be reached in ovarian masses [26,27]. Nevertheless, it has been associated to other biomarkers to improve the accuracy of the method for the differentiation of benign or malignant characteristics. In this context, it has been demonstrated that the combination of elevated levels of CA 15.3, CA 72.4 and CA 125 are predictive for malignant disease [28]. But differences exist considering tumor stage and tumor diameter, since serum levels of CA 125 and CA 19.9 were significantly different in patients with ovarian cancer at stages IA and IC [29].

The authors accompanied 373 pre-selected outpatient women with pelvic mass and found that the use of one of these tumor markers; CA 125, CA 15.3 or CA 19.9 showed varied sensitivity for malignancy, from 31.5% (CA 125) to 21% (CA 15.3 and CA 19.9), but the association of those reached 52.6% sensitivity. Besides, the use of Doppler and tumor markers increased sensitivity for detection of malignant tumors to 81.8%. Considering these findings, the authors recommended the use of a pelvic mass outpatient service for the follow-up of ovarian alterations detected by ultrasound exam. In this pre-selected group, ultrasound, Doppler and tumor markers should be added for an early diagnosis of ovarian neoplasia [17].

CA 19.9 was firstly identified in breast and gastrointestinal cancer, and together with CA 15.3 it helps to establish the nature of a pancreatic mass [30]. These biomarkers have also been used in ovarian carcinoma. In particular, CA 19.9 has the advantage to present high sensibility in mucinous tumor type, which frequently does not express CA 125. Serial measurements of CA 19.9, CA 15.3 and CA 72.4 can be an alternative to patients with negative CA 125 [24,31,32]. High serum levels of CA 19.9 can be found in mature cystic teratomas. It was recently demonstrated that increased levels of this marker, associated to elevated levels of CA 125, could be associated to bilateral tumor in this histological type [33].

Some additional information can be obtained in evaluating the pelvic masses through the performance of CA 72.4 [34]. In mucinous tumors, measurements of CA 72.4 are recommended in the differentiation between benign and malignant ones [31,35]. On the other hand, it has been shown that the positivity rate of CA 72.4 was significantly lower than CA 125 in patients with borderline tumor [36].

Biomarkers can also help in the diagnosis of the nature of pleural effusions and ascitic fluids. The concentrations of CEA, CA 125, CA 19.9, CA 15.3 and CA 72.4 in pleural effusions were significantly higher in the malignant group than in the benign one, except for CA 19.9, in which the levels were similar [37]. In this line, another possibility is the evaluation of the intracystic tumor microenvironment in patients with cystic ovarian tumors. In patients with epithelial malignant tumors, it was detected a high positivity of CA 15.3, CA 125, CA 19.9 and CEA in the serum and also in the intracystic fluid of the tumor [38]. The quantification of tumor markers in the cystic fluid of patients with benign and malignant ovarian tumors detected that elevated levels of CA 19.9 and progesterone were associated to benign tumors while local concentrations of CA 15.3 and β-hCG were increased for malignant compared to benign tumors [39]. It is well known that β-hCG is increased in gestational trophoblastic disease and besides, ß-hCG and AFP are useful in the diagnosis and follow-up of women with ovarian tumor of germinal origin [30,31]. Indeed, 80% patients with malignant ovarian tumors had β-hCG cystic levels higher than normal serum levels [39]. The significance of increased cystic fluid levels of tumor markers in patients with ovarian cancer remains to be further elucidated.

## Tumor Markers in the Follow-up of Patients with Ovarian Cancer

Considering that most cases of ovarian cancer are mainly diagnosed at advanced stages, the ceiling seems to be reached with chemotherapy. Instead of treating all patients according to standard guidelines, individualized molecular targeted treatment should be aimed for. This means that molecular profile of the distinct ovarian cancer subtypes should be established, although it is more likely that different ovarian cancer subtypes with extensive molecular heterogeneity exist [40].

CA 125 may have impact as prognostic marker. A retrospective study evaluating CA 125 as a prognostic factor in 82 patients demonstrated that this marker correlated well with the FIGO staging, but not with patient age, residual disease after surgery and free interval of the disease [41]. Others have showed that the complete surgical staging, histologic grade and the preoperative levels of CA 125 are independent prognostic factors and could be included as factors of decision in the performance of chemotherapy [42].

Preoperative CA-125 levels were found to be an independent predictor of survival in univariate and multivariate analyses, being that patients with levels <35 U/ml after two cycles of chemotherapy showed longer survival. The median preoperative CA 125 was 195 in high survival patients and 650 in low survival patients. Moreover, CA 125 levels correlated to responsiveness to chemotherapy [43]. In stage I epithelial ovarian cancer, patients with preoperative CA 125 levels <65 U/ml had significantly longer survival compared to those with serum CA 125 ≥65 U/ml, indicating that CA 125 may be useful for decision in respect to postoperative chemotherapy [44]. Still in this line, another study in suboptimal residual stage III and IV ovarian cancer showed that while pretreatment CA 125 levels did not correlate with survival, reduction in the serum CA 125 concentration over the initial two cycles of platinum-based chemotherapy was found to be a powerful independent predictor of survival [45].

Increased levels of tumor markers are indicative of recurrent disease, even before clinical demonstration of this recurrence. The risk of recurrent epithelial ovarian cancer in patients with serum levels of CA 125 lower than the normal (<35 mU/ml) was studied and it was found that a progressive increase of CA 125 levels, even low ones, could indicate recurrence of the disease [46]. Also, in women achieving a clinically-defined complete response to primary chemotherapy, the baseline CA 125 level before initiation of maintenance chemotherapy strongly predicted the risk of subsequent relapse [47].

CA 72.4 could complement CA 125 in the diagnosis and follow-up of patients with epithelial ovarian cancer [48]. Measurements of tumor markers in the follow-up of patients with borderline tumors can early detect the recurrence in small proportion of patients. For the follow-up of the mucinous borderline ovarian tumor, CA 19.9 should be of choice [49].

## New Tumor Markers

New biomarkers are needed for the detection of ovarian cancer that could complement the expression of CA 125. Osteopontin is one of the candidates identified by complementary DNA microarray techniques. Preoperative combined plasma osteopontin and CA 125 levels increased sensitivity in detecting ovarian cancer to 93.8%, compared to 84.4% with CA 125 alone [50]. Osteopontin associated to leptin and prolactin, trying to distinguish between normal women and ovarian cancer patients, showed 95% sensibility and specificity and 95% positive and negative predictive values [51].

Mesothelin is a cell surface protein which can be highly expressed in mesothelioma and ovarian cancer, being possible to be measured in serum samples. More important, its rapid reduction after treatment demonstrates that this protein can be useful in the monitoring of therapeutics. When associated CA 125 and mesothelin an increased sensibility in detecting ovarian cancer was observed [52].

Kallikreins are a family of steroid hormone-regulated secreted serine proteases, with several members associated with ovarian cancer. More specific, kallikreins 6 (KLK6) and 10 (KLK10) are elevated in tumor cells, serum and ascitic fluid of ovarian cancer patients and correlate with disease prognosis [53]. But tissue KLK8 has been indicated as an independent marker of favorable prognosis in ovarian cancer, considering that patients with KLK8-positive tumors has longer progression-free survival and overall survival compared to KLK8-negative patients [54].

Inhibin and macrophage colony stimulating factor (M-CSF) can be increased in ovarian cancer in a general way [31]. Serum inhibin and estrogen levels can be increased in tumors of the sex cord and from stromal origin [55,56]. YKL-40 can be a new marker for identifying ovarian cancer at early stages [57]. Oviductual glycoprotein is a new marker present in serous benign neoplasias and borderline tumors [58]. Octamer binding transcription factor 4 is a sensible marker and relatively specific in detecting dysgerminoma [59]. Gene-expression microarrays and proteomics are new alternatives in the management of ovarian masses [5,60].

## Conclusion

Despite new advances, the diagnosis of ovarian cancer is still late and the treatment in advanced stages is based on surgery of cytoreduction and chemotherapy. Combination of transvaginal ultrasound, Doppler and measurement of serum tumor markers is until now a good strategy for the diagnosis of ovarian neoplasia. Since CA 125 can be negative in ovarian cancer and positive in benign tumors, an alternative would be the combined assay with other tumor markers, which increases sensitivity for detection of malignancy. In the follow-up, tumor markers such as CA 125 has been considered as a factor of decision in the performance of chemotherapy and as an independent prognostic factor and predictor of survival. Although ovarian cancer is not very frequent, it is the main cause of death by gynecological cancer, which means that new alternatives must be searched in order to improve early diagnosis and survival.

## References

[1] Lai, LC; Cheong, SK; Goh, KL; Leong, CF; Loh, CS; Lopez, JB; Nawawi, H; Sivanesaratnam, V; Subramaniam, R; Clinical Practice Guidelines Committee on Tumour Markers of the Academy of Medicine of Malaysia. Clinical usefulness of tumour markers. *Malays J Pathol* 2003 25:83-105.

[2] Ugrinska, A; Bombardieri, E; Stokkel, MP; Crippa, F; Pawwels, EK. Circulating tumor markers and nuclear medicine imaging modalities breast, prostate and ovarian cancer. *Q J Nucl Med* 2002 46:88-104.

[3] Bast, RC; Klug, TL; St John, E; Jenison, E; Niloff, JM; Lazarus, H; Berkowitz, RS; Leavitt, T; Griffiths, CT; Parker, L; Zurawski, VR Jr; Knapp, RC. A radioimmunoassay using a monoclonal antibody to monitor the course of epithelial ovarian cancer. *N Eng J Med* 1983 309:883-7.

[4] Mongia, SK; Rawlins, ML; Owen, WE; Roberts WL. Performance characteristics of seven automated CA 125 assays. *Am J Clin Pathol* 2006 125:921-7.

[5] Rapkiewicz, AV; Espina, V; Petricoin EF 3rd; Liotta, LA. Biomarkers of ovarian tumours. *Eur J Cancer* 2004 40:2604-12.

[6] Moss, EL; Hollingworth, J; Reynolds, TM. The role of CA 125 in clinical practice. *J Clin Pathol* 2005 58:308-12.

[7] Matalliotakis, IM; Goumenou, AG; Mulayim, N; Karkavitsas, N; Koumantakis, EE. High concentrations of the CA-125, CA 19-9 and CA 15-3 in the peritoneal fluid between patients with and without endometriosis. *Arch Gynecol Obstet* 2005 271:40-5.

[8] Faggiano, P; D'Aloia, A; Brentana, L; Bignotti, T; Fiorina, C; Vizzardi, E; Dei Cas, L . Serum levels of different tumour markers in patients with chronic heart failure. *Eur J Heart Fail* 2005 7:57-61.

[9] Varol E, Ozaydin M, Dogan A, Kosar F. Tumour marker levels in patients with chronic heart failure. *Eur J Heart Fail* 2005; 7:840-3.

[10] Jemal, A; Murray, T; Ward, E; Samuels, A; Tiwari, RC; Ghafoor, A; Feuer, EJ; Thun, MJ. Cancer statistics, 2005. *CA Cancer J Clin.* 2005 55:10-30. Erratum in: *CA Cancer J Clin* 2005 55:259.

[11] Schwartz, DR; Kardia, SL; Shedden, KA; Kuick, R; Michailidis, G, Taylor, JM; Misek, DE; Wu, R; Zhai, Y; Darrah, DM; reed, H; Ellenson, LH; Giordano, TJ; Fearon, ER; Hanashi, SM; Cho, KR. Gene expression in ovarian cancer reflects both morphology and biological behavior, distinguishing clear cell from other poor-prognosis ovarian carcinomas. *Cancer Res* 2002 62:4722-9.

[12] Lu, KH; Patterson, AP; Wang, L; Marquez, RT; Atkinson, EN; Baggerly, KA; Ramoth, LR; Rosen, DG; Liu, J; Hellstrom, I; Smith, D; Hartmann, L; Fishman, D; Berchuck, A; Schmandt, R; Whitaker, R; Gershenson, DM; Mills, GB; Bast, RC Jr. Selection of potential markers for epithelial ovarian cancer with gene expression arrays and recursive descent partition analysis. *Clin Cancer Res* 2004 10:3291-300.

[13] Petricoin, EF; Ardekani, AM; Hitt, BA; Levine, PJ; Fusaro, VA; Steinberg, SM; Mills, GB; Simone, C; Fishman, DA; Kohn, EC; Liotta, LA. Use of proteomic patterns in serum to identify ovarian cancer. *Lancet* 2002 359:572-7.

[14] McIntosh, MW; Urban, N; Karlan, B. Generating longitudinal screening algorithms using novel biomarkers for disease. *Cancer Epidemiol Biomarkers Prev* 2002 11: 159-66.

[15] Smith, LH. Early clinical detection of ovarian cancer: a review of the evidence. *Expert Rev Anticancer Ther*, 2006 6:1045-52.

[16] U.S. Preventive Services Task Force. Screening for ovarian cancer: recommendation statement. *Ann Fam Med* 2004 2:260-2.

[17] Murta, EFC; Silva, CS; Gomes, RAS; Tavares-Murta, BM; Melo, ALKO. Ultrasonographic criteria and tumor marker assay are good procedures for the diagnosis of ovarian neoplasia in preselected outpatients. *Eur J Gynaecol Oncol* 2004 25:707-12.

[18] Murta, EFC; Nomelini, RS. Early diagnosis and predictors of malignancy in the evaluation of adnexal mass. *Curr Opinion Obstet Gynecol* 2006 18:14-9.

[19] Markar AP. Serum CA 125 le vel allows early identification of non responders during induction chemotherapy. *Gynecol Oncol* 1993 49:73-9.

[20] Vergote IB, Bormer OP, Abeler VM. Evaluation of serum CA125 levels in the monitoring of ovarian cancer. *Am J Obstet Gynecol* 1987 157: 88-92.

[21] Moss, EL; Hollingworth, J; Reynolds, TM. The role of CA125 in clinical practice. *J Clin Pathol* 2005 58:308-12.

[22] Kozak, KR; Amneus, MW; Pusey, SM; Su, F; Luong, MN; Luong, SA; Reddy, ST; Farias-Eisner, R. Identification of biomarkers for ovarian cancer using strong anion-exchange ProteinChips: potential use in diagnosis and prognosis. *Proc Natl Acad Sci USA* 2003 100:12343-8.

[23] Skates, SJ; Horick, N; Yu, Y; Xu, FJ; Berchuck, A; Havrilesky, LJ; de Bruijn, HW; van der Zee, AG; Woolas, RP; Jacobs, IJ; Zhang, Z; Bast, RC Jr. Preoperative sensitivity and specificity for early-stage ovarian cancer when combining cancer antigen CA-125II, CA 15-3, CA 72-4, and macrophage colony-stimulating factor using mixtures of multivariate normal distributions. *J Clin Oncol* 2004 22:4059-66.

[24] Woolas, RP; Conaway, FX; Jacobs, IJ. Combinations of multiple serum markers are superior to individual assays for discriminating malignant from benign pelvic masses. *Gynecol Oncol* 1995 59:111-6.

[25] Mancuso A, De Vivo A, Triolo O, Irato S. The role of transvaginal ultrasonography and serum CA 125 assay combined with age and hormonal state in the differential diagnosis of pelvic masses. *Eur J Gynecol Oncol* 2004 25:207-10.

[26] Erdogan, N; Ozcelik, B; Serin, IS; Akgun, M; Ozturk, F. Doppler ultrasound assessment and serum cancer antigen 125 in the diagnosis of ovarian tumors. *Int J Gynaecol Obstet* 2005 91:146-50.

[27] Roupa, Z; Faros, E; Raftopoulos, V; Tzavelas, G; Kotrotsiou, E; Sotiropoulou, P; Karanikola, E; Skifta, E; Ardavanis, A. Serum CA 125 combined with transvaginal ultrasonography for varian cancer screening. *In Vivo* 2004 18:831-6.

[28] Schutter, EM; Davelaar, EM; van Kamp, GJ; Verstraeten, RA; Kenemans, P; Verheijen, RH. The differential diagnostic potential of a panel of tumor markers (CA 125, CA 15-3, and CA 72-4 antigens) in patients with a pelvic mass. *Am J Obstet Gynecol* 2002 187:385-92.

[29] Muramatsu, T; Mukai, M; Sato, S; Tajima, T; Nagase, E; Ikeda, M; Goya, K; Shida, M; Hirasawa, T; Murakami, M; Shinozuka, T. Clinical usefulness of serum and immunohistochemical markers in patients with stage Ia and Ic ovarian cancer. *Oncol Rep* 2005 14:861-5.

[30] Perkins, GL; Slater, ED; Sanders, GK; Prichard, JG. Serum tumor markers. *Am Fam Physician* 2003 68:1075-82.

[31] Stenman, UH; Alfthan, H; Vartiainen, J; Lehtovirta, P. Markers supplementing CA 125 in ovarian cancer. *Ann Med* 1995 27:115-20.

[32] Gaducci, A; Cosio, S; Carpi, A; Nicolini, A; Genazzani, AR. Serum tumor markers in the management of ovarian, endometrial and cervical cancer. *Biomed Pharmacother* 2004 58:24-38.

[33] Dede, M; Gungor, S; Yenen, MC; Alanbay, I; Duru, NK; Hasimi, A. CA19-9 may have clinical significance in mature cystic teratomas of the ovary. *Int J Gynecol Cancer* 2006 16:189-93.

[34] Balbi, GC; Musone, R; Menditto, A; Balbi, F; Corcioni, C; Calabria, G; Maciariello, C; Balbi, C. Women with a pelvic mass: indicators of malignancy. *Eur J Gynaecol Oncol* 2001 22:459-62.

[35] Kikkawa, F; Kawai, M; Tamakoshi, K; Suganuma, N; Nakashima, N; Furuhashi, Y; Kuzuya, K; Hattori, S; Arii, Y; Tomoda, Y. Mucinous carcinoma of the ovary. Clinicopathologic analysis. *Oncology* 1996 53:303-7.

[36] Tamakoshi, K; Kikkawa, F; Shibata, K; Tomoda, K; Obata, NH; Wakahara, F; Tokuhashi, Y; Ishikawa, H; Kawai, M; Tomoda, Y. Clinical value of Ca125, CA19.9, CEA, CA72-4, and TPA in borderline ovarian tumor. *Gynecol Oncol* 1996 62:67-72.

[37] Ustun, H; Borazan, A; Bilgicli, N; Yilmaz, A. Diagnostic value of tumoural markers in pleural effusions. *Int J Clin Pract* 2004 58:22-5.

[38] Cherchi, PL; Capobianco, G; Ambrosini, G; Fadda, GM; Piga, MD; Ruiu, G; Fattorini, F; Dessole, S. Intracystic evaluation of tumor markers in benign and malignant ovarian pathology. *Eur J Gynaecol Oncol* 2002 23:163-5.

[39] Murta, BMT; Cunha, FQ; Miranda, R; Adad, SJ; Murta, EFC. Differential tumor microenvironment in human ovarian cystic tumors. *Tumori* 2004 90:491-7.

[40] Crijns, AP; Duiker, EW; de Jong, S; Willemse, PH; van der Zee, AG; de Vries, EG. Molecular prognostic markers in ovarian cancer: toward patient-tailored therapy. *Int J Gynecol Cancer* 2006 16:152-65.

[41] Rossi, AC; Di Vagno, G; Cormio, G; Cazzolla, A; Stefanelli, S; D'Elia, E; Selvaggi, L. A retrospective study of preoperative CA 125 levels in 82 patients with ovarian cancer. *Arch Gynecol Obstet* 2004 269:263-5.

[42] Paramasivam, S; Tripcony, L; Crandon, A; Quinn, M; Hammond, I; Marsden, D; Proietto, A; Davy, M; Carter, J; Nicklin, J; Perrin, L; Obermair, A. Prognostic importance of preoperative CA-125 in International Federation of Gynecology and Obstetrics stage I epithelial ovarian cancer: an Australian multicenter study. *J Clin Oncol* 2005 23:5938-42.

[43] Raspollini, MR; Amunni, G; Villanucci, A; Boddi, V; Taddei GL. COX-2 and preoperative CA-125 level are strongly correlated with survival and clinical responsiveness to chemotherapy in ovarian cancer. *Acta Obstet Gynecol Scand* 2006 85:493-8.

[44] Petri, AL; Hogdall, E; Christensen, IJ; Kjaer, SK; Blaakaer, J.; Hogdall, CK. Preoperative CA 125 as a prognostic factor in stage I epithelial ovarian cancer. *APMIS* 2006 114:359-63.

[45] Markman, M; Liu, PY; Rothenberg, ML; Monk, BJ; Brady, M; Alberts DS. Pretreatment CA-125 and risk of relapse in advanced ovarian cancer. *J Clin Oncol* 2006 24:1454-8.

[46] Santillan, A; Garg, R; Zahurak, ML; Gardner, GJ; Giuntoli, RL 2nd; Armstrong, DK; Bristow, RE. Risk of epithelial ovarian cancer recurrence in patients with rising serum CA-125 levels within the normal range. *J Clin Oncol* 2005 23:9338-43.

[47] Markman, M; Federico, M; Liu, PY; Hanningan, E; Alberts, DS. Significance of early changes in the serum CA-125 antigen level on overall survival in advanced ovarian cancer. *Gynecol Oncol* 2006 Apr 2; [Epub ahead of print].

[48] Fayed, ST; Ahmad, SM; Kassim, SK; Khalifa, A. The value of CA 125 and CA72-4 in management of patients with epithelial ovarian cancer. *Dis Markers* 1998 14:155-60.

[49] Engelen, MJ; de Bruijn, HW; Hollema, H; ten Hoor, KA; Willemse, PH; Aalders, JG; van der Zee, AG. Serum CA 125, carcinoembryonic antigen, and CA 19-9 as tumor markers in borderline ovarian tumors. *Gynecol Oncol* 2000 78:16-20.

[50] Nakae, M; Iwamoto, I; Fujino, T; Maehata, Y; Togami, S; Yoshinaga, M; Douchi, T. Preoperative plasma osteopontin level as a biomarker complementary to carbohydrate antigen 125 in predicting ovarian cancer. *J Obstet Gynaecol Res* 2006 32:309-14.

[51] Mor, G; Visintin, I; Lai, Y; Zhao, H; Schwartz, P; Rutherford, T; Yue, L; Bray-Ward, P; ward, DC. Serum protein markers for early detection of ovarian cancer. *Proc Natl Acad Sci USA* 2005 102:7677-82.

[52] McIntosh, MW; Drescher, C; Karlan, B; Scholler, N; Urban, N; Hellstrom KE; Hellstrom, I. Combining CA 125 and SMR serum markers for diagnosis and early detection of ovarian carcinoma. *Gynecol Oncol* 2004 95:9-15.

[53] Oikonomopoulou K, Scorilas A, Michael IP, Grass L, Soosaipillai A, Rosen B, Murphy J, Diamandis EP. Kallikreins as markers of disseminated tumour cells in ovarian cancer – a pilot study. *Tumour Biol* 2006 27:104-14.

[54] Borgono CA, Kishi T, Scorilas A, Harbeck N, Dorn J, Schmalfeldt B, Schmitt M, Diamandis EP. Human kallikrein 8 protein is a favorable prognostic marker in ovarian cancer. *Clin Cancer Res* 2006 12:1487-93.

[55] Robertson, DM; Pruysers, E; Burger, HG; Jobling, T; McNeilage, G; Healy, D. Inhibins and ovarian cancer. *Mol Cell Endocrinol* 2004 225:65-71.

[56] Duffy, MJ. Evidence for the clinical use of tumour markers. *Ann Clin Biochem* 2004 41:370-7.

[57] Chudecka-Glaz, A; Rzepka-Gorska, I; Kosmowska, B. Gonadotropin (LH, FSH) levels in serum and cyst fluid in epithelial tumors of the ovary. *Arch Gynecol Obstet* 2004 270:151-6.

[58] Woo, MM; Gilks, CB; Verhage, HG; Longacre, TA; Leung, PC; Auersperg, N. Oviductal glycoprotein, a new differentiation-based indicator present in early ovarian epithelial neoplasia and cortical inclusion cysts. *Gynecol Oncol* 2004 93:315-19.

[59] Cheng, L; Thomas, A; Roth, LM; Zheng, W; Michael, H; Karim, FW. OCT4: a novel biomarker for dysgerminoma of the ovary. *Am J Surg Pathol* 2004 28:1341-6.

[60] Huddleston, HG; Wong, KK; Welch, WR; Berkowitz, RS; Mok, SC. Clinical applications of microarray technology: creatine kinase B is an up-regulated gene in epithelial ovarian cancer and shows promise as a serum marker. *Gynecol Oncol* 2005 96:77-83.

In: Tumor Markers Research Focus
Editor: Deborah H. Chang, pp. 93-110
ISBN: 978-1-60021-544-5


*Chapter IV B*

# Biological Markers in Mammary Phyllodes Tumors

***Gary MK Tse[1]* and Puay Hoon Tan[2]***
[1]Deapartment of Anatomical and Cellular Pathology, Prince of Wales Hospital, Chinese University of Hong Kong, Hong Kong
[2]Department of Pathology, Singapore General Hospital, Singapore

## Abstract

Phyllodes tumors of the breast are biphasic lesions characterized by leaf like pattern arising from stromal expansion, with the stroma showing variable degree of cellularity and even sarcomatous changes. While most phyllodes tumors are benign, some may recur or metastasize, behaving in a malignant fashion. Conventionally, histological parameters of stromal cellularity, nuclear pleomorphism, stromal overgrowth, mitotic activity and margin configuration are used for grading, but to date, these criteria are not definitive. Recently, attempts have been made to evaluate the overexpression of various protein markers that have been proven to be useful in other human malignancies. p53 is a tumor suppressor gene located on 17p13, implicated in cell growth and division regulation, DNA repair and apoptosis. In phyllodes tumors, there is increased p53 protein expression in higher grade lesions compared to lower grade lesions. Hormonal receptor expression in phyllodes tumors is not well known. Estrogen and progesterone receptor expression was more common in the epithelial than the stromal component, and the epithelial expression decreased with increasing grade of the phyllodes tumors. Ki67 is a non histone nuclear protein that is present throughout the cell cycle, but it reaches a peak value during the G2M phase. It was reported that the Ki67 (proliferation) index increased progressively form benign to malignant phyllodes tumors. Furthermore, flow cytometry showed that benign phyllodes tumors were diploid, and aneuploidy was identified in some of the higher grade phyllodes tumors, paralleled by an S phase fraction increase from benign to malignant phyllodes tumors. Tumor angiogenesis assessed by microvessel density has been extensively investigated for carcinoma of the breast, and has been proposed as a prognostic factor in breast cancer. In phyllodes tumors, a progressive increase in microvessel density with increasing grade of phyllodes tumours has

* E-mail address:garytse@cuhk.edu.hk, Phone: (852)26322359, Fax: (852)26374858. Gary MK Tse, Senior Medical Officer, Department of Anatomical and Cellular Pathology, Prince of Wales Hospital, Chinese University of Hong Kong, Ngan Shing Street, Shatin, NT, Hong Kong

been demonstrated. Interestingly, this increase was independent of other traditional histologic criteria, suggesting that angiogenesis may be an important independent predictor for malignancy. c-kit (CD117) is a proto-oncogene that encodes a tyrosine kinase receptor and is now considered a diagnostic marker for gastrointestinal stromal tumors (GIST). It has been shown that there is a progressive increase in c-kit expression from benign to malignant phyllodes. The underlying mechanism for this differential c-kit expression remains uncertain, and is probably distinct from that of GIST. The potential of tyrosine kinase inhibitor as a treatment modality in malignant phyllodes tumors remains to be explored.

# Introduction

Phyllodes tumors and fibroadenomas are fibroepithelial tumors of the breast. While fibroadenoma is a common benign lesion, phyllodes tumor is uncommon. The real incidence of phyllodes tumors is difficult to estimate, but is probably less than 1% of all primary breast tumors. There appears to be an ethnic difference, with a higher incidence occurring in Asians. In general the patient age for phyllodes tumor is about 15-20 years older than that for fibroadenoma. Phyllodes tumor is characterized by proliferation of both epithelial and the stromal components, which are intimately related. The stromal component is thought to be derived from the interlobular specialized stroma, giving the characteristic myxoid like appearance (1).

# Histopathology of Phyllodes Tumors

Macroscopically, phyllodes tumor forms a firm lobulated mass with apparent circumscription (Figure 1). Its cut surface is yellowish tan, and may occasionally show compressed slit like spaces with frond like growths within it. Foci of haemorrhage or necrosis may be seen.

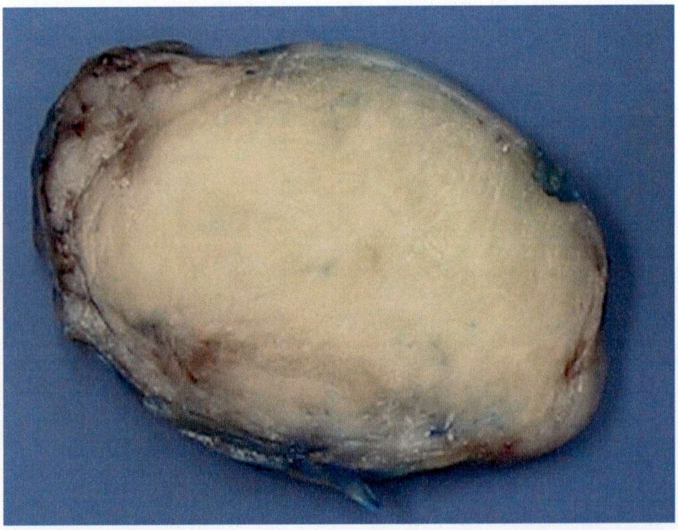

Figure 1. Macroscopic appearance of a phyllodes tumor, with a circumscribed lobulated margin and a pale yellowish-grey whorled cut surface.

Microscopically, phyllodes tumor shares with fibroadenoma the intimate proliferation of the stromal and epithelial components. Generally, in phyllodes tumors, the degree of stromal proliferation is more prominent, resulting in protrusion of stroma into epithelium-lined canaliculi, giving a leafy or fronded appearance, hence the name of phyllodes (leaf like, Figure 2).

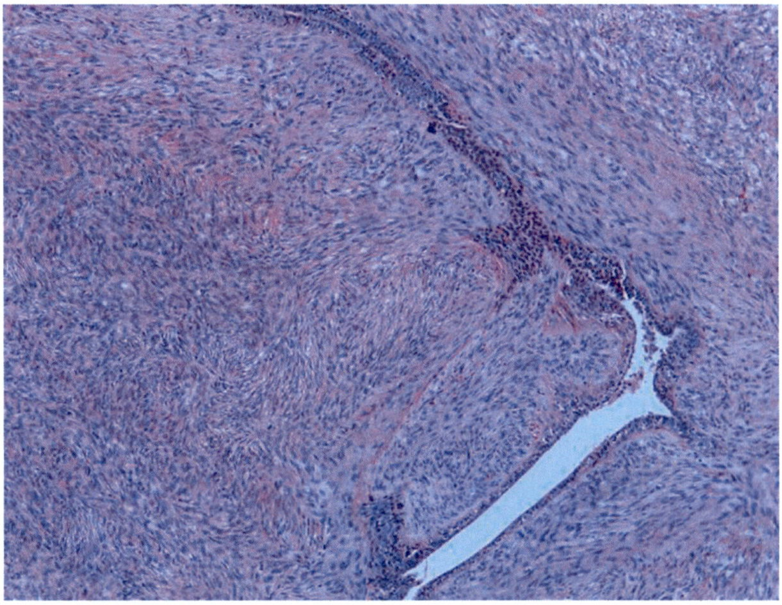

Figure 2. Microscopic appearance of phyllodes tumor, with compressed epithelium-lined cleft into which hypercellular stroma protrude.

The microscopic features of phyllodes tumors are very variable, and lie in a continuous spectrum from benign alterations at one end to malignant appearances at the other. In general, no single histological criterion can be used in the grading of phyllodes tumors. Instead several histological parameters are assessed, including stromal cellularity, stromal cell atypia, mitotic activity, stromal overgrowth (defined as the absence of epithelial elements in the expanded stroma within a low power microscopic field), whether the margin is rounded or infiltrative, necrosis, and malignant heterologous (osteosarcomatous or chondrosarcomatous) elements (2,3,4,5,6,7). Typically, a benign phyllodes tumor is diagnosed when the tumor shows low stromal cellularity, low mitotic count (less than 3-4 per 10 high power fields), a rounded margin, absence of stromal cell atypia or nuclear pleomorphism, absence of stromal overgrowth, and absence of necrosis or malignant heterologous elements. When there is stromal hypercellularity, significant stromal cell atypia or nuclear pleomorphism, high mitotic count (more than 10 per 10 high power fields), stromal overgrowth, infiltrative margins, presence of necrosis and / or malignant heterologous elements, a diagnosis of malignant phyllodes tumor is made. Many lesions however, possess some but not all of these features of malignancy, and they are labelled as of borderline malignancy. This division is arbitrary by nature, as the criteria are somewhat subjective. In fact, in different large series, the percentage of borderline malignant phyllodes tumors differs significantly (from 12% to up to 26%) (2,3,4,5,6,7).

While all grades of phyllodes tumors may recur, the malignant ones may also metastasize. In the literature, the recurrence rate of phyllodes tumors ranges from 10% to 25 % for benign phyllodes, up to 32% for phyllodes tumor of borderline malignancy, and up to 40% for frankly malignant phyllodes tumors. Distant metastasis has not been reported for benign phyllodes tumor, and the incidence is up to 22% in frankly malignant phyllodes tumors (3,5,7,8,9,10,11,12,13). Most local recurrences occur within two years after the initial presentation, and the recurrence may contain both epithelial and stromal components, or only the stromal component (7,13). Most distant metastases, occur in systemic organs, notably lung, and lymph node metastasis is exceedingly uncommon (9). Distant metastases may also be preceded by local recurrences (7). Another large series (3) with 57 recurrences (43 first, 9 second, 4 third and 1 fourth recurrences) did not demonstrate a definite relationship between the histological grade of the original and recurrent tumors. Progression from an initial lower grade tumor to higher grade recurrences was noted in 15 tumors (26%), regression from higher grade tumor to lower grade recurrences was noted in six tumors (11%), with the majority (36 recurrent tumors (63%)) being of the same grade as the original tumor, suggesting that grade progression was not necessary for recurrence, and that other factors like completeness of excision, may be of greater importance (3).

In addition to these, other incidental features may also occur in phyllodes tumors, including epithelial changes, stromal giant cells and pseudoangiomatous stromal hyperplasia, and these histological alterations have not been proven to affect disease outcome.

Epithelial hyperplasia within phyllodes tumors is very common, and can occur in up to 74% of the cases, most of which are of mild to moderate degree of epithelial hyperplasia (3). Atypical epithelial hyperplasia is less common, ranging form 1.5 % to 4% in these reports, and lobular neoplasia (encompassing atypical lobular hyperplasia and lobular carcinoma in situ) is noted in 0.5% to 5%. Ductal carcinoma in situ is most uncommon, occurring in less than 1% (3,7).

Multinucleated stromal giant cells have also been reported in fibroepithelial tumors of the breast including phyllodes tumors (3,14,15). The reported overall incidence of stromal giant cells ranged from 9% to 12%, with more being found in phyllodes tumors of higher grade (3,14). These giant cells tend to occur in tight aggregates in the subepithelial regions of high stromal cellularity. They possess five to eight nuclei that are arranged linearly to irregularly. There is no difference in morphology between these giant cells in phyllodes tumors of different grades, and their immunohistochemical profile has been shown to be similar to the adjacent stromal cells, implying that these giant cells have no independent bearing on prognosis (14,15).

The presence of pseudoangiomatous stromal hyperplasia (PASH) within the stroma of phyllodes tumours has been described in as many as 70% of phyllodes tumours when one low power field of characteristic slit like changes in the stroma was used as the cut off. Curiously PASH is shown to be inversely correlated to tumor grade, translating into its presence in a phyllodes tumor being less likely to be associated with malignancy (3).

The results of many large series studying the predictive value of histological parameters are conflicting and far from unanimous. In some series, only histological parameters including grade, stromal atypia, stromal hypercellularity, and margin status (3,9,16), or stromal overgrowth (17) are shown to be correlated to disease recurrence, whereas other authors also emphasized the importance of complete surgical excision at the initial time of treatment (5). Tumor necrosis and stromal elements other than fibromyxoid stroma were the only two identified independent prognostic factors in another large study (18), and tumor size and margin clearance were considered the only significant prognostic indicator by other groups (19). Many other authors did not find any role of histological parameters in tumor recurrences (4,8,11) or affecting the outcome (6,12,20). In another series (7), stromal overgrowth, high mitotic rate of >15 per 50 high power fields and stromal cytological atypia were identified in malignant phyllodes tumors that metastasized.

# Biological Markers in Phyllodes Tumors

## p53

Mutations of p53 are probably the most extensively studied in mammary phyllodes tumors. p53 is a tumor suppressor gene located on 17p13, and it has been implicated in the regulation of normal cell growth and division, DNA repair and apoptosis. It is found to be extensively altered in breast carcinoma. In phyllodes tumors, the results of p53 protein expression were variable. In general, there is increased p53 protein expression in higher grade phyllodes tumors compared to lower grade lesions by immunohistochemistry (4,21,22,23,24). The staining pattern in malignant phyllodes tumors, and very occasionally in borderline tumors, is characteristic, showing diffuse strong nuclear staining, particularly in the stromal cells that show a higher degree of atypicality and also in more cellular areas in the subepithelial location (Figure 3). Although it has been observed that p53 over expression was also present in epithelial cells as well as myoepithelial cells of phyllodes tumors, expression in these cell types tend to show a correlation with expression in stromal cells (24). Whether

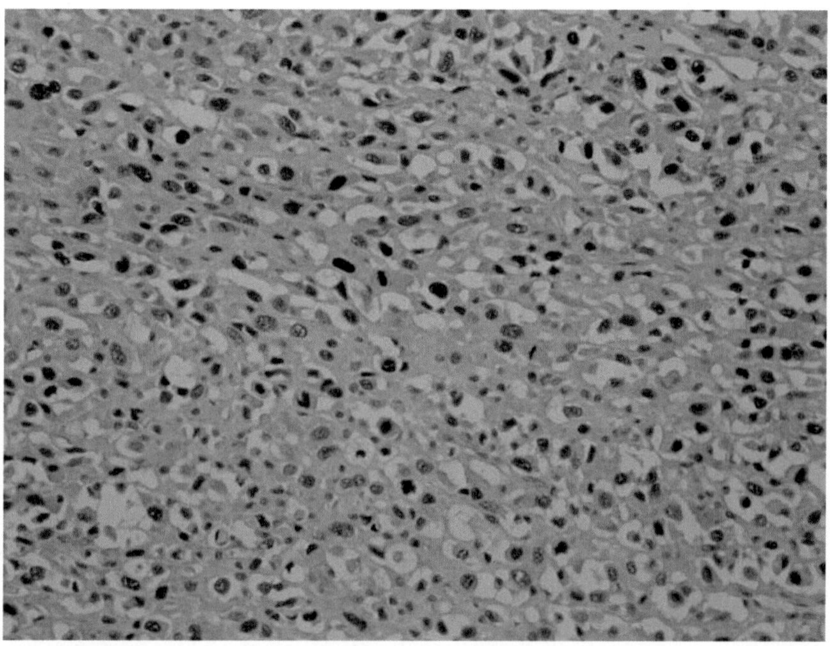

Figure 3. Immunohistoechemistry for p53 shows nuclear reactivity in stromal cells of a phyllodes tumor.

expression in epithelial and myoepithelial cells per se should be interpreted differently remains to be determined. The significance of stromal p53 over expression in the understanding of disease aetiology remains elusive. Some authors demonstrated that p53 expression is associated with tumor grade, prominent stromal overgrowth, stromal nuclear pleomorphism, high stromal mitotic count and an infiltrative margin (22), others showed correlation with mitotic count only, but not other histological parameters (4). These studies however, are unable to demonstrate the ability of p53 to independently predict outcome or recurrences (4,22,24).

## Hormonal Receptors

Evaluation of hormonal receptor status is now a standard procedure in the assessment of carcinoma of the breast, as this has bearing on both prognostication and prediction of response to adjuvant endocrine therapy. In phyllodes tumors, estrogen receptor alpha and progesterone receptors are detected, mainly within the epithelium, but not in the stroma. Progesterone receptor expression is common, estrogen receptor alpha expression is less common (25). Estrogen receptor alpha and progesterone receptor expression has been shown in 43% and 84% of the epithelium and less than 5% of stromal cells of phyllodes tumors (26). For epithelial estrogen receptor alpha, the expression was high in benign but low in borderline and malignant phyllodes. For epithelial progesterone receptor, the expression was high in both benign and borderline but low in malignant phyllodes. Furthermore, epithelial estrogen receptor alpha expression showed an inverse correlation with the stromal mitotic count, and overlapped with the stromal cell mitotic count in predicting the diagnosis. Another recent report demonstrated the presence of estrogen receptor beta in the stromal cells of phyllodes tumors, in contradistinction to the usual negativity for estrogen receptor alpha among the stromal cells. The over expression of estrogen receptor beta was demonstrated at both protein and mRNA levels, and those stromal cells that were estrogen receptor beta positive also expressed smooth muscle markers, indicative of a smooth muscle differentiation.

The observation of an inverse relationship of epithelial estorgen receptor alpha and progesterone receptor and tumor grade of the phyllodes tumors is particularly intriguing as it points to a significant role of the epithelium in triggering stromal proliferation. The expression of esteogen receptor beta in phyllodes tumors was mostly in patients who were older, suggesting that contrary to estrogen receptor alpha, the mechanism of phyllodes tumor progression may be estrogen receptor beta independent.

## Proliferation Markers

Ki67 (MIB1) is an immunohistochemical marker for cellular proliferation. It is a non histone nuclear protein that is present throughout the cell cycle, but it reaches a peak value during the G2M phase. In a study of MIB1 expression in phyllodes tumors, it was reported that the MIB1 indices were 5% and 15% respectively for benign and malignant phyllodes tumors (28). Furthermore, there was good correlation with conventional histologic grading of phyllodes tumors (Figure 4). Similar findings were echoed in another study involving 46 phyllodes tumors, with malignant phyllodes tumors showing a higher MIB1 expression than borderline and benign tumors. Within the benign group, the expression of MIB1 was related to stromal cellularity, with highly cellular lesions revealing higher MIB1 expression (29). The utility of MIB1 in predicting outcome is variable, with some studies confirming (30,31) and others refuting (28) its usefulness.

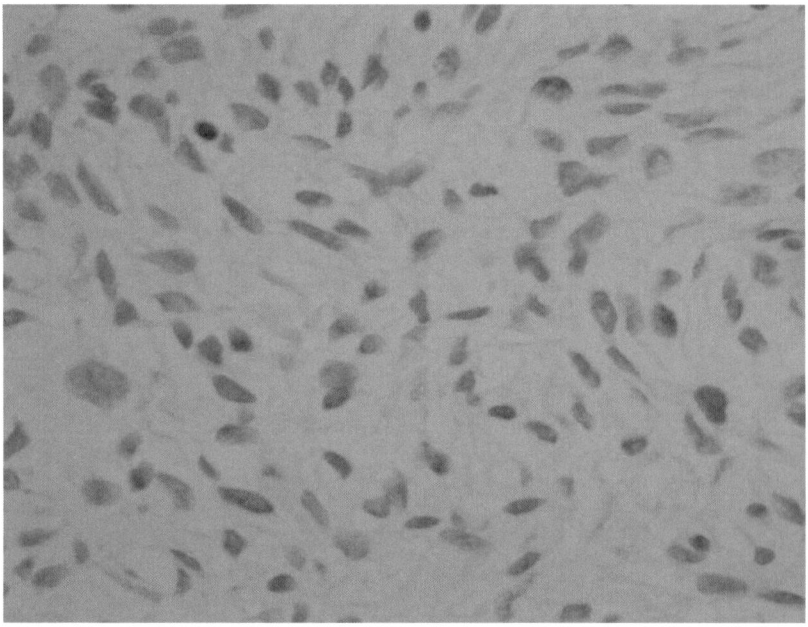

Figure 4. MIB1 immunostaining of stromal cell nuclei of a phyllodes tumor.

Measuring the DNA content and S phase fraction by flow cytometry is another approach taken to assess cellular proliferation. In general, benign phyllodes tumors are diploid, with aneuploidy identified in some of the borderline to malignant phyllodes tumors (30,31). The S phase fraction also shows a progressive increase from benign, borderline to malignant phyllodes (30). Furthermore, both DNA ploidy (31) and S phase fraction (30) have been reported as independent prognostic indicators in phyllodes tumors.

## Angiogenesis

Tumor angiogenesis as assessed by microvessel density has been under intensive investigation for its purported role as a prognostic factor in breast carcinoma including node negative cancers and ductal carcinoma in situ, and is thought to be related to tumor grade, vascular invasion, lymph node metastases and survival (32,33,34,35,36,37,38,39,40,41), although there are studies that failed to confirm the relationship with tumor parameters or outcomes (42,43,44,45,46). The relationship between angiogenesis and other biological prognostic markers including p53 (47,48,49,50), proliferative indices such as Ki67 (48) and cyclin D1 (49) was more variable. Among these, p53 was the most widely studied and there appears to be an association between p53 and angiogenesis (45,46,47). The association of angiogenesis with other factors had been inconsistent.

Vascular endothelial growth factor (VEGF) is a potent angiogenic peptide that stimulates angiogenesis. High VEGF level has been shown to be associated with decreased disease free and overall survival and lymph node metastasis (51,52,53,54,55), and a predictor of outcome after hormonal therapy (56) or chemotherapy in advanced disease (57). VEGF acts as a highly specific and potent mitogen for endothelial cells, inducing formation of new blood vessels and enhancing vascular permeability. Prominent members of VEGF include VEGF A,B,C and D. VEGF A is probably the most extensively studied, and is significantly related to the breast cancer (56,58). Expression of VEGF C and D had also been shown to be increased in breast cancer (59).

In phyllodes tumors, a progressive increase in microvessel density from benign to borderline to malignant lesions has been shown (60,61), and this is independent of mitotic count, nuclear pleomorphism and stromal overgrowth, suggesting that angiogenesis may be an important independent predictor of malignancy (60). There appears to be an association between microvessel density in phyllodes tumors and stromal cellularity, and also with p53 protein expression of stromal cells (60). The mechanism of increased angiogenesis is not fully understood, but preliminary evidence suggests a possible role of vascular endothelial growth factor (VEGF) (62).

## c-kit (CD117)

c-kit is a proto-oncogene that encodes a tyrosine kinase receptor and is now considered a diagnostic marker for gastrointestinal stromal tumors. In phyllodes tumors, a progressive increase in stromal cells of c-kit expression from benign to malignant phyllodes, ranging from

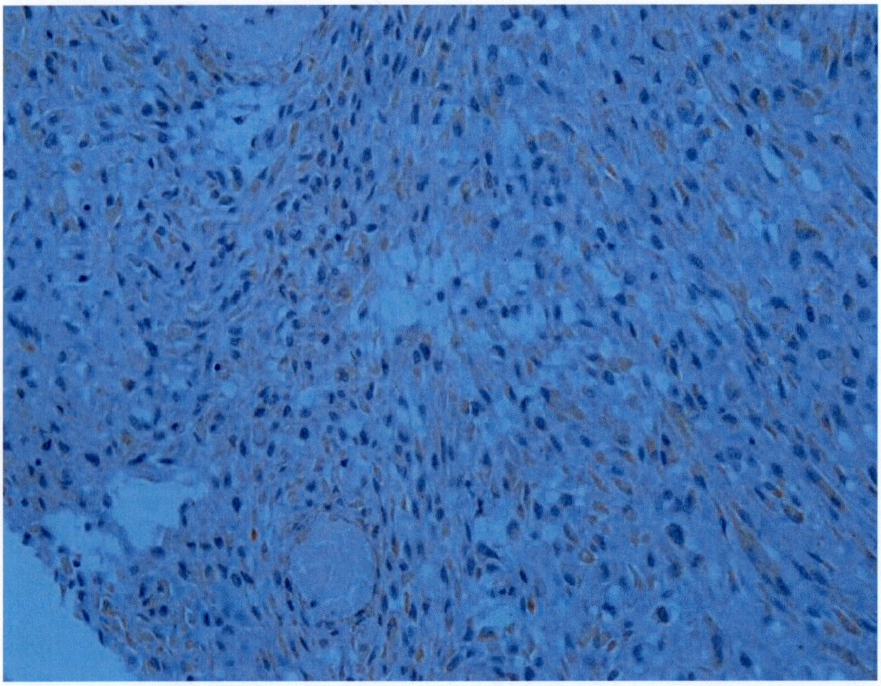

Figure 5. CD117 (c-kit) immunoreactivity within stromal cell cytoplasm of a phyllodes tumor.

5%-17% in benign lesions to 46%-50% in malignant ones (63,64) has been demonstrated by immunohistochemistry (Figure 5). Interestingly another study showed higher expression of c-kit in the epithelial than the stromal component (24). Nevertheless, the combined results of all these studies showed a correlation of c-kit expression with tumor grade in phyllodes tumors. In addition, there is early evidence that stromal c-kit expression may be related to recurrence (24). This is a significant finding, as so far no biological marker has been shown to be a predictor for recurrence. The underlying mechanism for c-kit expression remains uncertain, as known activation mutations in gastrointestinal stromal tumours in exons 8-15 and 17 of the c-kit gene have not been demonstrated by direct sequencing in the majority of c-kit overexpressed phyllodes tumors (63). The potential of tyrosine kinase inhibitor (imatinib mesylate / Gleevec / Glivec) as a treatment modality in malignant phyllodes tumors remains to be explored.

## Other Markers

### CD10 (CALLA)

CD10, or the common acute lymphoblastic leukaemia antigen (CALLA), is a cell surface neutral endopeptidase expressed by lymphoid precursor cells and some B lymphoid cells (65). It has long been used as a marker for leukaemia, Burkitt and follicular lymphomas (66,67). Recently CD10 was found in normal tissues including myoepithelial cells of breast and salivary glands, apocrine metaplastic cells and in situ adenocarcinoma of many organs including breast (68). Of interest, CD10 expression has also been reported in spindle cell neoplasms such as cutaneous dermatofibroma and dermatofibrosarcoma (69) and in endometrial stromal sarcoma (70-72). In fact, CD10 has been used as a diagnostic marker to differentiate endometrial stromal sarcoma from leiomyoma (71). CD10 expression in the breast is not well-documented, with only a few reports on its expression in myoepithelial cells (68,73) and its use as a myoepithelial marker to aid the diagnosis of problematic lesions (74). CD10 expression in breast stromal cell is even more sparsely addressed in the literature, with only a single report documenting the possible use of CD10 expression in the stroma of invasive carcinoma of the breast as an important predictor of clinical outcome (75). Although widely used in differential diagnosis of endometrial sarcoma, CD10 expression in mammary stromal neoplasms, particularly phyllodes tumours, had not been well-documented (76,77). The expression of CD10 has been reported to be significantly increased from a low 3% -6% expression in benign phyllodes tumors to a high 32% to 50% in borderline to frankly malignant phyllodes tumors (76,77). This however, remains a poorly evaluated marker, and its role in diagnosis or prognosis requires more extensive evaluation.

### Epithelial Growth Factor Receptor (EGFR)

EGFR expression has been reported in breast cancer (78) and this is thought to be important in early carcinogenesis. In phyllodes tumors, it has been described as being expressed in 19% of all tumors, with a progressive increase from benign to malignant phyllodes, reaching a high 63% in frankly malignant phyllodes tumors, predominantly in stromal cells. This expression was also reported to be correlated with p53, p16, c-kit, cyclin A and cyclin E (79). Further analysis of EGFR positive overexpressed cases showed whole gene and intron 1 amplification in the majority of the cases, indicating that gene amplification is the main mechanism. This observation has significant implications, raising the possibility of using tyrosine kinase inhibitor as a potential therapeutic agent in malignant cases.

## Hypoxia Inducible Factor 1 Alpha (HIF-1α)

It has recently been demonstrated that HIF-1α expression is of prognostic value in several types of cancer, including breast cancer (80). The two targets of HIF-1α are the vascular endothelial growth factor (VEGF) gene (81) and carbonic anhydrase 9 (CA9) gene (82), VEGF and microvessel proliferation in phyllodes tumors has been discussed in the earlier section. Upregulation of carbonic anhydrase 9 (CA9) gene expression was found to be dependent of HIF-1α, and the protein product, carbonic anhydrase IX (CAIX). CAIX has recently been shown to be related to poor outcome in breast cancer (83). It therefore seems that HIF-1α and its downstream targets play pivotal roles in the development and progression of cancer. In phyllodes tumors, both stromal and epithelial expression of HIF-1α are high, accounting for about 50% in a large series (84). Further analysis of that series showed the expression of HIF-1α correlated with the grade of the phyllodes tumor. Stromal expression of HIF-1α correlated positively with tumor grade. In the same study, expression of the downstream protein product CAIX, did not correlate with HIF-1α expression, suggesting that hypoxia may not be the underlying mechanism, as CAIX expression was known to be induced by hypoxia (85).

## Heparan Sulfate

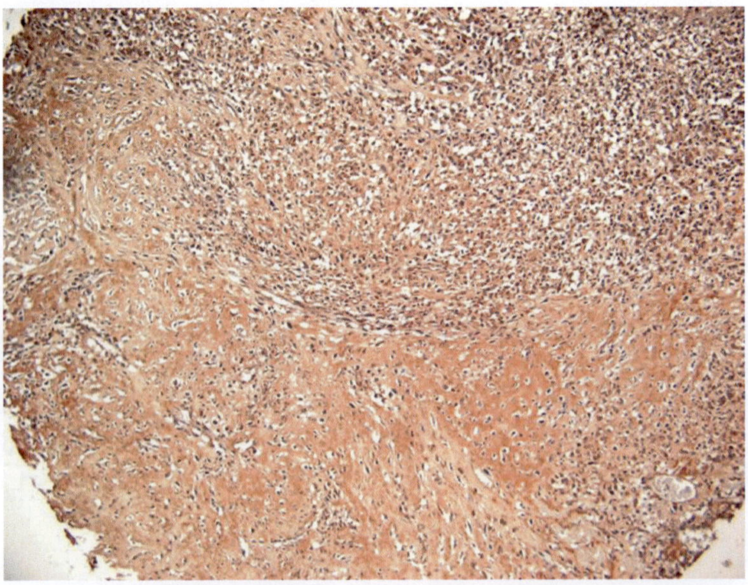

Figure 6. Heparan sulfate reactivity within the stroma of a malignant phyllodes tumor.

Heparan sulfate is an important biomolecule involved in maintaining cell–cell and cell–extracellular matrix adhesion, mediating receptor-ligand binding and regulating activities of growth and motility factors. Differential heparan sulfation patterns in breast cancer cells have been demonstrated, and several reports have also shown that syndecan 1 is an important heparan sulfate proteoglycan in cell signalling and tumor cell progression in breast cancer. Using a monoclonal antibody, 10E4 (known to detect mixed N-sulfated and N-acetylated heparan sulfate) to examine the localization of heparan sulfate in a tissue microarray series of 232 phyllodes tumors by immunohistochemistry, it was found that stromal 10E4 expression was significantly associated with tumor grade, stromal p53, and MIB1 expression in proliferating cells, suggesting that heparan sulfate may participate in malignant tumor growth (Figure 6). These molecules may act in concert in influencing cell cycle progression. It was suggested that heparan sulfate expression in breast phyllodes may assist in assignment of tumor grade and prediction of biologic behavior (86).

## Other Molecular Markers in Phyllodes Tumors

Comparative genomic hybridization (CGH) has been used to delineate the cytogenetic abnormalities of phyllodes tumors, and it has been reported that 1q gain, 3p loss, 7q gain, 6q loss and 3q loss are the most common changes detected. There is also evidence that 1q gain may be associated with recurrent disease in phyllodes tumors (87,88). 3p loss has been described in benign, atypical and malignant breast lesions, and one of the most commonly deleted regions has been mapped to the FHIT gene in the 3p12-14 region.

Clonality studies in phyllodes tumors showed that while the epithelial component is polyclonal, the stromal component is monoclonal (89,90), indicating that phyllodes tumor is a neoplastic stromal lesion. Recently there is new evidence that shows distinct clonality in both epithelial and stromal components of phyllodes tumors, implicating that the epithelial component may also be neoplastic (88). In addition, using single nucleotide polymorphism (SNP) array, primary phyllodes tumors and their recurrences were shown to share common regions of loss of heterozygosity (LOH) (91), confirming clonality of the primaries and their recurrences.

## Conclusion

The morphological features of phyllodes tumors have been well described in the literature, but determination of histologic grade still depends on a constellation of histologic criteria, resulting in some degree of non-uniformity in diagnosis. The prediction of outcome remains problematic, as the majority of phyllodes tumors behave in an indolent manner, and even for the malignant tumors, not all recur or metastasize. Some of the biological markers discussed herewith demonstrate some promises, either in assisting the grading of the tumor, or raising the potential of specific drug therapy. The etiology and progression of phyllodes tumors remain largely unknown, although recently an association between stromal beta-catenin with epithelial Wnt5a expression has been reported (92), and it is believed that in phyllodes tumor, the progression to malignancy results from stromal independence from the epithelium. This concept may represent a major step in our understanding of this group of biphasic lesions, and warrants further detailed studies.

# References

[1] Lerwill MF. Biphasic lesions of the breast. Sem Diagn Pathol 2004;21:48-56.

[2] Elston CW, Ellis IO. *The breast*. Systemic Pathology, 3rd, Vol 13, Edinburgh: Churchill Livingstone 2000; 147-186.

[3] Tan PH, Jayabaskar T, Chuah KL, Lee HY, Tan Y, Hilmy M, Hung H, Selvarajan S, Bay BH. Phyllodes tumours of the breast. The role of pathologic parameters. *Am J Clin Pathol* 2005;123:529-540.

[4] Tse GM, Putti TC, Kung FY, Scolyer RA, Law BK, Lau TS, Lee CS. Increased p53 protein expression in malignant mammary phyllodes tumours. *Mod Pathol* 2002;15: 734-740.

[5] Moffat CJ, Pinders SE, Dixon AR, Elston CW, Blamey RW, Ellis IO. Phyllodes tumours of the breast: a clinicopathologicla review of thirty-two cases. *Histopathology* 1995;27:205-218.

[6] Parkers SJ, Harries SA. Phyllodes tumours. *Postgrad Med J* 2001;77:428-435.

[7] Grimes MM. Cystosarcoma phyllodes of the breast: histological features, flow cytometric analysis, and clinical correlation. *Mod Pathol* 1992;5:232-239.

[8] Mokbel K, Price RK, Mostafa A, Wells CA, Carpenter R. Phyllodes tumour of the breast: a retrospective analysis of 30 cases. *Breast* 1999;8:278-281.

[9] Reinfuss M, Mitus J, Smolak K, Stelmach A. Malignant phyllodes tumours of the breast. A clinical and pathological analysis of 55 cases. *Eur J Cancer* 1993;29A:1252-1256.

[10] Staren ED, Lynch G, Boyle C, Witt TR, Bines SD. Malignant cystosarcoma phyllodes. *Am Surg* 1994;60:583-585.

[11] Ciatto S, Bonardi R, Cataliotti L, Cardona G. Phyllodes tumour of the breast: a multicenter series of 59 cases. Coordinating Center and Writing Committee of FONCAM (National Task Force for Breast Cancer), Italy. *Eur J Surg Oncol* 1992;18:545-549.

[12] Geisler DP, Boyle MJ, Malnar KF, McGee JM, Nolen MC, Fortner SM, Broughan TA. Phyllodes tumours of the breast: a review of 32 cases. *Am Surg* 2000;66:360-366.

[13] Bennett IC, Khan A, De Freitas R, Chaudary MA, Millis RR. Phyllodes tumours: a clinicopathological review of 30 cases. *Aust N Z J Surg* 1992;62:628-633.

[14] Tse GM, Law BK, Chan KF, Ma TK. Multinucleated stromal giant cells in mammary phyllodes tumours. *Pathology* 2001;33:153-156.

[15] Powell CM, Cranor ML, Rosen PP. Multinucleated stromal giant cells in mammary fibroepithelial neoplasms. A study of 11 patients. *Arch Pathol Lab Med* 1994;118: 912-916.

[16] Reinfuss M, Mitus J, Duda K, Stelmach A, Rys J, Smolak K. The treatment and prognosis of patients with phyllodes tumour of the breast: an analysis of 170 cases. *Cancer* 1996;77:910-916.

[17] Hawkins RE, Schofield JB, Fisher C, Wiltshaw E, McKinna JA. The clinical and histological criteria that predict metastases from cystosarcoma phyllodes. *Cancer* 1992;69:141-147.

[18] Cohn-Cedermark G, Rutqvist LE, Rosendahl I, Silfversward C. Prognostic factors in cystosarcoma phyllodes. A clinicopathologic study of 77 patients. *Cancer* 1991;68:2017-2022.

[19] Kapiris I, Nasiri N, A'Hern R, Healy V, Gui GP. Outcome and predictive factors of local recurrence and distant metastases following primary surgical treatment of high-grade malignant phyllodes tumours of the breast. *Eur J Surg Oncol* 2001;27:723-730.

[20] Keelan PA, Myers JL, Wold LE, Katzmann JA, Gibney DJ. Phyllodes tumour: clinicopathologic review of 60 patients and flow cytometric analysis in 30 patients. *Hum Pathol* 1992;23:1048-1054.

[21] Millar EK, Beretov J, Marr P, Sarris M, Clarke RA, Kearsley JH, Lee CS. Malignant phyllodes tumours of the breast display increased stromal p53 protein expression. *Histopathology* 1999;34:491-496.

[22] Feakins RM, Mulcahy HE, Nickols CD, Wells CA. p53 expression in phyllodes tumours is associated with histological features of malignancy but does not predict outcome. *Histopathology* 1999;35:162-169.

[23] Kuenen-Boumeester V, Henzen-Logmans SC, Timmermans MM, van Staveren IL, van Geel A, Peeterse HJ, Bonnema J, Berns EM. Altered expression of p53 and its regulated proteins in phyllodes tumours of the breast. *J Pathol* 1999;189:169-175.

[24] Tan PH, Jayabaskar T, Yip G, Tan Y, Hilmy M, Selvarajan S, Bay BH. p53 and c-kit (CD117) protein expression as prognostic indicators in breast phyllodes tumors: a tissue microarray study. *Mod Pathol* 2005;18:1527-1534.

[25] Umekita Y, Yoshida H. Immunohistochemical study of hormone receptor and hormone-regulated protein expression in phyllodes tumour: comparison with fibroadenoma. *Virchows Arch* 1998;433:311-314.

[26] Tse GM, Lee CS, Kung FY, Scolyer RA, Law BK, Lau TS, Putti TC. Hormonal receptors expression in epithelial cells of mammary phyllodes tumours correlates with pathologic grade of the tumour: a multicenter study of 143 cases. *Am J Clin Pathol* 2002;118:522-526.

[27] Sapino A, Bosco M, Cassoni P, Castellano I, Arisio R, Cserni G, Tos AP, Fortunati N, Catalano MG, Bussolati G. Estrogen receptor-beta is expressed in stromal cells of fibroadenoma and phyllodes tumors of the breast. *Mod Pathol* 2006;19:599-606.

[28] Kocova L, Skalova A, Fakan F, Rousarova M. Phyllodes tumour of the breast: immunohistochemical study of 37 tumours using MIB1 antibody. *Pathol Res Pract* 1998;194:97-104.

[29] Umekita Y, Yoshida H. Immunohistochemical study of MIB1 expression in phyllodes tumour and fibroadenoma. *Pathol Int* 1999;49:807-810.

[30] Niezabitowski A, Lackowska B, Rys J, Kruczak A, Kowalska T, Mitus J, Reinfuss M, Markiewicz D. Prognostic evaluation of proliferative activity and DNA content in the phyllodes tumour of the breast: immunohistochemical and flow cytometric study of 118 cases. *Breast Cancer Res Treat* 2001;65:77-85.

[31] el-Naggar AK, Ro JY, McLemore D, Garnsy L. DNA content and proliferative activity of cystosarcoma phyllodes of the breast. Potential prognostic significance. *Am J Clin Pathol* 1990;93:480-485.

[32] Weider NW, Semple JP, Welch WR, Folkman J. Tumor angiogenesis and metastasis - correlation in invasive breast carcinoma. *N Engl J Med* 1991;324:1-8.

[33] Horak E, Leek R, Klenk N, LeJeune S, Smith K, Stuart N, Greenall M, Stepniewska K, Harris AL. Angiogenesis, assessed by platelet/endothelial cell adhesion molecule antibodies, as indicator of node metastasis and survival in breast cancer. *Lancet* 1992;340:1120-1124.

[34] Weidner N, Folkman J, Pozza F, Bevilacqua P, Allred EN, Moore DH, Meli S, Gasparini G. Tumor angiogenesis: a new, significant, and independent prognostic indicator in early stage breast carcinoma. *J Natl Cancer Inst* 1992;84:1875-1887.

[35] Bosari S, Lee AKC, DeLellis RA, Wiley BD, Heatley GJ, Silverman ML. Microvessel quantitation and prognosis in invasive breast carcinoma. *Hum Pathol* 1992;23:755-761.

[36] Vincent-Salomon A, Carton M, Zafrani B, Freneaux P, Nicolas A, Massemin B, Fourquet A, Clough K, Pouillart P, Sastre-Garau X. Long term outcome of small size invasive breast carcinomas independent from angiogenesis in a series of 685 cases. *Cancer* 2001;92:249-256.

[37] Kato T, Kameoka S, Kimura T, Soga N, Abe Y, Nishikawa T, Kobayashi M. Angiogenesis as a predictor of long-term survival for 377 Japanese patients with breast cancer. *Breast Cancer Res Treat* 2001;70:65-74.

[38] de Jong JS, van Diest PJ, Baak JP. Hot spot microvessel density and the mitotic activity index are strong additional prognostic indicators in invasive breast cancer. *Histopathology* 2000;36:306-312.

[39] Heimann R, Ferguson D, Powers C, Recant WM, Weichselbaum RR, Hellman S. Angiogenesis as a predictor of long-term survival for patients with node-negative breast cancer. *J Natl Cancer Inst* 1996;88:1764-1749.

[40] Karaiossifidi H, Kouri E, Arvaniti H, Sfikas S, Vasilaros S. Tumor angiogenesis in node-negative breast cancer: relationship with relapse free survival. *Anticancer Res* 1996;16:4001-4002.

[41] Santinelli A, Baccarini M, Colanzi P, Fabris G. Microvessel quantitation in intraductal and early invasive breast carcinomas. *Anal Quant Cytol Histol* 2000;22:277-284.

[42] Medri L, Nanni O, Volpi A, Scarpi E, Dubini A, Riccobon A, Becciolini A, Bianchi S, Amadori D. Tumor microvessel density and prognosis in node-negative breast cancer. *Int J Cancer* 2000;89:74-80.

[43] Axelsson K, Ljung BM, Moore DH 2nd, Thor AD, Chew KL, Edgerton SM, Smith HS, Mayall BH. Tumor angiogenesis as a prognostic assay for invasive ductal breast carcinoma. *J Natl Cancer Inst* 1995;87:997-1008.

[44] Van Hoef ME, Knox WF, Dhesi SS, Howell A, Schor AM. Assessment of tumour vascularity as a prognostic factor in lymph node negative invasive breast cancer. *Eur J Cancer* 1993;29A:1141-1145.

[45] Morphopoulos G, Pearson M, Ryder WD, Howell A, Harris M. Tumour angiogenesis as a prognostic marker in infiltrating lobular carcinoma of the breast. *J Pathol* 1996;180:44-49.

[46] Nakopoulou L, Lekkas N, Lazaris AC, Athanassiadou P, Giannopoulou I, Mavrommatis J, Davaris P. An immunohistochemical analysis of angiogenesis in invasive breast cancer with correlations to clinicopathologic predictors. *Anticancer Res* 1999;19: 4547-4553.

[47] Gonzalez-Palacios F, Sancho M, Martinez JC, Bellas C. Microvessel density, p53 overexpression, and apoptosis in invasive breast carcinoma. *Mol Pathol* 1997;50: 304-309.

[48] Zolota V, Gerokosta A, Melachrinou M, Kominea A, Aletra C, Scopa CD. Microvessel density, proliferating activity, p53 and bcl-2 expression in in situ ductal carcinoma of the breast. *Anticancer Res* 1999;19:3269-3274.

[49] Heffelfinger SC, Yassin R, Miller MA, Lower EE. Cyclin D1, retinoblastoma, p53, and Her2/neu protein expression in preinvasive breast pathologies: correlation with vascularity. *Pathobiology* 2000;68:129-136.

[50] Tas F, Yavuz E, Aydiner A, Saip P, Disci R, Iplikci A, Topuz E. Angiogenesis and p53 protein expression in breast cancer: prognostic roles and interrelationships. *Am J Clin Oncol* 2000;23:546-53.

[51] Gasparini G. Prognostic value of vascular endothelial growth factor in breast cancer. Oncologist 2000;5 Suppl 1:37-44,.

[52] Manders P, Beex LV, Tjan-Heijnen VC, Geurts-Moespot J, Van Tienoven TH, Foekens JA, Sweep CG. The prognostic value of vascular endothelial growth factor in 574 node-negative breast cancer patients who did not receive adjuvant systemic therapy. *Br J Cancer* 2002;87:772-778.

[53] Gasparini G, Toi M, Gion M, Verderio P, Dittadi R, Hanatani M, Matsubara I, Vinante O, Bonoldi E, Boracchi P, Gatti C, Suzuki H, Tominaga T. Prognostic significance of vascular endothelial growth factor protein in node-negative breast carcinoma. *J Natl Cancer Inst* 1997;89:139-147.

[54] Nakamura Y, Yasuoka H, Tsujimoto M, Yang Q, Imabun S, Nakahara M, Nakao K, Nakamura M, Mori I, Kakudo K. Prognostic significance of vascular endothelial growth factor d in breast carcinoma with long-term follow-up. *Clin Cancer Res* 2003;9:716-721.

[55] Kinoshita J, Kitamura K, Kabashima A, Saeki H, Tanaka S, Sugimachi K. Clinical significance of vascular endothelial growth factor-C (VEGF-C) in breast cancer. Breast *Cancer Res Treat* 2001;66:159-164.

[56] Linderholm B, Grankvist K, Wilking N, Johansson M, Tavelin B, Henriksson R. Correlation of vascular endothelial growth factor content with recurrences, survival, and first relapse site in primary node-positive breast carcinoma after adjuvant treatment. *J Clin Oncol* 2000;18:1423-1431.

[57] Foekens JA, Peters HA, Grebenchtchikov N, Look MP, Meijer-van Gelder ME, Geurts-Moespot A, van der Kwast TH, Sweep CG, Klijn JG. High tumor levels of vascular endothelial growth factor predict poor response to systemic therapy in advanced breast cancer. *Cancer Res* 2001;61:5407-5414

[58] Linderholm BK, Lindahl T, Holmberg L, Klaar S, Lennerstrand J, Henriksson R, Bergh J. The expression of vascular endothelial growth factor correlates with mutant p53 and poor prognosis in human breast cancer. *Cancer Res* 2001;61:2256-2260

[59] Yang W, Klos K, Yang Y, Smith TL, Shi D, Yu D. ErbB2 overexpression correlates with increased expression of vascular endothelial growth factors A, C, and D in human breast carcinoma. *Cancer* 2002;94:2855-2861

[60] Tse GM, Lui PC, Scolyer RA, Putti TC, Kung FY, Law BK, Lau TS, Lee CS.. Tumour angiogenesis and p53 protein expression in mammary phyllodes tumours. *Mod Pathol* 2003;16:1007-1013.

[61] Tse GM, Ma TK, Chan KF, Law BK, Chen MH, Li KH, Chan EC, Mak MK. Increased microvessel density in malignant and borderline mammary phyllodes tumours. *Histopathology* 2001;38:567-570.

[62] Tse GM, Lui PC, Lee CS, Kung FY, Scolyer RA, Law BK, Lau TS, Karim R, Putti TC. Stromal expression of vascular endothelial growth factor correlates with tumour grade and microvessel density in mammary phyllodes tumours: a multicenter study of 185 cases. *Hum Pathol* 2004;35:1053-1057.

[63] Sawyer EJ, Poulsom R, Hunt FT, Jeffery R, Elia G, Ellis IO, Ellis P, Tomlinson IP, Hanby AM.. Malignant phyllodes tumours show stromal overexpression of c-myc and c-kit. *J Pathol* 2003;200:59-64.

[64] Tse GM, Putti TC, Lui PC, Lo AW, Scolyer RA, Law BK, Karim R, Lee CS. Increased c-kit (CD117) expression in malignant mammary phyllodes tumours. *Mod Pathol* 2004;17:827-831.

[65] Greaves MF, Hariri G, Newman RA, Sutherland DR, Ritter MA, Ritz J. Selective expression of the common acute lymphoblastic leukaemia (gp 100) antigen on immature lymphoid cells and their malignant counterparts. *Blood* 1983; 61:628-639.

[66] Gregory CD, Tursz T, Edwards CF, Tetaud C, Talbot M, Caillou B, Rickinson AB, Lipinski M. Identification of a subset of normal B cells with a Burkitt's lymphoma (BL)-like phenotype. *J Immunol* 1987; 139:313-318.

[67] Stein H, Lennert K, Feller AC, Mason DY. Immunohistological analysis of human lymphoma: correlation of histological and immunological categories. *Adv Cancer Res* 1984; 42:67-147.

[68] Chu P, Arber DA. Paraffin section detection of CD10 in 505 nonhematopoietic neoplasms. *Am J Clin Pathol* 2000; 113:374-382.

[69] Kanitakis J, Bourchany D, Claudy A. Expression of the CD10 antigen (neutral endopeptidase) by mesenchymal tumours of the skin. *Anticancer Res* 2000;20: 3539-3544.

[70] McCluggage WG, Sumathi VP, Maxwell P. CD10 is a sensitive and diagnostically useful immunohistochemical marker of normal endometrial stroma and of endometrial stromal neoplasms. *Histopathology* 2001;39:273-278.

[71] Chu PG, Arber DA, Weiss LM, Chang KL. Utility of CD10 in distinguishing between endometrial stromal sarcoma and uterine smooth muscle tumours: an immunohistochemical comparison of 34 cases. *Mod Pathol* 2001;14:465-471.

[72] Toki T, Shimizu M, Takagi Y, Ashida T, Konishi I. CD10 is a marker for normal and neoplastic endometrial stromal cells. *Int J Gynecol Pathol* 2002; 21:41-47.

[73] Mahendran R, McIlhinney R, O'Hare M, Monaghan P, Gusterson B. Expression of the common acute lymphoblastic leukaemia antigen (CALLA) in the human breast. *Mol Cell Probes* 1989;3:39-44.

[74] Moritani S, Kushima R, Sugihara H, Bamba M, Kobayashi TK, Hattori T. Availability of CD10 immunohistochemistry as a marker of breast myoepithelial cells on paraffin sections. *Mod Pathol* 2002;15:397-405.

[75] Iwaya K, Ogawa H, Izumi M, Kuroda M, Mukai K. Stromal expression of CD10 in invasive breast carcinoma: a new predictor of clinical outcome. *Virchows Arch* 2002; 440:589-593.

[76] Mechtersheimer G, Kruger KH, Born IA, Moller P. Antigenic profile of mammary fibroadenoma and cystosarcoma phyllodes. A study using antibodies to estrogen- and progesterone receptors and to a panel of cell surface molecules. *Pathol Res Pract* 1990; 186:427-438

[77] Tse GM, Tsang AK, Putti TC, Scolyer RA, Lui PC, Law BK, Karim RZ, Lee CS. Stromal CD10 expression in mammary fibroadenomas and phyllodes tumours. *J Clin Pathol* 2005;58:185-189.
[78] Tidow N, Boecker A, Schmidt H, Agelopoulos K, Boecker W, Buerger H, Brandt B. Distinct amplification of an untranslated regulatory sequence in the egfr gene contributes to early steps in breast cancer development. *Cancer Res* 2003 ;63:1172-1178
[79] Kersting C, Kuijper A, Schmidt H, Packeisen J, Liedtke C, Tidow N, Gustmann C, Hinrichs B, Wulfing P, Tio J, Boecker W, van Diest P, Brandt B, Buerger H. Amplifications of the epidermal growth factor receptor gene (egfr) are common in phyllodes tumors of the breast and are associated with tumor progression. *Lab Invest* 2006;86:54-61.
[80] Bos R, van der Groep P, Greijer AE, Shvarts A, Meijer S, Pinedo HM, Semenza GL, van Diest PJ, van der Wall E. Levels of hypoxia-inducible factor-1α independently predict prognosis in patients with lymph node negative breast cancer. *Cancer* 2003;97:1573–1581
[81] Forsythe JA, Jiang BH, Iyer NV, Agani F, Leung SW, Koos RD, Semenza GL. Activation of vascular endothelial growth factor gene transcription by hypoxia-inducible factor 1. *Mol Cell Biol.* 1996;16:4604–4613
[82] Wykoff CC, Beasley NJP, Watson PH, Turner KJ, Pastorek J, Sibtain A, Wilson GD, Turley H, Talks KL, Maxwell PH, et al. Hypoxia-inducible expression of tumor-associated carbonic anhydrases. *Cancer Res* 2000;60:7075–7083
[83] Chia SK, Wykoff CC, Watson PH, Han C, Leek RD, Pastorek JD, Gatter KC, Ratcliffe P, Harris AL. Prognostic significance of a novel hypoxia-regulated marker, carbonic anhydrase IX, in invasive breast cancer. *J Clin Oncol* 2001;19:3660–3668.
[84] Kuijper A, van der Groep P, van der Wall E, van Diest PJ. Expression of hypoxia-inducible factor 1 alpha and its downstream targets in fibroepithelial tumors of the breast. Breast Cancer Res 2005;7(5):R808-18. *Epub* 2005 Aug 5.
[85] Loncaster JA, Harris AL, Davidson SE, Logue JP, Hunter RD, Wykoff CC, Pastorek J, Ratcliffe PJ, Stratford IJ, West CM. Carbonic anhydrase (CA IX) expression, a potential new intrinsic marker of hypoxia: correlation with tumor oxygen measurements and prognosis in locally advanced carcinoma of the cervix. *Cancer Res* 2001;61:6394–6399.
[86] Koo CY, Bay BH, Lui PCW, Tse GMK, Tan PH, Yip GWC. Immunohistochemical expression of heparan sulfate correlates with stromal cell proliferation in breast phyllodes tumors. *Mod Pathol* in press.
[87] Lu YJ, Birdsall S, Osin P, Gusterson B, Shipley J. Phyllodes tumours of the breast analyzed by comparative genomic hybridization and association of increased 1q copy number with stromal overgrowth and recurrence. *Genes Chromosomes Cancer* 1997;20:275-281.
[88] Sawyer EJ, Hanby AM, Ellis P, Lakhani SR, Ellis IO, Boyle S, Tomlinson IP. Molecular analysis of phyllodes tumours reveals distinct changes in the epithelial and stromal components. *Am J Pathol* 2000;156:1093-1098.
[89] Noguchi S, Motomura K, Inaji H, Imaoka S, Koyama H. Clonal analysis of fibroadenoma and phyllodes tumour of the breast. Cancer Res 1993;53:4071-4074.

[90] Kuijper A, Buerger H, Simon R, Schaefer KL, Croonen A, Boecker W, van der Wall E, van Diest PJ. Analysis of the progression of fibroepithelial tumours of the breast by PCR-based clonality assay. *J Pathol* 2002;197:575-581.

[91] Wang ZC, Buraimoh A, Iglehart JD, Richardson AL. Genome-Wide analysis for loss of heterozygosity in primary and recurrent phyllodes yumor and fibroadenoma of breast using single nucleotide polymorphism arrays. *Breast Cancer Res Treat* 2006;97: 301-309.

[92] Sawyer EJ, Hanby AM, Rowan AJ, Gillett CE, Thomas RE, Poulsom R, Lakhani SR, Ellis IO, Ellis P, Tomlinson IP. The Wnt pathway, epithelial-stromal interactions, and malignant progression in phyllodes tumours. *J Pathol* 2002;196:437-444.

In: Tumor Markers Research Focus
Editor: Deborah H. Chang, pp. 111-119

ISBN: 978-1-60021-544-5


*Chapter V*

# Significance and Prognostic Value of Estradiol Modulating Enzymes in Breast Cancer

***Christian F. Singer*[1,2*]*, Daphne Gschwantler-Kaulich*[1]*,***
***Anneliese Fink-Retter*[1] *Ernst Kubista*[1,2]*, Klaus Czerwenka*[3]***
***and Gernot Hudelist*[1,4]**
[1]Division of Special Gynecology, Department of OB/GYN
[2]Ludwig-Boltzmann-Institute of Clinical Experimental Oncology,
Medical University of Vienna, Vienna, Austria
[3]Division of Gynecopathology, Medical University of Vienna, Vienna, Austria
[4]Department of OB/GYN, LKH Villach, Villach, Austria

## Abstract

Estradiol (E2) plays a key role in the development and progression of breast cancer. While in postmenopausal women systemic E2 levels are greatly diminished, intratumoral sex steroid concentrations remain high thus providing an estrogenic environment that is favourable for tumor growth. The local estrogen E2 concentration is essentially mediated by the concerted action of the four enzymes aromatase, 17β hydroxysteriod dehydrogenase type 1 (17βHSD1), estrogen sulfotransferase (EST) and steroid sulfatase (STS). While the enzymatic activity of aromatase and STS results in an increase of bioactive estradiol, 17βHSD2 and EST reduce local E2 levels by converting the hormone into biologically inactive estrogen sulfates or less active metabolites. The importance of aromatase has been identified early and has lead to extensive studies investigating the predictive and prognostic value of this enzyme. Considerably less is, however, is known about the other three enzymes. This is especially remarkable since it has been suggested that STS activity, which transforms estrone sulfates into the biologically active unconjugated E2, is in general 100-500 times higher than

* E-mail address: Christian.Singer@meduniwien.ac.at, Phone: +43 1 40400 2801, Fax: +43 1 40400 2323, Correspondence to: Christian F Singer, Division of Special Gynecology, University of Vienna Medical Center, Waehringer Guertel 18-20, 1090 Vienna, Austria.

aromatase activity, which converts androgens into estrogens. Several new compounds, such as dydrogesterone, sulfamates and tibolone, have been developed which are potent sulfatase inhibitors. In this article we describe the action and relevance of modulators of local E2 in breast cancer. We also discuss the prognostic value of intratumoral enzyme expression pattern and their potential use as predictors of response to endocrine antineoplastic therapies.

# The Intracrinology of Breast Cancer

The synthesis and metabolization of intratumoral estrogens are the result of a complex network of interactions of a number of enzymes that are physiologically expressed in human breast tissue. Among the CYP superfamily of estrogen-metabolizing enzymes, CYP19 or better know as aromatase is thought to play a key role by mediating the aromatization of androstenedione to estrone. The subsequent conversion of estrone by 17βHSD1 to E2 ultimately results in an elevation of local estrogen levels which are particularly relevant in postmenopausal patients with breast carcinoma. In breast cancer patients, intratumoral aromatase gene expression is increased in comparison to non-malignant tissues and aromatase mRNA levels have been shown to be significantly higher in the tumor-bearing quadrant, [1], [2]. Other investigators have matched the gene expression data by enzyme activity assays and have similarly demonstrated that intratumoral aromatase activity in breast cancer is generally increased in the majority of cases and is detectable in both, tumor epithelium and surrounding stroma [3], [4]. Interestingly, the cellular source of aromatase is still unclear: While mRNA expression of aromatase is detectable in both carcinoma and adjacent stromal cells, reported results of aromatase immunolocalization in breast cancers are varying considerably [5], [6]. Santen and other study groups [6], [7], [8], observed aromatase immunoreactivity predominantly in the stromal cells, while studies by Brodie et al. [9] and Esteban and colleagues [10] reported aromatase expression in epithelial components of breast tumors exclusively. Recently, Sasano et al. [8] validated several aromatase antibodies and showed that aromatase immunoreactivity was detected in various types of cells such as stromal cells, carcinoma cells and normal duct epithelial cells, thus adding to the confusion.

While aromatase is by far the most investigated molecule, other enzymes, such as the 17β-hydroxysteroid dehydrogenase (17β-HSD) isozymes, the estrogen sulfotransferase (EST), and the estrogen sulfatase (STS) also play key roles in the modulation of local estrogen concentrations:

The 17beta-hydroxysteroid dehydrogenase (17 β-HSD) interconverts estradiol (E2) and estrone (E1), thereby modulating local E2 levels. The enzyme exists in two isoforms: 17 β-HSD type 1, whose action mainly leads to a reduction of estrone (E1) to estradiol (E2), and 17β-HSD type 2, which essentially results in the oxidation of E2 to E1. While 17β-HSD type 1 is expressed in benign breast disorders, DCIS and in invasive ductal carcinoma, 17β-HSD type 2 activity is predominant in normal breast tissues [11]. The expression pattern of both aromatase and 17beta-HSD in breast carcinoma suggests that malignant tumors can effectively convert E1, produced as a result of in situ aromatization, to the biologically active E2, which, in turn, exerts estrogenic actions on tumor cells through estrogen receptor signalling [12].

The estrogen sulfotransferases (EST) convert estrogens to the biologically inactive estrone sulfates and can be separated into two isoforms: a) the EST-1, which is expressed in various breast cancer cells (e.g. MCF-7, ZR-75-1, T-47D) and which catalyzes the sulfation of 2-hydroxy-estrone and 2-hydroxy-estradiol, and b) the EST-2, which is responsible for the sulfonation of estradiol, estrone, and ethinyl estradiol [13], [14]. Both sulfotransferases are expressed in normal breast and in breast cancer, and while EST-1 gene expression in tumoral and peri-tumoral tissue is comparable, the tumoral expression pattern of EST-2 remains to be investigated [15].

Finally, steroid sulfatase (STS) hydrolyzes several sulfated steroids such as estrone sulfate, dehydroepiandrosterone (DHEA) sulfate, and cholesterol sulfate [16]. In breast carcinomas, STS expression catalyzes the conversion from estrone sulfate to estrone, which results in an increase in local estrogen concentration [17]. STS gene expression is significantly higher in breast carcinoma tissues than that in normal tissues [18], and the enzymatic activity of STS is consequently also detected in the vast majority of malignant breast cancers. In fact, in breast cancer, STS activity has even been described to be considerably higher than aromatase activity [16]. Both immunohistochemical findings and gene expression studies point to an epithelial source of STS, while intratumoral stroma does not appear to express the enzyme [17].

The expression of intratumoral aromatase, 17β-HSD type 1, EST and STS in human breast cancer vary considerably and are not necessarily inter-correlated. This not only implies an individual control of enzymatic gene expression and activity, but also suggests that patients differ by the source, quantity, and biologic activity of intratumoral estrogens.

## Prognostic and Predictive Value of the Hormone Receptor Status

Because of the widespread use of adjuvant tamoxifen and aromatase inhibitors (AIs), in most industrialized countries, an unbiased prognostic effect of estrogen receptor (ER) and progesterone receptor (PR) in untreated breast carcinoma is difficult to assess. There are, nevertheless, several older trial protocols that did not include adjuvant systemic treatment and that allow for an unbiased evaluation of the receptor status: The NSABP B-06 trial randomized women with early-stage breast cancer to mastectomy, lumpectomy alone, or lumpectomy followed by radiation therapy, all without adjuvant systemic treatment [19]. While women with ER-positive tumors had a 5-year disease-free survival (DFS) of 74% and an overall survival (OS) of 92%, women with ER-negative tumors had a significantly decreased 5-year DFS and OS of 66% and 82%, respectively. Interestingly, studies with follow-up periods extending beyond than 5 years suggest that the prognostic significance of hormone receptors does not persist long-term. Hilsenbeck et al. [20] have, for example, demonstrated an improved prognosis for ER-positive tumors during the first 3 years of follow, a beneficial effect that disappeared in subsequent years. While these results are somewhat difficult to interpret, it has been speculated that the presence of ER and PR characterizes a slow growing, yet more indolent tumor subtype rather than a more "benign" tumor entity.

While the prognostic value of the receptor status is still debated, there is no doubt that the presence of ER and PR is a powerful predictive factor for the likelihood of benefit from adjuvant tamoxifen: The 1998 Early Breast Cancer Trialists' Collaborative Group (EBCTCG) update of randomized trials involving adjuvant tamoxifen, included more than 37,000 women [21]. The data from this meta-analysis clearly demonstrate that adjuvant tamoxifen results in proportional reductions in the risk of recurrence and mortality of 47% and 26%, respectively in patients with ER-positive tumors. These endpoints translate to an absolute reduction in mortality of 5.6% for nodal-negative and of 10.9% for nodal-positive patients. Tamoxifen also led to a relative reduction of 47% in contralateral breast cancer. The use of AIs in large adjuvant trials (ATAC, BIG 1-98 and ABCSG/ARNO) results in an even further reduction in DFS and DDFS when compared to tamoxifen [21], [22], [23].

As expected, the benefit from endocrine therapies is exclusively limited to women with receptor-positive tumors which has led to the general recommendation to offer some kind of adjuvant endocrine treatment to hormone receptor-positive tumors unless otherwise contraindicated [24].

## Aromatase Expression and Malignant Behaviour

Aromatase is a key regulator of intratumoral estrogen levels and we have recently identified a differential aromatase and sulfotransferase protein expression pattern that is dependent of the spatial relation to a malignant breast tumor. Our results indicate a net increase in intra-tumoral active estrogen levels through increased stromal aromatization, while physiological local inactivation by sulfotransferase activity remains essentially [25]. While we found a significant correlation between aromatase and sulfotransferase, no such association was seen with the ER or PR status. While our findings somewhat contrast observations by Miller et al. [26] who reported a positive correlation between aromatase activity and ER, they are in line with several other publications which have similarly not found a consistent relationship between tumor aromatase and receptor status [10]. In addition, the level of aromatase expession in IDC was not correlated with other clinicopathological factors such as age, axillary lymph node status, tumor size, or histological grade [27], [28]. Interestingly, despite the efficacy of aromatase inhibitors in ER positive breast cancer in respect to the clinical outcome and despite the fact that aromatase activity in malignant breast tumors is increased [3], [29], [30], no significant association between aromatase activity and disease-free interval or overall survival has been reported so far [31], [32].

## Estrogen Sulfotransferase (EST) Expression and Clinical Outcome

EST enzymatic activity has been detected in breast carcinoma cells several years ago, and has also been found to correlated with the ER status [33], [34]. The EST activity in receptor positive tumors might actually be the consequence of a negative feed-back mechanism which leads to a reduction of the ligand at the receptor site and consequently results in a decrease in cellular estrogen sensitivity. This assumption is supported by *in vitro* models in which the transfection of an ER expressing tumor cell line (MCF-7) with EST resulted in a considerable reduction of estrogen-stimulated DNA synthesis or cell proliferation when compared to ununtransfected cells [35]. Conversely, the loss of EST in some breast tumors could result in a relevant increase in intratumoral estrogen concentrations that render an estrogen-sensitive tumor cell more malignant [35].

Suzuki et al. [15], [17] have recently reported that in a crude univariate analysis that EST immunoreactivity was inversely correlated with tumor size or lymph node status and associated with an improved prognosis. Results of multivariate analyses confirmed that EST immunoreactivity is an independent favourable prognostic factor for both recurrence and overall survival. In addition, EST expression was associated with lymph node status, which is still considered to be the the most robust and clinically relevant prognostic parameter for overall survival [15], [17].

## Prognostic Value of Intratumoral Steroid Sulfatase (STS)

The prognostic value of STS is still somewhat unclear: While Evans et al. [36] did not observe a significant association between STS activity and time to recurrence or OS in breast cancer patients, others have nevertheless found a direct correlation between STS mRNA expression and worse clinical outcome of patients [15], [37]. Utsumi et al. [18] have also observed increased levels of STS mRNA in tumors which developed lymph node metastases than in those without nodal involvement, and in patients who experienced a recurrence during the follow-up period. In their hands, high levels of STS mRNA turned out to be a significant predictor of reduced relapse-free survival when treated as a continuous variable while no significant association was seen between STS mRNA levels and overall survival. The discrepancy between these studies and the work by Evans et al. [36] is insofar interesting as STS activity has clearly been demonstrated to be correlated with the level of STS mRNA expression in breast cancer cells [38].

Recently, Suzuki et al. [32], [15] have compared STS mRNA expression with immunohistochemistry and enzyme activity. They found that all three were significantly associated and that immunohistochemistry was a valid method in the evaluation of STS expression. They also found STS protein to be confined to epithelial cells and was present in 74% of invasive ductal carcinomas. In their hands, immunohistochemical STS expression was correlated with tumor size, worsened prognosis and an increased risk of recurrence by univariate analysis, thus rendering STS immunohistochemistry a potent prognostic factor in human breast carcinoma.

## Prognostic Value of 17β-HSD1 and 17β-HSD2

While 17βHSD2 activity is predominant in breast tumors [11], 17βHSD1 appears to be specifically important in estrogen responsiveness, since this isozyme is significantly correlated with ERα and PR expression [39]. In addition, hormone-dependent cell lines preferentially express 17b-HSD1 while hormone-independent cell lines express 17β-HSD2 *in vitro* [40] . Miyoshi et al. [41] have reported increased 17β-HSD1 gene expression levels in postmenopausal women, and the increased intratumoral estradiol/estrone ratio in postmenopausal breast cancer patients suggests a role of 17β-HSD in maintaining an estrogen-rich environment in this population. Regardless of menopausal status, patients whose tumors are characterized by an increased 17b-HSD1 gene expression and / or a decreased 17b-HSD2 gene expression are associated with a higher risk of late relapse [42].

## Summary

Taken together, we have described the expression and prognostic relevance of the four enzymes that regulate local estrogen levels in both normal breast tissue and malignant breast epithelium. While aromatase, STS and 17β-HSD1 increase local estrogen levels, estrogen sulfotransferase (EST) and 17β-HSD2 activity results in a decrease of bioavailable hormone. It is thus evident that not only the amount of ER expression but also the expression and activity pattern of estrogen modifying enzymes is critical when the tumoral responsiveness to estrogens is evaluated. In addition, only a thorough understanding of the local estrogen synthesis and metabolization processes will enable us to develop novel endocrine strategies in the treatment of hormone-responsive breast cancer.

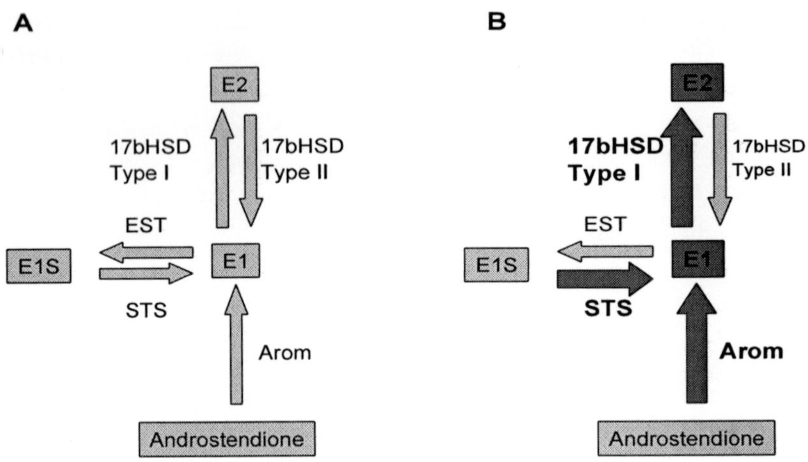


Figure. 1. Schematic representation of enzymes regulating local estrogen production in human normal breast (A) and in breast cancer tissue (B): Androstenedione and Estradiolsulfate (E1S) are major precursor substrates of local estrogen production in human breast tissue. Aromatase (Arom) converts androstenedione into E1 and STS mediates the conversion from E1S to E1. E1, is then converted to estradiol (E2) by 17β-HSD type I (17βHSD1), while 17β-HSD type II converts E2 to E1. Physiologically, EST and 17β–HSD2 [18] are expressed in several human tissues, most notably in the breast, controlling local E2 concentrations. However, in breast carcinoma, steroid sulfatase (STS), Aromatase (Arom) and 17β–HSD type I are overexpressed, while EST and 17_HSD2 tend to be decreased, thereby resulting in an increase in local E2 tissue concentrations.

# References


[1] T Utsumi, N Harada, M Maruta, Y Takagi: Presence of alternatively spliced transcripts of aromatase gene in human breast cancer. *J Clin Endocrinol Metab* 1996, 81:2344-9.

[2] SE Bulun, TM Price, J Aitken, MS Mahendroo, ER Simpson: A link between breast cancer and local estrogen biosynthesis suggested by quantification of breast adipose tissue aromatase cytochrome P450 transcripts using competitive polymerase chain reaction after reverse transcription. *J Clin Endocrinol Metab* 1993, 77:1622-8.

[3] P Bolufer, E Ricart, A Lluch, C Vazquez, A Rodriguez, A Ruiz, F Llopis, J Garcia-Conde, R Romero: Aromatase activity and estradiol in human breast cancer: its relationship to estradiol and epidermal growth factor receptors and to tumor-node-metastasis staging. *J Clin Oncol* 1992, 10:438-46.

[4] A Purohit, DY Wang, MW Ghilchik, MJ Reed: Regulation of aromatase and sulphatase in breast tumour cells. *J Endocrinol* 1996, 150 Suppl:S65-71.

[5] H Sasano, H Nagura, N Harada, Y Goukon, M Kimura: Immunolocalization of aromatase and other steroidogenic enzymes in human breast disorders. *Hum Pathol* 1994, 25:530-5.

[6] RJ Santen, J Martel, M Hoagland, F Naftolin, L Roa, N Harada, L Hafer, R Zaino, SJ Santner: Stromal spindle cells contain aromatase in human breast tumors. *J Clin Endocrinol Metab* 1994, 79:627-32.

[7] KC Shenton, M Dowsett, Q Lu, A Brodie, H Sasano, NP Sacks, MG Rowlands: Comparison of biochemical aromatase activity with aromatase immunohistochemistry in human breast carcinomas. *Breast Cancer Res Treat* 1998, 49 Suppl 1:S101-7; discussion S109-19.

[8] H Sasano, DP Edwards, TJ Anderson, SG Silverberg, DB Evans, RJ Santen, P Ramage, ER Simpson, AS Bhatnagar, WR Miller: Validation of new aromatase monoclonal antibodies for immunohistochemistry: progress report. *J Steroid Biochem Mol Biol* 2003, 86:239-44.

[9] AM Brodie, Q Lu, BJ Long, A Fulton, T Chen, N Macpherson, PC DeJong, MA Blankenstein, JW Nortier, PH Slee, et al: Aromatase and COX-2 expression in human breast cancers. *J Steroid Biochem Mol Biol* 2001, 79:41-7.

[10] JM Esteban, Z Warsi, M Haniu, P Hall, JE Shively, S Chen: Detection of intratumoral aromatase in breast carcinomas. An immunohistochemical study with clinicopathologic correlation. *Am J Pathol* 1992, 140:337-43.

[11] M Miettinen, M Mustonen, M Poutanen, V Isomaa, M Wickman, G Soderqvist, R Vihko, P Vihko: 17Beta-hydroxysteroid dehydrogenases in normal human mammary epithelial cells and breast tissue. *Breast Cancer Res Treat* 1999, 57:175-82.

[12] H Sasano, T Suzuki, T Nakata, T Moriya: New development in intracrinology of breast carcinoma. *Breast Cancer* 2006, 13:129-36.

[13] G Chetrite, E Le Nestour, JR Pasqualini: Human estrogen sulfotransferase (hEST1) activities and its mRNA in various breast cancer cell lines. Effect of the progestin, promegestone (R-5020). *J Steroid Biochem Mol Biol* 1998, 66:295-302.

[14] AA Adjei, BA Thomae, JL Prondzinski, BW Eckloff, ED Wieben, RM Weinshilboum: Human estrogen sulfotransferase (SULT1E1) pharmacogenomics: gene resequencing and functional genomics. *Br J Pharmacol* 2003, 139:1373-82.

[15] T Suzuki, T Nakata, Y Miki, C Kaneko, T Moriya, T Ishida, S Akinaga, H Hirakawa, M Kimura, H Sasano: Estrogen sulfotransferase and steroid sulfatase in human breast carcinoma. *Cancer Res* 2003, 63:2762-70.

[16] MJ Reed, A Purohit, LW Woo, SP Newman, BV Potter: Steroid sulfatase: molecular biology, regulation, and inhibition. *Endocr Rev* 2005, 26:171-202.

[17] T Suzuki, Y Miki, T Nakata, Y Shiotsu, S Akinaga, K Inoue, T Ishida, M Kimura, T Moriya, H Sasano: Steroid sulfatase and estrogen sulfotransferase in normal human tissue and breast carcinoma. *J Steroid Biochem Mol Biol* 2003, 86:449-54.

[18] T Utsumi, N Yoshimura, M Maruta, S Takeuchi, J Ando, K Maeda, N Harada: Significance of Steroid Sulfatase Expression in Human Breast Cancer. *Breast Cancer* 1999, 6:298-300.

[19] B Fisher, JH Jeong, S Anderson, J Bryant, ER Fisher, N Wolmark: Twenty-five-year follow-up of a randomized trial comparing radical mastectomy, total mastectomy, and total mastectomy followed by irradiation. *N Engl J Med* 2002, 347:567-75.

[20] SG Hilsenbeck, PM Ravdin, CA de Moor, GC Chamness, CK Osborne, GM Clark: Time-dependence of hazard ratios for prognostic factors in primary breast cancer. *Breast Cancer Res Treat* 1998, 52:227-37.

[21] Tamoxifen for early breast cancer: an overview of the randomised trials. Early Breast Cancer Trialists' Collaborative Group. *Lancet* 1998, 351:1451-67.

[22] D Koeberle, B Thuerlimann: Letrozole as adjuvant endocrine therapy in postmenopausal women with breast cancer. *Expert Rev Anticancer Ther* 2006, 6:5-10.

[23] R Jakesz, W Jonat, M Gnant, M Mittlboeck, R Greil, C Tausch, J Hilfrich, W Kwasny, C Menzel, H Samonigg, et al: Switching of postmenopausal women with endocrine-responsive early breast cancer to anastrozole after 2 years' adjuvant tamoxifen: combined results of ABCSG trial 8 and ARNO 95 trial. *Lancet* 2005, 366:455-62.

[24] B Thurlimann, HJ Senn: [Consensus Meeting of the 9th International Conference on Primary Therapy of Early Breast Cancer (St. Gall, January 26-29, 2005)]. *Gynakol Geburtshilfliche Rundsch* 2005, 45:143-6.

[25] C Singer, A Fink-Retter, D Gschwantler-Kaulich, T Thalhammer, G Hudelist, R Mueller, K Czerwenka and E Kubista: Selective spatial up-regulation of intratumoral stromal aromatase in breast cancer patients: evidence for imbalance of local estrogen metabolism. *Endocrine-Related Cancer*, accepted 2006

[26] WR Miller: Aromatase activity in breast tissue. *J Steroid Biochem Mol Biol* 1991, 39:783-90.

[27] Z Zhang, H Yamashita, T Toyama, Y Omoto, H Sugiura, Y Hara, X Wu, S Kobayashi, H Iwase: Quantitative determination, by real-time reverse transcription polymerase chain reaction, of aromatase mRNA in invasive ductal carcinoma of the breast. *Breast Cancer Res* 2003, 5:R250-6.

[28] Z Zhang, H Yamashita, T Toyama, Y Hara, Y Omoto, H Sugiura, S Kobayashi, N Harada, H Iwase: Semi-quantitative immunohistochemical analysis of aromatase expression in ductal carcinoma in situ of the breast. *Breast Cancer Res Treat* 2002, 74:47-53.

[29] A Lipton, RJ Santen, SJ Santner, HA Harvey, SI Sanders, YL Matthews: Prognostic value of breast cancer aromatase. *Cancer* 1992, 70:1951-5.

[30] MC Silva, MG Rowlands, M Dowsett, B Gusterson, JA McKinna, I Fryatt, RC Coombes: Intratumoral aromatase as a prognostic factor in human breast carcinoma. *Cancer Res* 1989, 49:2588-91.

[31] PC de Jong, MA Blankenstein, JW Nortier, PH Slee, J van de Ven, JM van Gorp, JR Elbers, ME Schipper, GH Blijham, JH Thijssen, et al: The relationship between aromatase in primary breast tumors and response to treatment with aromatase inhibitors in advanced disease. *J Steroid Biochem Mol Biol* 2003, 87:149-55.

[32] T Suzuki, Y Miki, Y Nakamura, T Moriya, K Ito, N Ohuchi, H Sasano: Sex steroid-producing enzymes in human breast cancer. *Endocr Relat Cancer* 2005, 12:701-20.

[33] L Tseng, J Mazella, LY Lee, ML Stone: Estrogen sulfatase and estrogen sulfotransferase in human primary mammary carcinoma. *J Steroid Biochem* 1983, 19:1413-7.

[34] JB Adams, T Pewnim, DP Chandra, L Archibald, MS Foo: A correlation between estrogen sulfotransferase levels and estrogen receptor status in human primary breast carcinoma. *Cancer Res* 1979, 39:5124-6.

[35] JL Falany, N Macrina, CN Falany: Regulation of MCF-7 breast cancer cell growth by beta-estradiol sulfation. *Breast Cancer Res Treat* 2002, 74:167-76.

[36] TR Evans, MG Rowlands, M Law, RC Coombes: Intratumoral oestrone sulphatase activity as a prognostic marker in human breast carcinoma. *Br J Cancer* 1994, 69: 555-61.

[37] Y Miyoshi, A Ando, S Hasegawa, M Ishitobi, T Taguchi, Y Tamaki, S Noguchi: High expression of steroid sulfatase mRNA predicts poor prognosis in patients with estrogen receptor-positive breast cancer. *Clin Cancer Res* 2003, 9:2288-93.

[38] JR Pasqualini, C Maloche, M Maroni, G Chetrite: Effect of the progestagen Promegestone (R-5020) on mRNA of the oestrone sulphatase in the MCF-7 human mammary cancer cells. *Anticancer Res* 1994, 14:1589-93.

[39] T Suzuki, T Moriya, N Ariga, C Kaneko, M Kanazawa, H Sasano: 17Beta-hydroxysteroid dehydrogenase type 1 and type 2 in human breast carcinoma: a correlation to clinicopathological parameters. *Br J Cancer* 2000, 82:518-23.

[40] JR Pasqualini: The selective estrogen enzyme modulators in breast cancer: a review. *Biochim Biophys Acta* 2004, 1654:123-43.

[41] Y Miyoshi, A Ando, E Shiba, T Taguchi, Y Tamaki, S Noguchi: Involvement of up-regulation of 17beta-hydroxysteroid dehydrogenase type 1 in maintenance of intratumoral high estradiol levels in postmenopausal breast cancers. *Int J Cancer* 2001, 94:685-9.

[42] C Gunnarsson, BM Olsson, O Stal: Abnormal expression of 17beta-hydroxysteroid dehydrogenases in breast cancer predicts late recurrence. *Cancer Res* 2001, 61:8448-51.

In: Tumor Markers Research Focus
Editor: Deborah H. Chang, pp. 121-133

ISBN: 978-1-60021-544-5


*Chapter VI*

# Current and Emerging Biomarkers in Prostate Cancer

***Edward N. Rampersaud, Leon Sun and Judd W. Moul****
Duke Prostate Center and Division of Urology, Department of Surgery, Duke University Medical Center, Durham, North Carolina

## Abstract

The American Cancer Society estimates that in the United States, 234,460 new cases of prostate cancer will be diagnosed in 2006. Although 80% of diagnosed patients will eventually die from an unrelated reason, prostate cancer still accounts for the second highest cause of cancer-related deaths in men in the United States, with 27,350 deaths estimated for 2006. This has produced much interest in the early diagnosis and treatment of clinically pertinent cases in which the length or quality of life would be greatly impacted by the natural course of prostate cancer.

From 1988 to the present, the availability of clinically practical screening tests has been limited to the digital rectal exam (DRE), the serum prostate specific antigen (PSA) test, and transrectal ultrasound (TRUS)-guided prostate biopsy. Early in the PSA era, which revolutionized the diagnosis of prostate cancer, many prostate biopsies were performed simply for elevated values. These patients yielded many positive pathologic findings and went on to receive treatment by way of radical prostatectomy, radiation therapy, and hormone suppression therapy. However, with the knowledge that upwards of 80% of patients diagnosed with prostate cancer will eventually die of a cause unrelated to their slowly progressive cancer, interest was turned to detection of more "clinically relevant" cancers, those cancers that would potentially impact the quality and length of a patient's life. More sensitive methods of detecting serum PSA levels and extrapolative derivatives of this biomarker such as PSA doubling time (PSA DT), PSA velocity (PSAV), PSA density

* E-mail address: judd.moul@duke.edu, Tel: 919-684-5057, Fax: 919-684-8794. Judd W. Moul, MD, Professor and Chief, Division of Urologic Surgery and Duke Prostate Center, Duke University Medical Center, Box 3707, Durham, NC 27710

(PSAD), percentage free PSA, and the use of the PSA nadir after primary treatment have progressively furnished superior detection and treatment modalities of prostate cancer [1]. The Surveillance, Epidemiology, and End Results (SEER) program has demonstrated that advances in screening and detection of prostate cancer over the past 20 years have yielded diagnosis at progressively lower levels of prognostic risk. For many patients, this has afforded curative treatment and a decrease in prostate cancer specific mortality. The proportion of patients with low-risk disease defined as those with a PSA≤10 ng/mL, Gleason pathologic grade less than 7 (without any grade 4 or 5 component), and clinical stage T1 or T2a disease has increased from 31% of patients in 1990 to 47% of patients in 2001. In contrast, the high-risk diagnoses (PSA>20ng/mL, Gleason sum > 7, or clinical stage T3 or T4) has decreased from 41% to 15% of prostate cancer diagnoses [2]. The American Cancer Society estimates that this downward risk migration with earlier treatment is the reason for the 3.5% yearly decrease in the death rate noted in recent years. This positive news is contrasted by the unfortunate fact that some patients may be subjected to unnecessary invasive procedures with their numerous possible complications. Efforts are being directed to develop algorithms and screening tests with greater sensitivity and specificity for clinically relevant prostate cancer to decrease unnecessary biopsies and treatment and to also decrease overall healthcare costs.

Modern advances in the fields of genomics and microarray technology have allowed the medical community to embrace the possibility of diagnosis and treatment of diseases even before their clinical presentations. This is of immense clinical interest in oncology, as the ability to effect change on tumor biology at a cellular level would revolutionize the treatment of all types of cancer. These advances are beginning to elucidate biomarkers that could potentially be used to diagnose, as well as follow current treatment in numerous types of cancer, including prostate cancer.

## Current Clinical Markers

In 1979 Wang et al. published their findings of a monomeric protein isolated from prostatic tissue [3]. Antisera developed to this protein were found to be nonreactive with epitopes from other tissues, hence prostate *specific* antigen (PSA). Although, immunohistochemical and immunoassay methods later detected PSA in female and male periurethral glands, anal glands, apocrine sweat glands, apocrine breast cancers, salivary gland neoplasms, and human breast milk, none of these findings have shown to affect the use of the PSA in the diagnosis or treatment of prostate cancer. Currently, use of the serum PSA and derivatives of the PSA serve as the backbone of clinical biomarkers currently in use for prostate cancer diagnosis, treatment, and monitoring.

### Age Adjusted PSA

The production of PSA by the prostate is linearly proportional to the volume of glandular tissue. As benign prostatic hyperplasia (BPH) is considered part of the normal aging process, it is reasonable to assume that these first order kinetics result in higher PSA values; and that the normal values for patients of varying ages would be different. The findings of one cross-sectional population study of PSA values in patients not found to have prostate cancer are in Table 1 [4].

**Table 1.**

| Age | 40-49 | 50-59 | 60-69 | 70-79 |
|---|---|---|---|---|
| PSA (ng/mL) | 0.0-2.5 | 0.0-3.5 | 0.0-4.5 | 0.0-6.5 |
| PSAD (ng/mL/mL) | 0.0-0.08 | 0.0-0.10 | 0.0-0.11 | 0.0-0.13 |

These data are currently used as a guide in clinical judgment to decide who may benefit from biopsy for detection of potentially relevant prostate cancer.

## PSA Kinetics

Much interest has been generated in the area of PSA kinetics, the observed phenomenon of changing PSA values over time and its relationship to the initial presence of prostate cancer or its recurrence. These kinetics specifically refer to PSA doubling time (PSA DT) and PSA velocity (PSAV). PSA DT is calculated as the time required to observe a doubling effect on the PSA measured in months, with a minimum of 3 months separating the measurements, and with each having a value of at least 0.2ng/mL. The PSAV is calculated as a change in PSA (measured in ng/mL) over time (usually annually). PSA recurrence, also known as biochemical failure, is the presence of an increasing or higher-than expected level of PSA in a patient after definitive therapy for prostate cancer has been completed. This includes patients who have received radical prostatectomy as well as those who have completed radiation therapy as their primary treatment modality. PSA recurrence often indicates the presence of cancer recurrence or unrecognized metastasis. Educated attempts are made to divide the recurrences into one of two main groups: those having a local recurrence from residual tumor post-treatment, or those with metastatic disease. Whereas patients with local recurrence may benefit from localized salvage therapies, those with metastatic disease are unlikely to profit. Pretreatment PSA kinetics are being examined and dissected in the hopes of predicting which patients are likely to have distant versus local recurrence, as well as attempting to discern which of those patients are most likely to experience an impact to the quality or length of their lives as a result of prostate cancer specific mortality.

## PSA Doubling Time (PSA DT)

For PSA DT's of less than 3 months, the median survival from time of recurrence is approximately 6 years, whereas survival is greater than a decade from those patients with PSA DT's greater than 12 months. [5]. As such, much interest has been directed at using the PSA DT as a marker for tumor aggression, and its implication on cancer specific mortality. It has been demonstrated that a shorter PSA DT indicates a potentially higher stage or more aggressive cancer [5]. The use of the PSA DT has also become more relevant in directing the care of patients who suffer a PSA failure after radical prostatectomy. A PSA DT of less than 3 months has been associated with a significantly shorter time to prostate cancer-specific mortality. [6]. This information could be used to direct those who would benefit from postoperative salvage radiation and systemic therapy. As an extension to the use of the post-treatment PSA DT, the question is raised as to whether or not it would be possible to predict which patients would suffer from PSA failure with unfavorable PSA DT before primary treatment was instituted. A preoperative PSA velocity greater than 2.0 ng/mL/yr and a Gleason score ≥7 appear to be significantly associated with a postoperative PSA DT of less than 3 months [6]. Similar findings have been reported in patients who initially were treated with radiotherapy. A PSA DT < 3 months and initial Gleason scores of 8-10 independently predicted prostate cancer-specific mortality, with a 5 year survival of 25% if both factors were present [7]. As these results portend a poorer prognosis, perhaps patients with PSAV ≥ 2.0 ng/mL/yr and Gleason score > 7 would benefit from salvage radiotherapy with systemic therapy sooner than waiting for the PSA DT calculation.

## PSA Velocity (PSAV)

Early studies investigating the use of PSAV debated the significance of the value being able to predict pathologic stage, Gleason score, and chances of biochemical recurrence. More recent retrospective analyses have begun to demonstrate its potential value. In a series of 1095 patients that underwent radical prostatectomy (RP), D'Amico, *et al.* found that an annual PSAV ≥ 2.0 ng/mL/yr provided a predictive indicator for time to recurrence, prostate cancer specific mortality, and death from any cause. It was also significantly associated with distant metastasis, higher-grade disease, and advanced pathological stage. Men with annual PSAV ≥ 2.0 ng/mL/yr were 10 times more likely to suffer prostate cancer specific mortality than those patients with PSAV < 2.0 ng/mL/yr [8]. Patel, *et al.* also demonstrated the use of PSAV ≥ 2 ng/mL/yr as a poor prognostic indicator for recurrence [9]. In a multivariate analysis on 31 of 202 patients who had relapsed after radical prostatectomy, only preoperative PSAV ≥ 2.0 ng/mL/yr and biopsy Gleason score served as significant indicators of future biochemical failure [9]. These data could provide possible validation for preemptively treating patients with a higher likelihood of biochemical recurrence. Patients with poorer prognostic PSAV could also be enrolled in longitudinal studies that examined outcomes for patients who underwent systemic treatment for presumed later recurrence prior to PSA failure.

## PSA Density (PSAD)

The PSAD is calculated by dividing the PSA by the volume of the gland. Although preoperative volume determination is more accurate using computed tomography, currently the most clinically efficient method of determining prostate volume is with the use of three-dimensional transrectal ultrasound. There is still debate as to the utility of PSAD in predicting clinically relevant prostate cancer. The PSAD is proposed to be clinically pertinent by attempting to negate the effect increased gland volume has on the PSA value (Table 1). This would theoretically offset the fact that older patients tend to have larger prostates in the natural course of benign hyperplasia. It is also postulated that since cancerous glandular tissue produces PSA at logarithmic rates, that the PSAD would be even more sensitive and specific than the PSA alone in distinguishing prostate cancer [10]. The suggested upper limit for PSAD to distinguish cancer from BPH is 0.15 ng/mL per milliliter volume of prostate [11].

Postoperatively the use of the preoperative PSAD in predicting biochemical recurrence has been debated. The use of PSAD relative to preoperative PSA alone does not appear to provide statistically significant improvement in predicting postoperative PSA failure [12].

## Free to Total PSA Ratio (Percentage Free PSA)

There is continued effort in prostate cancer screening to decrease both costs of screening and those undergoing prostate biopsy while retaining adequate sensitivity. Benefit-cost analyses have demonstrated that even relatively small increases of 5% in the specificity of prostate cancer detection produce approximately 50% reductions in the net cost per individual screened [13]. The majority of PSA in serum is bound to protease inhibitors alpha$_1$-antichymotrypsin and alpha$_2$-macroglobulin. It has been described that patients with prostate cancer display a lower level of unbound PSA in relation to total PSA [14]. Use of the percentage-free PSA as a more reliable predictor for patients with prostate cancer is still debatable. Approximately 10% of patients present with total PSA 4.0-10.0 ng/mL, but these patients represent approximately one third of all biopsies [15]. Several series from the Catalona group found that a cutoff of $\leq$ 25% free PSA in patients with total PSA 4.0 – 10.0 ng/mL would detect 95% of cancers and spare 20% of patients with benign prostatic hyperplasia from unnecessary biopsy [15]. Although several studies contradict some of these findings, there is enough compelling data to warrant subgroup analyses in multicenter database pooling.

## PSA Nadir

The PSA nadir is often used as a benchmark after primary treatment, a level above which often indicates biochemical failure. The theoretical goal after prostatectomy is a PSA level that is undetectable using standard assays. This threshold is commonly 0.2ng/mL. The half-life of PSA undergoing first order clearance kinetics is 3.2 days with clearance to baseline sometimes requiring several weeks due to ongoing inflammation after certain procedures [16]. Many times, the clinical practice is to measure the PSA 2 months after prostatectomy to gauge the PSA nadir. With this value the PSA is measured regularly to note, if any, a rise that may indicate biochemical failure. Multiple factors play into what the PSA nadir will ultimately be. After a prostatectomy, some glandular tissue may remain at the bladder neck contributing to a low level PSA post operatively, there may be residual disease that remains in the prostatectomy bed as a result of direct extension, or there may be occult metastatic disease present that continues to produce the antigen. After radiation therapy, some glandular tissue may be missed as a result of averaging technique. The importance of measuring a PSA nadir has also been demonstrated in patients who receive primary androgen suppression therapy [17]. New interest has been given to the use of the PSA nadir after treatment for PSA recurrence. In patients who have received primary treatment with radical prostatectomy or radiation therapy and then suffered PSA failure, the treatment of choice is often androgen suppression therapy (AST). Recent data from Stewart *et al.* has pointed to the use of 0.2 ng/mL as the threshold for concern after AST. After 8 months of AST, a PSA nadir greater than 0.2 ng/mL predicted prostate cancer specific mortality in 75% of patients [18]. Of 224 patients who had a pre-AST doubling time of less than 3 months, 68 (30%) of them did not ultimately have a PSA nadir ≤ 0.2 ng/mL. For this group of patients, the 7-year estimate of prostate cancer specific mortality was 72% (95% CI, 45% to 99%) compared with 4% (95% CI, 0% to 27%) for those patients with PSA nadir that was ≤ 0.2 ng/mL [18]. Newer assays to measure serum PSA are becoming more sensitive and accurate. As these tests become more refined and materialize into clinical use investigation will be needed to perceive if an even lower PSA nadir becomes the clinical standard.

## Molecular Markers

Although the use of the PSA and its derivatives is of great use in clinical urology, recently concluded prospective trials have demonstrated their limitations. As such, there remains a very strong interest in the development of more predictive biomarkers and the tests required to detect them. A notable shift from the traditional blood-based human biological specimens such as serum and plasma has characterized the noteworthy advances in prostate screening tools currently being developed around the world. Attention has been drawn to the recent advances in microarray technology and its ability to study molecular events involved in many types of cancer. As would be expected, a number of genetic abnormalities are noted in prostate cancer cells. Unfortunately, many of these cellular derangements occur in other types of cancer as well, and may point to common mechanism further down the chain of events that eventually lead to abnormal cell cycle timelines. The p53 and p21 tumor suppressor genes, c-met and HER2/neu oncogenes, and various transcription factors have been implicated.

Prostate specific tumor markers are also being investigated. Prostate-specific membrane antigen (PMSA), prostate mucin antigen, hepsin, and a protein named DD3 are all being investigated as markers to be used in the future

### uPM3/DD3

A very promising biomolecular test for prostate cancer, the uPM3 (DiagnoCure, Quebec, Canada) test is conducted on urine specimens from men after prostate massage during digital rectal examination (DRE) [19]. This particular method of extracting a test specimen for laboratory examination takes advantage of the discharging of epithelial prostatatic cellular material revealed in the urine after manipulation of the prostate gland. DD3, a prostate cancer-specific protein is demonstrated to be strongly over-expressed in more than 95% of both primary prostate cancer specimens as well as metastatic prostate cancer specimens [20]. As compared to benign prostate tissue, DD3 mRNA transcription is noted to be up-regulated 66-fold in malignant prostate tissue that hints to a diagnostic potential for this non-protein coding gene [21].

mRNA transcripts of the DD3 gene were originally isolated from prostate cell lysates gathered from urinary sediments of men after attentive digital rectal examination using a time-resolved florescence-based quantitative reverse transcription-polymerase chain reaction (RT-PCR) assay [21] . The DD3 mRNA remains untranslated, and the function of the mRNA is unknown.

Using measured PSA transcripts to correct for the number of prostate cells in the urinary specimen, an optimal cut-off value for this DD3-based RT-PCR assay garnered a specificity of 83% and a negative predictive value of 90%. Going one step further, the uPM3 test was developed utilizing a nucleic acid sequence-based amplification assay (NASBA) that simultaneously quantifies both DD3 mRNA transcripts and PSA mRNA transcripts and uses the relative expression levels between the two to determine the presence of disease [19, 22]. In a single institution study, the uPM3 test had an overall sensitivity of 82% and specificity of 76% [22]. In men with serum PSA levels between 4-10ng/ml, the uPM3 test predicted the presence of prostate cancer in 84% of the biopsy-proven cases and correctly identified 80% of the men who had a negative biopsy result. In a multi-center study involving five institutions, uPM3 demonstrated an astounding 89% overall specificity and a positive predictive value of 75% superior to serum PSA (38% in the study population) [19]. Most promising was the noted maintenance of high specificity of the test observed in men with PSA < 4ng/ml (91%) and in those with PSA between 4-10ng/ml (91%) suggesting that this new molecular urine test may serve as an important adjunct to current methods of prostate cancer diagnosis.

One disadvantage of the uPM3 test is in the defining of "attentive" DRE. The technique for expressing prostatic secretions into the urine would no doubt vary among urologists and its effects on the results of the uPM3 test have not been carefully studied demanding a need for standardization of prostate gland manipulation performed prior to collection of the specimen. Another important issue to be considered is increasing the adequacy rate, the portion of assessable specimens with an adequate number of prostate cells in the voided specimen for the assay, which for the initial studies ranged from 79-86% [19, 22]. Developers of this promising urine-based molecular test are currently addressing these and other minor disadvantages.

## Serum Protein Profiling

The technique of utilizing serum protein profiles as resolved by mass spectrometry as a diagnostic tool for prostate cancer and as a platform for the discovery of prostate cancer biomarkers has garnered much attention due to very promising results that have been tempered by close scrutiny and criticism by the scientific community. Serum protein profiling using surface enhanced laser/desorption ionization time-of-flight mass spectrometry (SELDI-TOF-MS) profiling relies on affinity-based chromatographic separation of proteins in minute amounts of serum applied to arrays that are subjected to matrix assisted laser desorption/ionization time-of-flight mass spectrometry (MALDI-TOF-MS) producing mass spectral profiles dependent on proteins found in the sera [19, 22]. Bioinformatics analyses of these serum proteomic signatures generate classification algorithms predictive of diseases ranging from ovarian, prostate and breast cancer in blinded serum samples with very favorable accuracy [23]. Deriving diagnostic information from patterns of proteins hidden in human serum elucidated through SELDI-TOF-MS for detection of prostate adenocarcinoma was first reported by Adam *et al.*, wherein serum protein signatures generated from a copper-metal affinity array (Ciphergen Biosystems, Fremont, CA) was used to generate decision tree algorithms which could accurately identify prostate cancer patients with a sensitivity of 83% and specificity of 97% [24] Comparable successes were reported by other institutions that employed modifications in their methodologies such as utilizing other protein array types and methods of spectral data analyses [25].

The popularity elicited when serum protein profiling was first introduced has led to close scrutiny by critics of serum protein profiling technology [26]. Much of the criticism focused on controlling potential sources of bias in the experiments as well as drifting mass calibration of the mass spectrometer used. To address these issues, a multi-center trial consisting by eight institutions was constructed and aimed at validating the utility of serum SELDI-TOF-MS profiling and assessing the reproducibility of this technology [27]. The initial phase of validation focused on standardization of serum processing and optimization of spectral data generated in all mass spectrometers consistently throughout the study while providing quality assurance between all laboratories. Robotic handling was carried out to minimize human error and further enhance mass spectral quality and reproducibility. The reproducibility of serum SELDI-TOF-MS profiles across laboratories was found to be closely comparable with acceptably low variability [28]. This reduction of variation was successfully preserved across all institutions over a 6-month period and was attributed to strict adherence to standard operating procedures while maintaining optimal calibration of instruments. This multi-center trial has now progressed to its second phase wherein serum samples from multiple institutions will be utilized to refine the classification algorithms generated from serum protein profiles.

Efforts to further improve on serum protein profiling technology range from improvements in instrumentation to identification of candidate biomarkers as a means of validation. Higher resolution mass spectrometers such as the QSTAR (Applied Biosystems, Foster City, CA), a hybrid quadruple time-of-flight mass spectrometer have expanded the number of candidate biomarkers by resolving a greater number of datapoints compared to SELDI-TOF-MS. Serum profiles generated with the QSTAR was shown discriminate men with elevated PSA due to benign conditions from men with prostate cancer even when PSA levels fall within the diagnostic gray zone of 2.5-15 ng/ml [29].

Critics of serum protein profiling technology have pushed for identification of candidate protein markers derived from studies to validate the results. By employing liquid chromatography, gel electrophoresis and tandem mass spectrometry, an isoform of Apolipoprotein A-II (ApoA-II) was identified as one of the discriminatory SELDI-TOF-MS proteins by one of the pioneering laboratories [30]. This finding not only validated the technique of serum protein profiling by showing a correlation between serum levels of ApoA-II and its corresponding peak on the protein spectral profile but it also yielded a novel biomarker which could detect prostate cancer in patients whose PSA is within normal limits (0-4 ng/ml). Another laboratory reported serum amyloid A as a potential biomarker for metastatic prostate cancer using SELDI-TOF-MS as an initial screening tool then employing two-dimensional gel electrophoresis, in-gel trypsin digestion, and tandem mass spectrometry for protein identification [31]. Breakthroughs in engineering exhibited by constant upgrading of mass spectrometry platforms giving rise to high-performance hardware resources capable of fairly rapid protein identification will lead to the development of a platform that provides very high resolution, robust spectra and easy identification of protein markers, which does not sacrifice ease of use and portability, seems to be the compromise that will eventually translate into clinical practice.

## AMACR / Autoantibody Signatures

Among the prostate cancer markers recently discovered through tissue and gene microarray technology, alpha methylacyl-CoA racemase (AMACR) appears to be overexpressed in malignant prostate epithelial cells and has the potential to yield a novel clinically usable test for diagnosis of prostate cancer [32]. Western blot analysis for AMACR in urine specimens following transrectal ultrasound-guided prostate biopsy and was detected in the urine of all patients with biopsy-confirmed prostate cancer in a pilot study [33]. Similar to the uPM3 test, mRNA transcripts of the AMACR gene have been measured in prostatic secretions in urine voided after prostatic massage using quantitative RT-PCR [34]. Relative AMACR value scores calculated by normalizing AMACR transcript levels with PSA mRNA transcript measurements correlated well with disease status correctly identifying all cancer-free participants including men with benign prostatic hyperplasia in this preliminary investigation.

The presence of autoantibodies to AMACR protein has also been investigated in its ability to detect adenocarcinoma of the prostate. Screening through protein microarrays and later development of high-throughput immunoblot analysis and enzyme linked immunosorbent assays for sera using AMACR as a target molecule yielded positive results [35]. In this study, immune response against AMACR was observed to be more sensitive (77.8%) and specific (80.6%) than PSA in distinguishing sera from prostate cancer patients relative to control specimens. Furthermore, by assaying for autoantibodies directed at Huntingtin Interacting Protein-1 (HIP-1), another bait molecule, reactivity of sera also correlated well with the presence of prostate cancer [36]. Interestingly, when the humoral response information from HIP-1 is supplemented to the AMACR autoantibody assay, the overall specificity of the combined test may be increased further up to 97%.

Studies on AMACR and HIP-1 have led to a more global approach of autoantibody profiling to amplify otherwise undetectable molecular signals which are characteristic of disease and may prove to be diagnostic for prostate malignancy [37]. To assay for autoantibodies in serum, phage protein microarrays were developed using a phage-display library derived from prostate cancer tissue. By iterative purification and isolation of phages carrying high affinity and specificity for autoantibodies and by subjecting humoral response information to bioinformatics analyses, a 22-phage-peptide detector elicited an autoantibody signature predictive of disease. In a blinded validation, 49 of 60 (81.6%) prostate cancer serum samples and 60 of 68 (88.2%) controls were correctly identified according to their autoantibody signature. This humoral reactive panel even performed better than serum PSA in this investigation. Further refinements to the technology along with prospective trials and evaluation of these autoantibody signatures in subjects with inflammatory conditions such as prostatitis, rheumatic and autoimmune disease should be forthcoming.

## ERG / Biomarker Panel

Combining multiple biomarkers may provide a synergistic solution in attaining a truly superior diagnostic specificity for prostate cancer. Following microarray analysis of micro-dissected prostate cancer tissue samples, ETS-related gene (ERG) was recently reported as the most frequently over-expressed proto-oncogene in the transcriptome of malignant prostate epithelial cells [38]. ERG codes for transcription factors which through molecular signaling regulate cellular differentiation and proliferation [39]. Recurrent fusion of ERG with another gene, TMPRSS2, was also reported to be associated with prostate cancer validating ERG as a potential biomarker for prostate cancer and implicating these genes in carcinogenesis and possible clinical use in molecular diagnostics [40]. By taking advantage of the high sensitivity of AMACR and the impressive specificity of DD3 for prostate cancer, researchers demonstrated that the combined quantitative expression analysis in a novel three-gene panel (ERG + AMACR + DD3) can detect virtually all malignant prostate specimens [38]. This discovery emphasizes the advantage of multiplexing biomarkers to optimize the accuracy of prostate cancer detection. Investigators are on the cusp of translating these preliminary results and developing this biomarker panel into a new screening tool for prostate cancer.

### Key Issues for Future Biomarker Study

Emerging technologies comprise the cutting-edge in non-invasive prostate cancer diagnostics. As the call is made for the development of methods to discern clinically relevant prostate cancer from those patients with indolent tumors that would minimally impact quality or length of life without treatment, it is not enough for screening tests to merely ascertain the presence of disease. The necessity for earliest possible diagnosis should be balanced against the potential morbidities of over-diagnosis and over-treatment. It is of paramount importance that a diagnostic test be able to elucidate the aggressive potential of a particular tumor as well as to identify men who would benefit more from surveillance rather than repeated prostate biopsies. The information supplied by future diagnostic procedures should also be able to stratify patients according to risk for recurrence after treatment bringing the practice of treatment for prostate cancer, whether surgical or non-surgical, closer to the ideal therapy tailored to the individual patient. As the sensitivities and specificities of these newer tests are being compared to our current benchmark of PSA and its derivatives in combination with prostate biopsy, consideration will be needed to determine how close to our current methodologies is close enough. Whether measured by cost, morbidity, or lives saved or lost in comparison to the current standard of care, these analyses should be conducted separate from further development of these novel technologies. Without question however, is that the use of innovative biological specimens, engineered technological advances and new paradigms incorporating multiplexed biomarker assays are forging the superior and more clinically relevant prostate cancer tests of the future.

## References

[1] D'Amico AV, Chen MH, *et al.* Identifying patients at risk for significant versus clinically insignificant postoperative prostate-specific antigen failure. *J Clin Oncol.* Aug 1;23(22):4975-9 (2005).

[2] Cooperberg MR, Lubeck DP, *et al.* Time trends in clinical risk stratification for prostate cancer: implications for outcomes (data from CaPSURE). *J Urol.* Dec; 170:S21-S27 (2003).

[3] Wang MC, Valenzuela LA, *et al.* Purification of a human prostate specific antigen. *Invest Urol.* Sep;17(2):159-63 (1979).
[4] Oesterling, Joseph E.; Jacobsen, *et al.* Serum prostate-specific antigen in a community-based population of healthy men: establishment of age-specific reference ranges. *JAMA* 270(7), 860-4 (1993).
[5] D'Amico AV, Moul JW, *et al.* Surrogate marker for prostate cancer specific mortality following radical prostatectomy or radiation therapy. *J Natl Cancer Inst.* 95:1376-83 (2003).
[6] D'Amico AV, Chen MH, *et al.* Identifying patients at risk for significant versus clinically insignificant postoperative prostate-specific antigen failure. *J Clin Oncol.* 23(22):4975-79 (2005).
[7] Zhou P, Chen MH, *et al.* Predictors of prostate cancer-specific mortality following radical prostatectomy or radiation therapy. *J Clin Oncol.* Oct 1;23(28):6992-8 (2005).
[8] D'Amico AV, Chen MH, *et al.* Preoperative PSA Velocity and the Risk of Death from Prostate Cancer after Radical Prostatectomy. *NEJM* July 8;351(2):125-136 (2004).
[9] Patel DA, Presti JC Jr, *et al.* Preoperative PSA velocity is an independent prognostic factor for relapse after radical prostatectomy. *J Clin Oncol.* Sep 1;23(25):6157-62 (2005).
[10] Benson MC, McMahon DJ, *et al.* An algorithm for prostate cancer detection in a patient population using prostate-specific antigen density. *World J Urol.* 11:206–13 (1993).
[11] Cooner WH (contributor). Early diagnosis of prostate cancer. *Campbell's Urology.* 6th ed, update 4. Philadelphia, Pa: WB Saunders Co, (1992).
[12] Freedland SJ, Kane CJ, *et al.* Comparison of preoperative prostate specific antigen density and prostate specific antigen for predicting recurrence after radical prostatectomy: results from SEARCH database. *J Urol.* Mar;169:969-73 (2003).
[13] Littrup PJ, Kane RA, Mettlin CJ *et al.* Economic considerations of prostate cancer: the role of detection specificity and biopsy reduction. *Cancer.* Dec 15;74(12):3146-58 (1994).
[14] Stenman UH, Hakama M, Knekt P *et al.* Serum concentrations of prostate specific antigen and its complex with alpha 1-antichymotrypsin before diagnosis of prostate cancer. *Lancet* 344:1594-98 (1994).
[15] Catalona WJ, Partin AW, Slawin KM *et al.* Use of the percentage of free prostate-specific antigen to enhance differentiation of prostate cancer from benign prostatic disease: a prospective multicenter clinical trial. *JAMA* 279:1542-47 (1998).
[16] Oesterling JE, Chan DW, Epstein JI *et al.* Prostate specific antigen in the preoperative and postoperative evaluation of localized prostatic cancer treated with radical prostatectomy. *J Urol* 139:766 (1988).
[17] Kwak C, Jeong SJ *et al.* Prognostic significance of the nadir prostate specific antigen level after hormone therapy for prostate cancer, *J Urol,* 168:995-1000 (2002).
[18] Stewart AJ, Scher HI, Chen MH *et al.* Prsotate-specific antigen nadir and cancer-specific mortality following hormonal therapy for prostate-specific antigen failure. *J Clin Oncol,* 23(27), 6556-60 (2005).
[19] Fradet Y, Saad F, Aprikian A *et al.* uPM3, a new molecular urine test for the detection of prostate cancer. *Urology,* 64(2),311-315 (2004).
[20] de Kok JB, Verhaegh GW, Roelofs RW *et al.* DD3(PCA3), a very sensitive and specific marker to detect prostate tumors. *Cancer Research.* 62(9), 2695-2698 (2002).

[21] Hessels D, Klein Gunnewiek JM, van Oort I *et al.* DD3(PCA3)-based molecular urine analysis for the diagnosis of prostate cancer. *European Urology.* 44(1), 8-15 (2003).

[22] Tinzl M, Marberger M, Horvath S *et al.* DD3PCA3 RNA analysis in urine--a new perspective for detecting prostate cancer. *European Urology.* 46(2),182-186 (2004)

[23] Li J, Zhang Z, Rosenzweig J *et al.* Proteomics and bioinformatics approaches for identification of serum biomarkers to detect breast cancer. *Clinical Chemistry.* 48(8), 1296-1304 (2002).

[24] Petricoin EF 3rd, Ornstein DK, Paweletz CP *et al.* Serum proteomic patterns for detection of prostate cancer. *J Natl Cancer Inst.* 94(20), 1576-1578 (2002).

[25] Li J, White N, Zhang Z *et al.* Detection of prostate cancer using serum proteomics pattern in a histologically confirmed population. *J Urol.* 171(5), 1782-1787 (2004).

[26] Baggerly KA, Morris JS, Coombes KR. Reproducibility of SELDI-TOF protein patterns in serum: comparing datasets from different experiments. *Bioinformatics.* 20(5), 777-785 (2004).

[27] Grizzle WE, Adam BL, Bigbee WL *et al.* Serum protein expression profiling for cancer detection: validation of a SELDI-based approach for prostate cancer. *Dis Markers.* 19(4-5), 185-195 (2003-2004).

[28] Semmes OJ, Feng Z, Adam BL *et al.* Evaluation of serum protein profiling by surface-enhanced laser desorption/ionization time-of-flight mass spectrometry for the detection of prostate cancer: I. Assessment of platform reproducibility. *Clin Chem.* 51(1), 102-112 (2005).

[29] Ornstein DK, Rayford W, Fusaro VA *et al.* Serum proteomic profiling can discriminate prostate cancer from benign prostates in men with total prostate specific antigen levels between 2.5 and 15.0 ng/ml. *J Urol.* 172(4 Pt 1), 1302-1305 (2004).

[30] Malik G, Ward MD, Gupta SK *et al.* Serum levels of an isoform of apolipoprotein A-II as a potential marker for prostate cancer. *Clin Cancer Res.* 11(3), 1073-1085 (2005).

[31] Le L, Chi K, Tyldesley S *et al.* Identification of serum amyloid A as a biomarker to distinguish prostate cancer patients with bone lesions. *Clin Chem.* 51(4), 695-707 (2005).

[32] Rubin MA, Zhou M, Dhanasekaran SM *et al.* alpha-Methylacyl coenzyme A racemase as a tissue biomarker for prostate cancer. *JAMA.* 287(13), 1662-1670 (2002).

[33] Rogers CG, Yan G, Zha S *et al.* Prostate cancer detection on urinalysis for alpha methylacyl coenzyme a racemase protein. *J Urol.* 172(4 Pt 1), 1501-1503 (2004).

[34] Zielie PJ, Mobley JA, Ebb RG *et al.* A novel diagnostic test for prostate cancer emerges from the determination of alpha-methylacyl-coenzyme a racemase in prostatic secretions. *J Urol.* 172(3), 1130-1133 (2004).

[35] Sreekumar A, Laxman B, Rhodes DR *et al.* Humoral immune response to alpha-methylacyl-CoA racemase and prostate cancer.[see comment] *J Natl Cancer Inst.* 96(11), 834-843 (2004).

[36] Bradley SV, Oravecz-Wilson KI, Bougeard G *et al.* Serum antibodies to huntingtin interacting protein-1: a new blood test for prostate cancer. *Cancer Res.* 65(10), 4126-4133 (2005).

[37] Wang X, Yu J, Sreekumar A *et al.* Autoantibody signatures in prostate cancer. *N Engl J Med.* 353(12), 1224-1235 (2005).

[38] Petrovics G, Liu A, Shaheduzzaman S *et al.* Frequent overexpression of ETS-related gene-1 (ERG1) in prostate cancer transcriptome. *Oncogene.* 24(23), 3847-3852 (2005).

[39] Oikawa T, Yamada T. Molecular biology of the Ets family of transcription factors. *Gene.* 303, 11-34 (2003).

[40] Tomlins SA, Rhodes DR, Perner S *et al.* Recurrent fusion of TMPRSS2 and ETS transcription factor genes in prostate cancer. *Science.* 310(5748), 644-648 (2005).

In: Tumor Markers Research Focus
Editor: Deborah H. Chang, pp. 135-142
ISBN: 978-1-60021-544-5


*Chapter VII*

# Free to Total PSa Ratio Is Not Clinically Useful as An Independent Determinant of Prostate Biopsy

***Stefano Ciatto[1*], Tiziana Rubeca[1], Francesca Martinelli[1], Giovanni Pontenani[1], Claudio Lombardi[2] and Simonetta Di Lollo[3]***
[1]Centro per lo Studio e la Prevenzione Oncologica, Florence
[2] Department Urology, Torre Galli Hospital, Florence
[3] Institute of Pathology, University, Florence

## Abstract

**Aim**: To assess the validity of free to total (F/T) prostate specific antigen ratio as a predictor of prostate biopsy outcome, and its usefulness in improving biopsy positive predictive value.
Material and methods: A consecutive series of 1,093 prostate biopsies performed during 2002-2005 was considered. Variables tested as possible predictors were age, findings at palpation (DRE) and ultrasonography (TRUS), total PSA, and F/T. Association to biopsy outcome (cancer vs non-cancer) was investigated by univariate and multivariate analysis.
**Results**: All tested variables showed a statistically significant and independent association to biopsy outcome, either at univariate or multivariate analysis. Nevertheless, no variable had a good performance as a biopsy indicator: depending on the considered variable, from 3.4 to 7 cancers would be missed to spare 10 benign biopsies. Using 0.12, 0.15 or 0.20 cut off for F/T would spare 77.3, 64.4 or 43.1% of benign biopsies but would miss 54.0, 35.6 or 21.0 % of cancers, respectively. Cost-benefit ratio was slightly better, though still clinically unacceptable, among random biopsies with negative DRE and TRUS, in the 4-10 ng/ml total PSA range: missed cancers varied from 2 to 1.2 per 10 spared benign biopsies, depending on F/T cut off value.
**Conclusion**: Although it may contribute to diagnostic suspicion, F/T should neither discount a biopsy indicated for suspicious DRE or TRUS, nor determine random biopsies prompted by PSA elevation.

[*] E-mail address: s.ciatto@cspo.it, Tel +39 055 5012275, Fax +39 055 5001623, Correspondence to: Stefano Ciatto, MD, Centro per lo Studio e la Prevenzione Oncologica, viale A. Volta 171, I-50131, Florence Italy

**Key words**: prostate specific antigen, prostate cancer, diagnosis

# Introduction

Prostate core biopsy is usually performed for suspicion arising at digital rectal examination (DRE), and/or transrectal ultrasonography (TRUS)[1,2] and/or in presence of prostate specific antigen (PSA) abnormal values. A substantial proportion of biopsy are negative, as criteria adopted to indicate biopsy are poorly specific. This is the case for both DRE and TRUS, but particularly for PSA, as the currently adopted PSA cut off prompting random biopsy (4 ng/ml or higher) is poorly specific, being reached in approximately 10-15% of healthy men over 50 years of age. New biopsy criteria, associated with a higher positive predictive value (PPV) for cancer would be welcome. Several methods of adjusting PSA value, such as density [1,3], velocity [4,5], and age-adjusted reference ranges [6,7], have been tested, but they failed the purpose, as they are not cost effective (excess reduction of sensitivity, to reduce unnecessary benign biopsies).

The ratio of free to total PSA (F/T) is associated to prostate cancer, and has also been suggested as a further criterion to indicate biopsy, particularly in the 4-10 ng/ml total PSA range, but the optimal cut off for F/T to be use for this purpose is controversial [1,8-10].

At the Centro per lo Studio e la Prevenzione Oncologica (CSPO) of Florence prostate biopsy is currently performed since 1991, prompted by DRE, TRUS and PSA abnormalities in subjects referred by general or urological practices to the outpatient clinic [2] or within a controlled randomised clinical trial of PSA screening running at CSPO since 1996 [11]. Since 2002 F/T has been determined for study purpose, immediately prior to biopsy. A large biopsy series is now available and has been evaluated to assess the accuracy of F/T to predict cancer and its clinical usefulness as an indicator for biopsy.

# Material and Methods

A total of 1,093 biopsies were performed consecutively at CSPO from January 2002 to December 2005. Strong suspicion at DRE (nodule or circumscribed increased consistence) and/or at TRUS (circumscribed or asymmetric hypoechoic area) usually prompted directed biopsy, whereas total PSA elevation ($\geq$ 4 ng/ml), either isolated or associated with uncertain findings at DRE/TRUS, prompted sextant random biopsy (+/- additional directed). Patients age ranged from 43 to 95 years (average=71.5, SD=7.9).

F/T was tested immediately prior to biopsy at CSPO laboratory using the Hybritech Tandem®–MP PSA and Tandem®–MP free PSA kit (Beckman Coulter Inc., USA). The Tandem PSA assay is a solid phase, two-site immunoenzymetric assay. Blood samples react with a solution of two PSA-specific monoclonal antibodies. After the formation of a solid phase/capture antibody/PSA/labelled antibody sandwich, microplates are washed to remove unbound labelled antibody and are incubated with an enzyme substrate. The amount of substrate turnover is determined by measuring the quenched reaction absorbance at 450 nm in a microplate reader. Absorbance is proportional to sample PSA concentration. PSA concentration is determined by PSA and Zero Calibrator/Diluent calibrators concurrent testing. Since 2003 total and free PSA were tested using the Access Hybritech PSA kit (Beckman Coulter Inc., USA) The Access Hybritech PSA assay is a two-site immunoenzymatic ("sandwich") assay. A sample is added to a reaction vessel with mouse monoclonal anti- PSA alkaline phosphatase conjugate, and paramagnetic particles coated with a second mouse monoclonal anti-PSA antibody. The PSA in the sample binds to the immobilized monoclonal anti – PSA on the solid phase while, at the same time , the monoclonal anti- PSA alkaline phosphatase conjugate reacts with different antigenic sites on the sample PSA. After incubation in a reaction vessel, materials bound to the solid phase are held in a magnetic field while unbound materials are washed away.Then, the chemiluminescent substrate Lumi-Phos* 530 is added to the vessel and light generated by the reaction is measured with luminometer. The light production is directly proportional to the concentration of PSA in the sample. The amount of analyte in the sample is determined from a stored, multi-point calibration curve. External quality control is provided by Nijmegen University St Radboud Medical Centre (LWBA QA Scheme for Hormones, Vitamins and Tumour markers).

US guided biopsies in the study were all performed with a transperineal approach (local anaesthesia, no antibiotic prophylaxis) by the same team (SC, CL, PZ), having a large (>1500 biopsies) previous experience. Side effects (haematuria, spermaturia) were neligible and well tolerated: one case had a moderate perineal-prostate infection, requiring no hospitalisation. A single pathologist (SDL) read all biopsies.

We assessed the performance of different possible biopsy indicators, namely: age (continuos), DRE and TRUS report (negative/benign vs. suspicious), PSA (4 and 10 ng/ml cut off were separately tested), and F/T (0.12, 0.15 and 0.20 cut off were separately tested). We determined the accuracy (sensitivity, specificity, positive predictive value = PPV, negative predictive value = NPV) of these variables, and their association to biopsy outcome (malignant vs. other) was assessed by univariate (Pearson $\chi^2$ statistic), and multivariate analysis (logistic regression, Stata 7.0 software). Statistical significance of observed differences was set at $p<0.05$. As the role of F/T to indicate biopsy is less relevant in presence of very high PSA value, and/or strong suspicion at DRE/TRUS (all these conditions are associated to a high positive predictive value (PPV) for cancer and no further selection to biopsy is needed), analysis was performed only on the subset of random biopsies, performed in absence of DRE/TRUS abnormalities and in the 4-10 ng/ml PSA range, as such a presentation is commonly associated to a low PPV, and the need for further selection to biopsy is evident, particularly in a possible future population based screening scenario.

## Results

Overall, biopsy revealed cancer in 501 (45.8%), high grade prostatic intraepithelial neoplasia (HPIN) in 35 (3.2%) , atypical adenomatous hyperplasia (AAH) in 9 (0.8%), and benign hyperplasia in 548 cases (50.1%), respectively.

Table 1 shows the distribution of biopsy outcome (cancer vs. other) according to studied variables. Age was significantly associated to biopsy results, cancer prevalence being 38.1 or 53.0% below or over 70 years ($p = 10^{-6}$). Significant association to biopsy outcome was observed also for DRE (suspicious vs. negative/benign: $p = 10^{-6}$), TRUS (suspicious vs. negative/benign: $p = 10^{-6}$), total PSA (<4 vs. 4> ng/ml: $p = 10^{-6}$; <10 vs 10> ng/ml: $p = 10^{-6}$), and F/T (0-0.12 vs. >0.12: $p = 10^{-6}$; 0-0.15 vs. >0.15: $p = 10^{-6}$; 0-0.20 vs. >0.20: $p = 10^{-6}$). DRE was less sensitive (54.8 vs 74.4%) but more specific (82.4 vs. 53.3%) as compared to TRUS. The corresponding PPV and NPV values were 72.5 and 68.3% for DRE, or 57.4 and 71.1% for TRUS, respectively. Total PSA with a 4 ng/ml cut off was highly sensitive (90.8 vs. 53.4%) but had an unacceptable low specificity (22.4 vs. 73.9%) when compared to a cut off of 10 ng/ml. Similarly, F/T increased sensitivity (56.2, 70.8, or 83.2%) but decreased its specificity (72.9, 57.0, or 35.8%) when the cut off varied from 0.12 to 0.15 to 0.20..

**Table 1. Distribution of studied cases by age and diagnostic variable and according to biopsy outcome.**

| Variable | Values | Biopsy outcome | | SENS | SPEC | PPV | NPV |
|---|---|---|---|---|---|---|---|
| | | Cancer (%) | Benign | | | | |
| Age | <60 | 28 (41.1) | 40 | - | - | - | - |
| | 60-69 | 148 (37.6) | 245 | | | | |
| | 70-79 | 234 (47.6) | 257 | | | | |
| | >79 | 91 (64.5) | 50 | | | | |
| DRE | Suspicious | 275 (72.5) | 104 | 54.8 | 82.4 | 72.5 | 68.3 |
| | Negative/benign | 226 (31.6) | 488 | | | | |
| TRUS | Suspicious | 373 (57.4) | 276 | 74.4 | 53.3 | 57.4 | 71.1 |
| | Negative/benign | 128 (28.8) | 316 | | | | |
| Total PSA (ng/ml) | <4 | 46 (25.6) | 133 | 90.8 | 22.4 | 49.7 | 74.3 |
| | ≥4 | 455 (49.7) | 459 | | | | |
| Total PSA (ng/ml) | <10 | 233 (34.7) | 438 | 53.4 | 73.9 | 63.5 | 65.2 |
| | ≥10 | 268 (63.5) | 154 | | | | |
| F/T | 0-0.12 | 282 (63.8) | 160 | 56.2 | 72.9 | 63.8 | 66.3 |
| | >0.12 | 219 (33.6) | 432 | | | | |
| F/T | 0-0.15 | 355 (58.2) | 254 | 70.8 | 57.0 | 58.2 | 69.8 |
| | >0.15 | 146 (30.1) | 338 | | | | |
| F/T | 0-0.20 | 417 (52.3) | 380 | 83.2 | 35.8 | 52.3 | 71.6 |
| | >0.20 | 84 (28.3) | 212 | | | | |
| Total | - | 501 (100.0) | 592 | - | - | - | - |

SENS = sensitivity, SPEC = specificity, PPV = positive predictive value, NPV = negative predictive value, F/T = free to total PSA ratio

Table 2 shows the results of multivariate analysis of the association of studied variables to biopsy result. As observed at univariate analysis, age , DRE, TRUS, total PSA (cut off 4 ng/ml), and F/T (cut off 0.12) showed an independent significant association p = 0.000). Other F/T cut off values were also significantly associated to biopsy outcome, though with a lower odds ratio as compared to 0.12 cut off (data nor reported).

**Table 2. Results of multivariate analysis of the association of different variables to biopsy outcome (Odds ratio = probability of cancer at biopsy)**

| Variable | Odds ratio | 95% confidence interval | P value |
|---|---|---|---|
| Age (by incremental year) | 1.04 | 1.02-1.06 | 0.000 |
| DRE : negative/benign | 1.00 | - | - |
| suspicious | 3.74 | 2.72-5.15 | 0.000 |
| TRUS : negative/benign | 1.00 | - | - |
| susoicious | 2.02 | 1.48-2.75 | 0.000 |
| PSA : <4 ng/ml | 1.00 | - | - |
| ≥4 ng/ml | 2.54 | 1.69-3.82 | 0.000 |
| F/T : 0-0.12 | 1.00 | - | - |
| >0.12 | 2.92 | 2.20-3.87 | 0.000 |

F/T: Free to total PSA ratio

Table 3 shows the results of using each studied variable as a determinant for biopsy, presented as the ratio of missed cancers to spared benign biopsies. Missed cancers to spare 10 benign biopsies would be 7.0 or 6.1 for age >60 or >70 years, 5.0 for DRE, 4.0 for TRUS, 3.4 or 5.3 for total PSA ≥4 or ≥10 ng/ml, 5.0, 4.3 or 3.9 for a F/T of 0-0.12, 0-0.15, or 0-0.20, respectively.

**Table 3. Benign biopsies (number and % of total benign biopsies) which would be spared and cancer (number and % of total cancer biopsies) which would be missed if each studied variable would act as biopsy indicator**

| Variable prompting biopsy | spared benign biopsies | | missed cancers | | missed cancers/ |
|---|---|---|---|---|---|
| | nr | % | nr | % | 10 spared biopsies |
| Age ≥60 | 40 | 6.7 | 28 | 5.5 | 7.0 |
| Age ≥70 | 285 | 48.1 | 176 | 35.1 | 6.1 |
| DRE suspicious | 488 | 82.4 | 226 | 45.1 | 5.0 |
| TRUS suspicious | 316 | 53.3 | 128 | 25.5 | 4.0 |
| Total PSA ≥4 ng/ml | 133 | 22.4 | 46 | 9.1 | 3.4 |
| Total PSA ≥10 ng/ml | 438 | 73.9 | 233 | 46.5 | 5.3 |
| F/T 0-0.12 | 432 | 72.9 | 219 | 43.7 | 5.0 |
| F/T 0-0.15 | 338 | 57.0 | 146 | 29.1 | 4.3 |
| F/T 0-0.20 | 212 | 35.8 | 84 | 16.7 | 3.9 |

F/T: Free to total PSA ratio

Table 4 shows the accuracy of F/T using different cut off values within the subset of 218 sextant random biopsies, performed in absence of DRE or TRUS abnormalities, in the 4-10 ng/ml total PSA range. A significant association to biopsy outcome was confirmed for F/T (0-0.12 vs. >0.12: p=0.08; 0-0.15 vs. >0.15: p=0.03; 0-0.20 vs. >0.20: p=0.05), sensitivity was 38.0 %, 57.1 % or 80.9 % for a F/T cut off value of 0.12, 0.15 or 0.20, respectively. Corresponding values were 77.7 %, 62.2 %, or 36.0 % for specificity, 29.0 %, 26.6 %, or 23.2 % for PPV, and 82.9 %, 85.8 %, or 88.7 % for NPV. Had F/T being used as a determinant for biopsy, from 2 to 1.2 cancers would have been missed, depending of the adopted F/T cut off, to spare 10 benign biopsies.

**Table 4. Distribution of studied cases by F/T and biopsy outcome, among 217 random biopsies, with negative DRE and TRUS, in the 4-10 ng/ml total PSA range**

| Variable | Values | Biopsy outcome | | SENS | SPEC | PPV | NPV |
|---|---|---|---|---|---|---|---|
| | | Cancer (%) | Benign | | | | |
| F/T | 0-0.12 | 16 (29.0) | 39 | 38.0 | 77.7 | 29.0 | 82.9 |
| | >0.12 | 28 (17.0) | 136 | | | | |
| F/T | 0-0.15 | 24 (26.6) | 66 | 57.1 | 62.2 | 26.6 | 85.8 |
| | >0.15 | 18 (14.1) | 109 | | | | |
| F/T | 0-0.20 | 34 (23.2) | 112 | 80.9 | 36.0 | 23.2 | 88.7 |
| | >0.20 | 8 (11.2) | 63 | | | | |
| Total | - | 42 (19.3) | 175 | - | - | - | - |

SENS = sensitivity, SPEC = specificity, PPV = positive predictive value, NPV = negative predictive value, F/T = free to total PSA ratio

# Discussion

The present consecutive biopsy series is rather large, biopsies were performed by a unique team, slides were read by the same pathologist, PSA was determined with the same method in the same lab, and F/T was determined in a blind fashion, i.e. it did not influence biopsy indication: all these conditions should minimize possible confounding effects, and allow for a reliable analysis of the value of F/T as a possible determinant of biopsy. We used a transperineal approach, less common than the transrectal one, but equally (if not more) effective [12]. Sextant biopsy sensitivity may be regarded to as suboptimal as compared to sampling a higher number of cores[13], but has been shown to be anyhow associated with a high risk (at least 50%) of overdiagnosis [14]. Our decision to maintain classic sextant biopsy as a current option was taken in attempt to minimize overdiagnosis, and should not represent a major bias of the study: we are aware that sampling more cores would yield a higher cancer detection rate, but would also likely increase overdiagnosis. Adopting a more aggressive biopsy procedure might also have biased the study, which is aimed at evaluating a method to reduce unnecessary biopsies, as overdiagnosed cancer biopsies might be considered to be detected unnecessarily. Moreover, to our knowledge there is no literature evidence that F/T performance has improved by adopting extended instead of classic sextant biopsy.

Both univariate and multivariate analysis confirmed for all studied variables an independent significant association to biopsy outcome. The ideal biopsy indicator should reduce as much as possible the frequency of benign biopsies while delaying no cancer biopsy: according to this criterion, none of the studied variables showed had a good performance. The proportion of spared benign biopsies and of delayed cancer biopsies when using each variable as a biopsy indicator is summarized in Table 3: depending on the variable, from 3.4 to 7 cancer biopsies would be delayed to avoid 10 benign biopsies, a unacceptable cost benefit ratio, considering that a benign biopsy has a limited physical [15-17], psychological and economical cost. F/T was not better than other variables: using a 0.12, 0.15 or 0.20 cut off fof F/T would avoid 72.9, 57.0, or 35.8% of benign biopsies but would delay 43.8, 29.2, or 16.8% of cancer biopsies, respectively.

The present is a consecutive biopsy series including two different sub-populations, carrying a substantially different probability of a positive biopsy: a) subjects selected to biopsy for clinical suspicion at DRE and/or TRUS and/or with major PSA elevation (10 ng/ml or higher) and b) normal subjects selected to random biopsy only for moderately elevated PSA (4-10 ng/ml), in absence of DRE and TRUS abnormalities, a subset more representative of a possible screening scenario. In fact the latter subset has a much lower PPV for cancer (19.3%) as compared to the former (52.3%), due to the relatively higher specificity of a supicious DRE/TRUS finding and or major PSA elevations. The need to improve PPV and to spare unnecessary benign biopsies is particularly evident in the latter subset, and the benefit of using F/T as a biopsy determinant might be expected to be higher: in fact, the cost-benefit ratio was slightly better than in the overall series (1.2 to 2 cancers per 10 spared biopsies), but it was still clinically unacceptable.

The study confirmed a significant association of F/T to a positive biopsy outcome but was associated to suboptimal sensitivity or specificity, with a unacceptable ratio of missed cancers to spared benign biopsies, would F/T be used as a biopsy determinant, using a defined cut off value, both in the overall series and in the subset of PSA driven random biopsies. We are used to employ quantitative lab assays with a reference cut off for clinical purpose and to guide decisions. This seems not to be reliable for F/T (and total PSA, to some extent), which might be "wisely" used. as they contribute to create a complex patient's scenario, to influence, but not to determine the final decision of taking a biopsy in a simple "yes or no" cut-off based fashion. Although it may contribute to diagnostic suspicion, F/T should neither discount a biopsy indicated because of suspicion arising at DRE or TRUS, nor determine random biopsy in the 4-10 ng/ml PSA range.

# References


[1] Ciatto S, Bonardi R, Lombardi C, Cappelli G, Castagnoli A, D'Agata A, Zappa M, Gervasi G: Predicting prostate biopsy outcome by findings at digital rectal examination, transrectal ultrasonography, PSA, PSA density and free-to-total PSA ration in a population-based screening setting. *Int. J. Biol. Markers* 2001; 16: 179-82.

[2] Ciatto S, Bonardi R, Gervasi G, Lombardi C, Di Lollo S, Zappa M: Transperineal sonography guided biopsy of the prostate: critical review of 1107 cases. *Radiol. Med.* 2002; 103: 219-24.

[3] Benson KC, Wang IS, Olsson CA: The use of prostate specific antigen density to enhance the predictive value of intermediate levels of serum prostate specific antigen, *J. Urol.* 1992; 147: 817-21.

[4] Carter HB, Pearson JD, Metter EJ, Brant LJ, Chan DW, Andres R, Fozard JL, Walsh PC: Longitudinal evaluation of prostate specific antigen levels in men with and without prostate disease. *J.A.M.A.* 1992; 267: 2215-20.

[5] Ciatto S, Bonardi R, Lombardi C, Zappa M, Gervasi G, Cappelli G: Analysis of PSA velocity in 1666 healthy subjects undergoing total PSA determination at two consecutive screening rounds. *Int. J. Biol. Markers* 2002; 17: 79-83.

[6] Oesterling JE, Cooner WH, Jacobsen SJ, Guess HA, Lieber MM: Influence of patient age on the serum PSA concentration. *Urol. Clin. N. Am.* 1993; 20: 671-80.

[7] Ciatto S, Bonardi R, Mazzotta A, Santoni R: Reliability of volume or age-adjusted prostate specific antigen to improve diagnostic accuracy. *Int. J. Biol. Markers* 1995; 10: 226-8.

[8] Lilja H, Bjork T, Abrahamsson PA: Improved separations between normals, benign prostatic hyperplasia and carcinoma of the prostate by measuring free, complexed and total concentrations of prostate specific antigen, *J. Urol.* 1994;1 51: 400A.

[9] Catalona WG, Smith S, Wolfer RL: Evaluation of percentage of free serum prostate specific antigen to improve specificity of prostate cancer screening. *J.A.M.A.* 1995; 274: 1214-20.

[10] Oesterling JE, Jacobsen SJ, Klee GG: Free, complexed and total serum prostate specific antigen: the establishment of appropriate reference ranges for their concentration and ratios. *J. Urol.* 1995; 154: 1090-5.

[11] de Koning HJ, Auvinen A, Berenguer-Sanchez A, Calais da Silva F, Ciatto S, Denis L, Gohagan JK, Hakama M, Hugosson J, Kranse R, Nelen V, Prorok PC, Schroeder FH: Large-scale randomised prostate cancer screening trials ; program performance in the ERSPC and PLCO trials. *Int. J. Cancer* 2002; 97: 237-44.

[12] Vis NA, Boerma MO, Ciatto S, Hoedemaeker RF, Schroeder FH, van der Kwast T: Detection of prostate cancer: a comparative study of the diagnostic efficacy of sextant transrectal versus sextant transperineal biopsy. *Urology* 2000; 56: 617-21.

[13] Eskew LA, Bare RL, McCulloch DL:. Systematic 5 region prostate biopsy is superior to sextant method for diagnosing carcinoma of the prostate. *J. Urol.* 1997; 157: 199-203.

[14] Draisma G, Boer R, Otto SJ, van der Cruijsen IW, Damhuis RAM, Schroder FH, de Koning HJ: Lead Times and Overdetection Due to Prostate-Specific Antigen Screening: Estimates From the European Randomized Study of Screening for Prostate Cancer. *J. Natl. Cancer Inst.* 2003; 95: 868-78.

[15] Makinen T, Auvinen A, Hakama M, Stenman UH, Tammela TLJ: Acceptability and complications of prostate biopsy in population-based PSA screening versus routine clinical practice: a prospective, controlled study, *Urology* 2002; 60: 846-50.
[16] Raaijmakers R, Kirkels W.J, Roobol M.J, Wildhagen M, Schroeder FH: Complication rates and risk factors of 5802 transrectal ultrasound guided sextant biopsies of the prostate within a population-based screening program. *Urology* 2002; 60: 826-30.
[17] Rietbergen JBW, Kruger AE, Kranse R, Schroeder FH: Complications of transrectal ultrasound (TRUS) guided systematic sextant biopsies of the prostate: Evaluation of complication rates and risk factors within a population based screening program. *Urology* 1997; 49: 875-80.

In: Tumor Markers Research Focus
Editor: Deborah H. Chang, pp. 143-157
ISBN: 978-1-60021-544-5


*Chapter VIII*

# Title Cancer-Testis Antigens as Biomarkers for the Diagnosis and Treatment of Hepatocellular Carcinoma: Usefulness and Validation in the Light of Cancer Complexity

***Fabio Grizzi***[1,2*]

[1]Laboratories of Quantitative Medicine, Istituto Clinico Humanitas IRCCS, Via Manzoni 56, 20089 Rozzano, Milan, Italy

[2]"Michele Rodriguez" Foundation – Scientific Institute for Quantitative Measures in Medicine, Milan, Italy

## Abstract

Despite advances in our cellular and molecular knowledge, hepatocellular carcinoma (HCC) remains one of the major public health problems throughout the world. It is now known to be highly heterogeneous: it encompasses various pathological entities and a wide range of clinical behaviors, and is underpinned by a complex array of gene alterations that affect supra-molecular processes. Surgical resection is currently the most effective treatment strategy, but many cases are unsuitable for surgery because of the presence of intrahepatic or distant metastases at the time of diagnosis, and so it is therefore extremely important to recognize the disease and any recurrence as early as possible.

Four categories of HCC tumour markers have been proposed: a) onco-fetal and glycoprotein antigens; b) enzymes and iso-enzymes; c) cytokines and d) genes. A family of tumour-associated antigens called cancer-testis (CT) antigens has recently been identified and their encoding genes have been extensively investigated. CT antigens are expressed in a limited number of normal tissues as well as in malignant tumors of unrelated histological origin (including the liver), and are being vigorously pursued as targets for therapeutic cancer vaccines. They are also being evaluated because of their role in oncogenesis and the recapitulation of portions of the germ line gene-expression programme, which might contribute characteristic features to the neoplastic phenotype such as immortality,

* E-mail address: fabio.grizzi@humanitas.it

invasiveness, immune evasion, hypomethylation and metastatic capacity. Given that cancers are being recognized as increasingly complex (an intrinsic property of every human neoplasia), we here review the role of CT antigens as liver tumour biomarkers and their validation process, and discuss why they may improve the effectiveness of screening HCC patients and help in determining the risk of developing HCC.

# Introduction

Hepatocellular carcinoma (HCC) represents the fifth most common cancer worldwide [1], it is the most common primary cancer associated with hepatitis B (HBV) and hepatitis C virus (HCV) chronic infections, alcohol abuse or in developing countries with food contaminated with *Aspergillus flavus* fungus [1,3]. The incidence of HCC has been rising in the last two decades in Europe, United states and Japan [4]. Furthermore, it is the second common cause of death in China, where its mortality rate is 20.37/100 thousand [5].

Despite advances in our cellular and molecular knowledge HCC remains one of the major public health problems throughout the world. It is now known to be highly heterogeneous: it encompasses various pathological entities and a wide range of clinical behaviors, and is underpinned by a complex array of gene alterations that affect supra-molecular processes [6].

A variety of genomic and molecular alterations have been identified in fully developed HCC and to a lesser extent in morphologically defined precancerous lesions [6-8]. However, this database has been obtained largely in a shatter and uncoordinated manner, typically in investigations in which aberrations in single genes have been analyzed in a group of HCC from humans and experimental animals [6]. Although these data all seems to be helpful, they have not led to a coherent understanding of the complex mechanisms underlying HCC development, or to the identification of critical genomic and/or molecular aberrations that improve the carefulness of diagnosis or therapeutic interventions.

HCC is a non-linear complex disease that emerges from multiple spontaneous and/or inherited mutations that induce dramatic changes in expression patterns of genes and proteins that function in networks controlling critical cellular events [9-12].

Therefore, it is compulsory to identify HCC and the recurrence at its earlier period. A number of serum markers have been proposed and currently used as an effective method for detecting HCC for a long time [5]. Four categories of HCC tumour markers have mainly been proposed and currently applied in the clinical practice. In addition, a family of tumour-associated antigens called *cancer-testis (CT) antigens* has recently been identified and their encoding genes have been extensively investigated. CT antigens are expressed in a limited number of normal tissues as well as in malignant tumors of unrelated histological origin, and are being vigorously pursued as targets for therapeutic cancer vaccines.

Given that cancers are being recognized as increasingly complex (an intrinsic property of every human neoplasia), we here review the role of CT antigens as liver tumour biomarkers and their validation process, and discuss why they may improve the effectiveness of screening HCC patients and help in determining the risk of developing HCC.

# HCC Biomarkers: From Biochemistry to Genomics

In general terms four categories of HCC tumour markers have been proposed and currently applied: *(a)* onco-fetal and glycoprotein antigens; *(b)* enzymes and iso-enzymes; *(c)* cytokines and *(d)* genes. However, a truthful specific biomarker for early detection, diagnosis or clinical outcome/prognosis of HCC is still undiscovered.

## Onco-fetal Antigens and Glycoprotein Antigens

(1) *Alpha-fetoprotein (AFP)* is a fetal $\alpha_1$-globulin synthesized primarily by the fetal liver, yolk sac and gut, in the first trimester of pregnancy [13-15]. In normal conditions, its serum concentration falls quickly after birth and its synthesis in adult humans is repressed. Today, AFP represents the most useful tumor marker in screening HCC patients. Although some discrepancies, the serum concentration of 500 μg/L is the widely used cut-off value to differentiate HCC patients from healthy human beings. Lower levels may be detected in patients with chronic liver disease but with no evidence of HCC.

(2) *Glypican-3 (GPC3)* is a heparan sulfate proteoglycan anchored to the plasma membrane [5, 16] and may be secreted. GPC3 mRNA and protein are expressed in >80% of human HCC but not in normal tissues except for placenta and fetal liver [17]. Recently, Nakatsura and Nishimura described GPC3 as a novel tumor marker for human HCC [18]. It was found in sera from 40-50% of HCC patients, although it was not detected in sera from patients with liver cirrhosis or chronic hepatitis, or in sera from healthy individuals [18].

## Enzymes and Iso-enzymes

(1) *Gamma-glutamyl transferase (GGTII)* is mainly secreted in serum by macrophagic Kupffer cells and endothelial cells of bile ducts and its activity increases in tissues with HCC [5]. Sensitivities of GGTII have been reported to be 74.0% in detecting HCC and 43.8% in detecting small HCC [19].

(2) *Alpha-l-fucosidase (AFU)* is a glycosidase primarily found in lysosome and involved in the degradation of a variety of fucose-containing fucoglycoconjugates [20]. The alterations of AFU catalytic activity in human cells, tissues and body fluids have a diagnostic value for human tumors including primary HCC [5,21-23], colorectal cancer [24] and ovarian cancer [25].The deficiency of AFU activity in female sera is probably a hereditary condition related to higher risk of ovarian cancer [20]. The persistently elevated AFU level in sera of patients with liver cirrhosis contributes to early detection of HCC [5,20].

(3) *Des-gamma-carboxyprothrombin (DCP)* is a well recognized tumor marker for HCC. It is an abnormal product from liver carboxylation disturbance during the formation of thrombogen, and acts as an autologous mitogen for HCC cell lines [5,26]. DCP was more sensitive and specific than AFP for differentiating HCC from nonmalignant chronic liver disease [27].

## Citokines

(1) *Vascular endothelial growth factor (VEGF)* is a secreted homodimeric cytokine that positively regulates tumor neovascularization [5,28]. It has been recently shown that angiogenesis is a fundamental process occurring during liver carcinogenesis, that the expression of VEGF in cancerous tissues of HCC was higher than that in normal liver tissue, and that HCC patients with over-expression of VEGF have a lower survival rate [29,30].

(2) *Interleukin-8 (IL-8)* is a multifunctional CXC chemokine that affects human neutrophil functions, including chemotaxis, enzyme release, and expression of surface adhesion

molecules [5]. IL-8 seems to have also direct effects on tumor and vascular endothelial cell proliferation, angiogenesis, and tumor migration. Recently, Kubo *et al* have shown that the expression of IL-8 in human HCC has more relevance to metastatic potential, such as vessel invasion, than to angiogenesis or cell proliferation [31]. Moreover, significant correlations of serum IL-8 levels with tumor size and tumor stage suggest that IL-8 may be directly or indirectly involved in the progression of HCC. These findings indicate that serum IL-8 may be a useful biological marker of tumor invasiveness and an independent prognostic factor for patients with HCC [32,33].

(3) *Transforming growth factor-beta 1 (TGF-β1)* is a negative growth factor which correlates with cellular immunosuppression during the progression of HCC. Its serum level in HCC patients has been shown to be elevated compared with those in healthy adults and patients with non-malignant hepatopathy [5,34]. In the liver, endogenous factors, such as TGF-β1 may be involved in induction of apoptosis. In HCC, birth and death rates of cells are several times higher than in surrounding liver. Consequently, tumor promoters may act as survival factors, *i.e.*, inhibit apoptosis preferentially in precancerous and even in malignant liver cells, thereby stimulating selective growth of precancerous lesions [35].

(4) *Tumor-specific growth factor (TSGF)* is a product synthesized and released by malignant cells. It results in blood capillary amplification surrounding the tumor, into peripheral blood during its growing period. Thus, the higher presence in serum of TSGF can be used as diagnostic marker in detecting HCC. Its sensitivity can reach 82% at the cut-off of 62 UI/mL [5,36]. TSGF is the first kind of tumor marker *in vitro* which was primarily obtained the approval by Chinese government to land the market, there was no any reports about it in abroad before [36].

It is important to underline that the quantification of cytokines in serum/plasma, collected prior to the clinical recognition of HCC, may provide insights into the nature of a host immune system environment that contributes to cancer development and/or growth. Such studies need to be designed with knowledge of the biology of the cytokines to be measured, and of the limitations inherent in the measurement of these molecules. Also, many cytokines are labile and/or are produced locally in immune system organs and not distributed systemically, so they cannot be detected in serum/plasma.

## Genes

(1) *Alpha-fetoprotein mRNA (AFP mRNA)* It has recently been demonstrated that AFP mRNA expression detected by reverse-transcription polymerase chain reaction (RT-PCR) in peripheral blood 1 week after surgery correlated with the recurrence of HCC and was a good predictor for tumor recurrence [37]. In 1994, Matsumura *et al.* first reported that single HCC cell in circulation could be detected by means of RT-PCR, targeting AFP mRNA [38]. Subsequently, many investigators reported the value of AFP mRNA as a predictor for HCC recurrence, but the results are rather controversial. This may be due to the blood-borne dispersion of both tumor cells and normal liver cells during surgical manipulation and the mis-transcription of AFP mRNA by peripheral mononuclear cells, which may damage the specialty and prognostic value of AFP mRNA.

(2) *Gamma-glutamyl transferase mRNA (GGT mRNA)* can be detected in the serum and liver tissues of healthy adults or patients with HCC, nonmalignant hepatopathy, hepatic benign tumor, and secondary tumor of the liver [5]. It can be divided into three types: fetal liver

*(type A)*, HepG2 cells *(type B)* and placenta *(type C)*. Type A is predominantly expressed in normal liver tissues or liver tissues without malignant hepatopathy, benign tumor or secondary liver cancer. On the contrary type B is commonly found in cancerous tissues of HCC. Sheen *et al.* have demonstrated that patients of HCC with type B gamma-GTP mRNA both in cancer and in non-cancerous tissue had a worse outcome, earlier recurrence, and more post-recurrence death [39].

*(3) Human telomerase reverse transcriptase mRNA (hTERT mRNA)* It has originally been reported to be detectable in the serum of patients with breast cancer. However, recent data have demonstrated that liver carcinogenesis may involve increased h-TERT [40], that the induction of hTERT mRNA is an important early event, and that its measurement by RT-PCR is a useful tool to detect precancerous tendencies in hepatic nodules. However, hTERT gene dosage is not the main mechanism regulating hTERT expression in hepatocarcinogenesis [41].

It can be said that other biomarkers have been proposed and preliminarily applied in the early detection of HCC. AFP and DCP are currently the most useful serum tumor markers for detection of HCC, and the simultaneous determination of these markers might improve the accuracy, especially in differentiating HCC from precancerous lesions, and nonmalignant hepatopathy.

A family of *tumour-associated antigens* (TAAs) has recently been identified and their encoding genes have been extensively investigated. Among them CT antigens are expressed in a limited number of normal tissues as well as in malignant tumors of unrelated histological origin, and are being vigorously pursued as targets for new therapeutic strategies. They are also being evaluated because of their role in oncogenesis and the recapitulation of portions of the germ line gene-expression programme, which might contribute characteristic features to the neoplastic phenotype such as immortality, invasiveness, immune evasion, hypomethylation and metastatic capacity.

## The Discovery of Tumour-Associated Antigens

One of the most controversial issues in immunology for over a century has been whether an effective immune response can be elicited against malignant tumors [42]. Based on recent immunological developments, there is no doubt that the immune system can recognize and eliminate malignant cells. In 1967 Frank Macfarlane Burnet introduced a general hypothesis suggesting that lymphocytes are continually patrolling tissues and eliminating transformed cells, presumably via recognition of TAAs, a process he called "immunosurveillance" [43].

The immune system is capable of discriminating between benign and malignant cells based on specific recognition of aberrantly expressed proteins or peptide fragments from these proteins in the context of major histocompatibility complex.

Thus, the proteins encoded by abnormally expressed genes of a tumour cell may represent potential targets for immune cells, serving as tumour-associated rejection or regression antigens. With the exception of melanoma, few candidate TAAs have been defined for human malignancies [44].

Since the first cloning of a human TAA, called melanoma antigen-1 (MAGE-1), the identification of TAAs capable of inducing an immune response in cancer patients and the development of vaccines targeting these antigens, has represented formidable tasks confronting tumour immunologists [45].

The majority of melanoma antigens have been identified by screening cDNA libraries with melanoma-specific cytotoxic T lymphocytes (CTL) isolated from melanoma patients. The introduction of a genetic approach of T-cell epitope cloning and subsequently an innovative method through the *serological analysis of recombinant tumor cDNA expression libraries with autologous serum (SEREX)* has greatly expanded the identification of a promising class of TAAs called CT antigens. Many TAAs have been identified using a genetic approach in which a cDNA library from tumour cell mRNA is generated in a eukaryotic expression system. Bacterial generated pools of cDNA, containing between 50-200 individual clones, are co-transfected with a construct encoding the appropriate MHC I gene into a highly transfectable eukaryotic cell line. The cells transfected with the cDNA pools are then investigated for their ability to stimulate cytokine release from tumour reactive CTL [46]. Single clones are isolated and the peptide epitopes derived from these antigens are identified through the use of HLA peptide-binding motif algorithms [47]. SEREX is a valid alternative molecular approach for TAAs discovery. Unlike molecular approaches that attempt to ascribe immunity to cloned genes, SEREX employs patient sera and autologous tumors to identify TAAs that have elicited high titer IgG antibodies in patients demonstrating immunity to the antigen. This approach has identified a number of gene products that have a know or suspected relevance to tumour development as well as other antigens that may be potential targets for cancer vaccines. Some of the TAAs discovered using SEREX that may be useful, as vaccines include antigens cloned from small cell carcinoma, colon cancer and breast cancer.

Another method used in the search for TAAs is *acid elution of peptides from tumour-cell surface MHC I molecules*. Pools of peptides are produced, fractioned with high pressure liquid chromatography, and sequenced [47,48]. The peptides are subsequently tested for their ability to sensitise targets to enable recognition by specific T cells.

TAAs that are over-expressed or up-regulated in cancer cells can also be identified by analysis of differentially expressed genes in tumour cells compared to their counterpart normal cells.

*Serial analysis of gene expression (SAGE)* is a useful approach to determine the expression of a high number of genes simultaneously. There are many benefits to SAGE, firstly the ability to evaluate the expression pattern of many genes in a quantitative manner without prior sequence information. SAGE can determine the abundance of mRNAs and can also detect small differences in expression levels between samples. The SAGE method is based on two main concepts: *a)* a short sequence tag consisting of 9-10 base pairs (bp) is used to identify a transcript; *b)* serial units of short sequence tags allow the efficient analysis of transcripts by the sequencing of multiple tags with a single clone.

Since the introduction of differential display by Liang and Pardee [49], the rate at which differentially expressed genes have been identified has dramatically increased. The abundance of genes is a result of the simplicity and sensitivity of differential display and also the capability of this method to compare multiple RNA samples in order to distinguish between up-regulated and down-regulated genes without knowing their sequences. Differential display employs PCR and DNA gel electrophoresis: compared to other methods, it is more sensitive and only a few picograms of total RNA is needed, and results are highly reproducible from run to run (>90%).

# Cancer-Testis Antigens as a New Class of Biomarkers

CT antigens represents a category of tumour antigens with normal expression restricted to male germ cells in the testis but not in adult somatic tissues [50]. Since the restricted CT expression profile, the presence of multi-gene family, and the X chromosomal location of all the SEREX identified antigens, has been proposed the term of CT antigen to encompass the heterogeneous group of antigens.

Although, earlier studies of CT antigens defined common features of these antigens, namely the cancer/testis-restricted expression profile, presence of multi-gene families, mapping to the X chromosome, and immunogenicity in cancer patients, subsequently additional features have been identified. Among them: *(a)* heterogeneous protein expression in cancer; *(b)* correlation of mRNA expression with tumour progression and with tumors of higher malignant potential; *(c) in vitro* activation by hypomethylation and/or histone deacetylation.

Actually, 44 distinct CT "gene" or "antigen" families have been reported in literature. Certain CT gene families contain multiple members, as well as splice variants and today a total of 89 distinct transcripts are know to be encoded by CT genes [51]. Examples of widely characterized CT antigen families include MAGE, B melanoma antigen (BAGE) and G melanoma antigen (GAGE). In addition the CT antigens from melanoma (SSX2), oesophageal cancer (NY-ESO-1), and renal cancer (SCP-1) were identified by SEREX analysis.

By comparing CT antigen expression data the following comments have been made [52]:

(1) the expression frequency of a single CT antigen is variable in different tumors type;
(2) the frequency of different CT antigen expression in a single tumour type is highly variable;
(3) there is a tendency for CT antigen expression to be clustered, *i.e.* certain tumour specimens are found to express multiple CT antigens simultaneously, whereas other tumour will be totally negative for CT antigens.

Excluding nervous system tumors and pancreatic cancers, which have been insufficiently studied with regard to CT transcript expression, the tumour types can be distinct in three groups based on the number of CT genes expressed and their expression frequency:

(1) *high CT expressors*: tumors which express more than 50% of the CT-antigens;
(2) *moderate CT expressors*: tumors which express between 30-50% of the CT transcripts;
(3) *low CT expressors*: tumors which express less than 30% of the CT transcripts.

It is necessary to emphasize that these data are taken from mRNA expression frequencies, which do not necessarily directly correlate with protein expression frequencies. Discrepancies between gene and protein expression frequencies may reflect variations in tissue sampling, tumour heterogeneity or different level of sensitivity of detection.

The expression of these antigens may however correlate with advanced stage and grade of tumors, and the presence of spontaneous immune reactivity to these antigens has been shown to correlate with improved prognosis in some studies.

## Expression of Cancer-Testis Antigens in HCC

A number of CT antigens have been found expressed with a high percentage and specificity in HCC and their products are promising targets for antigen-specific immunotherapy of this tumor. Moreover, the high frequent co-expression of multiple members of CT antigens in HCC provides possibility of polyvalent vaccinations for HCC.

Zhao *et al* reported that of 105 HCC tissues, MAGE1, SSX-1, CTp11 and HCA587 mRNA expressions were detectable in 75.2%, 72.4%, 62.9% and 56.2% of HCC samples, respectively [52]. About 93.3%, 72.4%, 48.6% and 37.1% of HCC tissues positively expressed at least one, two, three, and four members of CT antigens, respectively. Conversely, only SSX-1 could be detectable in 2.9% of the corresponding adjacent non-HCC tissues in which no metastatic lesion was found. Interestingly, in that study the serum AFP was normal (< 20 ng/mL) or slightly elevated (< 40 ng/mL) in 30.0% of HCC patients. In these patients, 91% had MAGE-1, SSX1, CTp11 or HCA587 transcripts in their HCC tissues, suggesting applying their mRNAs as tumour-specific markers to detect HCC cells in circulation might be an adjuvant diagnostic tool [52].

The expression of the CT antigens mRNA was also investigated by Wu *et al.* in the tissues of HCC and corresponding peripheral blood of 37 patients with HCC [53]. Fifteen samples of cirrhotic tissues and 15 normal tissues were examined with the same method. Two kinds of CT antigens (SSX-2 and SSX-5) showed high-specific and high-frequent expression in HCC tissues, but neither of them could be detected in adjacent non-HCC tissues. In corresponding peripheral blood of HCC tissues, the positive expression rate of the SSX-2 and SSX-5 mRNA was not very high. No relationship was found between the expression of CT antigens and clinical indicators such as age, sex, tumor size, TNM staging, serum AFP level and infection with hepatitis virus [53]. In 15 patients with cirrhosis and 15 other non-tumor patients, none of the SSX-2 and SSX-5 mRNA was detected in liver tissue or peripheral blood. High frequency and specificity of CT antigens in HCC indicates that their products may be new potential promising targets for antigen-specific immunotherapy of HCC. Moreover, the high frequent co-expression of the two genes in HCC provides a possibility of polyvalent vaccinations for this neoplasia. Specific expression of CT antigens was observed in AFP-negative HCC, suggesting the application of their mRNA as tumor markers to detect circulating HCC cells, as adjuvant diagnostic tool, and as indicators of recurrence and prognosis. Peng *et al.* found that the expression of MAGE-A3, SSX-1, SSX-2, SSX-4, MAGE-B2, MAGE-C1, and MAGE-C2 correlated significantly with older age [54]. Moreover, the expressions of MAGE-A4 and SCP-1 were related to AFP abnormality, and the expression of NY-ESO-1 was related to early tumor stage [54]. There was no correlation observed between the expression of CT antigens and the sex, HBV infection or tumor size [54].

In search for genes associated with HCC by cDNA microarray, Yin *et al.* found that the transcription of TSPY, "testis-specific protein Y-encoded", was up-regulated in HCC, and that TSPY is a novel CT antigen which might be serve as a potential candidate in vaccine strategy for immunotherapy in HCC patients [55].

NY-ESO-1 and LAGE-1 are expressed in a high percentage of HCC, especially in cases with metastasis [56]. It is thus possible that also NY-ESO-1/LAGE-1 might serve as targets for antigen-specific immunotherapy in HCC and NY-ESO-1 peptide vaccination may be of use for patients with advanced HCC [56]. Positive rate of NY-ESO-1 mRNA was 27.4% in HCC; it was higher in HCC with tumor embolus of portal vein than in HCC without tumor embolism (40.0% *versus* 18.9%). Positive rate of NY-ESO-1 protein was 18.9% in HCC tissue microarray; it was significantly higher in HCC with metastasis than in HCC without metastasis (29.6% *versus* 11.5%,). Positive rates of NY-ESO-1 mRNA and protein were 28.3% and 19.1% respectively in

HBsAg positive HCC, and were 29.5% and 20.7% respectively in HCC with AFP of > 20 ng/ml. Both NY-ESO-1 mRNA and protein were not detected in adjacent normal liver tissue [57].

Recently, Shi *et al.* identified another antigen of great interest called transgelin 2 [58]. The over-expression of transgelin 2 mRNA in a large per cent (69%) of HCC points to its potential as a diagnostic marker for this cancer.

Li *et al* showed that in HCC specimens the HCA587 (the HCA587 gene, identified by SEREX from a HCC patient, encodes a new member of CT antigens) protein was expressed in 37.1% samples. The expressed protein was either detected in the cytoplasm or nucleus depending on the individual samples. More importantly, there appears to be correlation between the tumor differentiation of HCC and HCA587 protein expression, ie, the lower differentiation, the higher percentage of protein expression [59].

From the data of Luo *et al.* it appears that about >80% of the patients with HCC would be eligible for specific immunotherapeutic approaches with at least one CT antigen in ways similar to those currently being evaluated in malignant melanomas, which express CT antigens at a similar frequency as HCC [60]. While all patients with a tumor expressing a given CT antigen would be candidates for vaccine strategies using whole antigenic proteins, the percentage of patients eligible for peptide-specific vaccination would be much lower, since it requires antigenic peptides with binding motifs restricted to specific MHC alleles.

# Conclusion

It is indubitable that there is a growing interest in identifying diagnostic tools that could complement standard histopathologic evaluation to determine the presence of cancer cells in tissues [61]. In particular, a pressing need exists for biomarkers useful for early cancer detection, accurate pretreatment staging, prediction of response to treatment, and monitoring of disease progression [62].

The availability of a suitable serological marker to distinguish between HCC and benign liver lesions would be very useful for early diagnosis. The only serological marker currently widely used for the diagnosis of HCC is AFP. However, the sensitivity of this marker is limited. Given the high heterogeneity of HCC, it is currently thought that an optimal serological test for HCC will be based on the simultaneous measurement of two or three highly specific serological markers [16].

Although several studies have proposed many serum markers, everyone agrees that it is difficult to accurately diagnose early HCC. But early detection is still the only way to improve mortality – the disease is nearly always fatal once the tumors are no longer amenable to surgical or ablative approaches [63] In an effort to find a more reliable serum test for early HCC the National Cancer Institute has launched a 2-year study to validate the usefulness of DCP as a molecular marker [63]. In Japan, where HCV causes 80% of HCC and HBV causes another 10%, have been implemented guidelines describing an ideal screening program for high-risk patients. The program consists of checking the tumor markers AFP and DCP every month, performing abdominal ultrasonography every 3 months, and performing abdominal computed tomography every 6 months.

There is growing evidence for a link between the immune system and the control of cancer. Emerging evidence indicate, however, that some of the results are not generalizable, and the markers would need to be studied for each tumor type. Since the markers studied to date are not universally prognostic, further details in approaches for studying these markers are warranted. Although a number of CT antigens have been discovered and it has been suggested that some of them could be helpful in the early detection of HCC, the complexity of human beings leads us to reflect on the need to establish compelling new criteria for validating their real applicability.

*Biological complexity* can be intuitively appreciated – at least in terms of *morphological* or *behavioral* complexity, or the variety of cell types in an organism – but the term itself is notoriously difficult to define [64].

Human beings are complex hierarchical systems consisting of a number of levels of anatomical organization (genes, cells, tissues, organs, apparatuses, and organism) that interrelate differently with each other to form networks of growing complexity [10, 64-66].

The concept of anatomical entities as hierarchy of graduated forms, and the increasing number of known structural variables, have highlighted new properties of organized biological matter and raised a series of intriguing questions.

In order to understand biology at the system level, we need to examine the structure and dynamics of the functions of organisms rather than the characteristics of their constitutive isolated parts [64].

The expression of TAA in biological materials has mainly been studied at the level of gene expression and gene level measurement by RT-PCR analysis and the quantitative real-time PCR (qrt-PCR) technology [67,68]. However, the information provided by these approaches is limited by the fact that the phenomena observed at each level of anatomical organization have properties that do not exist at a lower or higher level: RT-PCR and qrt-PCR may offer a satisfactory qualitative/quantitative description of small-scale structures, but this is likely to be irrelevant when it comes to large-scale features.

The above considerations, in conjunction with the complexity of tumor-host interactions within the tumor microenvironment caused by temporal changes in tumor phenotypes and an array of immune mediators expressed in the tumor microenvironment might clarify the limited reliability and applicability of current molecular biomarkers.

Recently we have described a system level-based approach for validating the appropriateness of using CT antigens for diagnostic and clinical purposes, which includes the following never defined before key points:

(1) *discriminating* the cell types expressing the candidate antigen on the basis of the morphological visualization of all of the parts making up the organ under investigation;
(2) *discriminating* the candidate antigen's sub-cellular localization (at the level of cell nucleus, cytoplasm and/or plasma membrane) by ultra-structural morphological visualizations;
(3) *mapping* candidate antigen expression in all of the organs making up the apparatuses;
(4) *mapping* candidate antigen exprcssion in all of the apparatuses making up the living organism;
(5) *estimating* the percentage of normal cells and their neoplastic counterparts expressing the candidate antigen;
(6) *evaluating* the dynamics of candidate antigen expression at the level of the cell cycle, the physiological status of the organism and the process of aging.

Despite the rapid advances that have been made in the fields of molecular and cellular biology, there is no doubt that cancer is still a very complex disease: it can be hypothesized that each tumour is unique, and that the spectrum of biological changes determining human tumors is infinitely variable [10]. Carcinogenesis is a *dynamic process* that depends on a large number of *variables* and is regulated at *multiple spatial* and *temporal scales*, thus making it one of the most complex phenomena in biology. Carcinogenesis is a non-linear process, whose behavior does not follow clearly predictable and repeatable pathways. Periods of inactivity may be punctuated by sudden change, apparent patterns of behavior may disappear and new patterns surprisingly emerge [10]. Such behavior emerges in complex systems, and are permanently sensitive to small perturbations. This chaotic behavior does not indicate a lack of order. Rather, the order is difficult or impossible to describe in simple terms and requires complex narrative description. Cancer is determined by a number of processes and controls operating over much broader scales, and by factors such as structural controls that may operate at scales ranging from molecular to environmental. This *multiple scale causality* not only recognizes multiple processes and controls acting at multiple scales but, unlike a strict reductionist approach, may also recognize the fact that relevant "first principles" may reside at scales other than the smallest micro-scales. In other words, the observed phenomenon at each scale has structural and behavioral properties that do not exist at lower or higher organizational levels [10].

Viewing cancer as a system that is dynamically complex in time and space will probably reveal more about its underlying behavioral characteristics. This way of thinking may further help to clarify concepts, interpret new and old experimental data, indicate alternative experiments and categorize the acquired knowledge on the basis of the similitude and/or shared behaviors of very different tumors. It is encouraging that mathematics, theoretics, biology and medicine continue to contribute together towards a common quantitative understanding of cancer complexity. In order to advance our knowledge in a currently widely debated field of investigation such as that of biomarkers in HCC, a clearer distinction must be made between *in vitro* laboratory results (the discovery and validation of possible biomarkers) and their real application (*in vivo* validation), and it is necessary to adopt a more complete experimental approach that forcefully includes both morphological and molecular techniques. Finally, the analysis of these markers could be useful in identifying patients that are most likely to benefit from immune intervention strategies.

## References

[1] Zerbini A, Pilli M, Ferrari C, Missale G. Is there a role for immunotherapy in hepatocellular carcinoma? *Dig Liver Dis*. 2006, 38, 221-225.

[2] Jemal A, Murray T, Ward E, Samuels A, Tiwari RC, Ghafoor A, Feuer EJ, Thun MJ. Cancer statistics, 2005. *CA Cancer J Clin.* 2005, 55, 10-30.

[3] Jaskiewicz K, Stepien A, Banach L. Hepatocellular carcinoma in a rural population at risk. *Anticancer Res.* 1991, 11, 2187-2189.

[4] Tanaka Y, Hanada K, Mizokami M, Yeo AE, Shih JW, Gojobori T, Alter HJ. A comparison of the molecular clock of hepatitis C virus in the United States and Japan predicts that hepatocellular carcinoma incidence in the United States will increase over the next two decades. *Proc Natl Acad Sci U S A.* 2002, 99, 15584-15589.

[5] Zhou L, Liu J, Luo F. Serum tumor markers for detection of hepatocellular carcinoma. *World J Gastroenterol.* 2006, 12, 1175-1181.

[6] Thorgeirsson SS, Lee JS, Grisham JW. Functional genomics of hepatocellular carcinoma. *Hepatology* 2006, 43, S145-150.

[7] Llovet JM, Burroughs A, Bruix J. Hepatocellular carcinoma. *Lancet* 2003, 362: 1907-1917.

[8] Kojiro M. Histopathology of liver cancers. *Best Pract Res Clin Gastroenterol.* 2005, 19, 39-62.

[9] Grizzi F, Russo C, Portinaro N, Hermonat PL, Chiriva-Internati M. Complexity and cancer. *Gastroenterology* 2004, 126, 630-631.

[10] Grizzi F, Chiriva-Internati M. Cancer: looking for simplicity and finding complexity. *Cancer Cell Int.* 2006, 6, 4

[11] Lee JS, Thorgeirsson SS. Genome-scale profiling of gene expression in hepatocellular carcinoma: classification, survival prediction, and identification of therapeutic targets. *Gastroenterology* 2004, 127, S51-55.

[12] Thorgeirsson SS, Grisham JW. Molecular pathogenesis of human hepatocellular carcinoma. *Nat Genet.* 2002, 31, 339-346.

[13] Terentiev AA, Moldogazieva NT. Structural and functional mapping of alpha-fetoprotein. *Biochemistry (Mosc).* 2006, 71, 120-132.

[14] Canick JA, MacRae AR. Second trimester serum markers. *Semin Perinatol.* 2005, 29, 203-208.

[15] Ding X, Yang LY, Huang GW, Yang JQ, Liu HL, Wang W, Peng JX, Yang JQ, Tao YM, Chang ZG, Ling XS. Role of AFP mRNA expression in peripheral blood as a predictor for postsurgical recurrence of hepatocellular carcinoma: a systematic review and meta-analysis. *World J Gastroenterol.* 2005, 11, 2656-2661.

[16] Gebo KA, Chander G, Jenckes MW, Ghanem KG, Herlong HF, Torbenson MS, El-Kamary SS, Bass EB. Screening tests for hepatocellular carcinoma in patients with chronic hepatitis C: a systematic review. *Hepatology* 2002, 36, S84-92.

[17] Filmus J, Capurro M. Glypican-3 and alphafetoprotein as diagnostic tests for hepatocellular carcinoma. *Mol Diagn.* 2004, 8, 207-212.

[18] Nakatsura T, Nishimura Y. Usefulness of the novel oncofetal antigen glypican-3 for diagnosis of hepatocellular carcinoma and melanoma. *BioDrugs* 2005, 19, 71-77.

[19] Cui R, He J, Zhang F, Wang B, Ding H, Shen H, Li Y, Chen X. Diagnostic value of protein induced by vitamin K absence (PIVKAII) and hepatoma-specific band of serum gamma-glutamyl transferase (GGTII) as hepatocellular carcinoma markers complementary to alpha-fetoprotein. *Br J Cancer.* 2003, 88, 1878-1882.

[20] Haydon GH, Hayes PC. Screening for hepatocellular carcinoma. *Eur J Gastroenterol Hepatol.* 1996, 8, 856-860.

[21] Li C, Qian J, Lin JS. Purification and characterization of alpha-L-fucosidase from human primary hepatocarcinoma tissue. *World J Gastroenterol.* 2006, 12, 3770-3775.

[22] Giardina MG, Matarazzo M, Varriale A, Morante R, Napoli A, Martino R. Serum alpha L-fucosidase. A useful marker in the diagnosis of hepatocellular carcinoma. *Cancer* 1992, 70, 1044-1048.

[23] Deugnier Y, David V, Brissot P, Mabo P, Delamaire D, Messner M, Bourel M, Legall JY. Serum alpha-L-fucosidase: a new marker for the diagnosis of primary hepatic carcinoma? *Hepatology* 1984, 4, 889-892.

[24] Ayude D, Fernandez-Rodriguez J, Rodriguez-Berrocal FJ, Martinez-Zorzano VS, de Carlos A, Gil E, Paez de La Cadena M. Value of the serum alpha-L-fucosidase activity in the diagnosis of colorectal cancer. *Oncology* 2000, 59, 310-316.

[25] Abdel-Aleem H, Ahmed A, Sabra AM, Zakhari M, Soliman M, Hamed H. Serum alpha L-fucosidase enzyme activity in ovarian and other female genital tract tumors. *Int J Gynaecol Obstet* 1996, 55, 273-279.

[26] Suzuki M, Shiraha H, Fujikawa T, Takaoka N, Ueda N, Nakanishi Y, Koike K, Takaki A, Shiratori Y. Des-gamma-carboxy prothrombin is a potential autologous growth factor for hepatocellular carcinoma. *J Biol Chem.* 2005, 280, 6409-6415.

[27] Marrero JA, Su GL, Wei W, Emick D, Conjeevaram HS, Fontana RJ, Lok AS. Des-gamma carboxyprothrombin can differentiate hepatocellular carcinoma from nonmalignant chronic liver disease in american patients. *Hepatology* 2003, 37: 1114-1121.

[28] Semela D, Dufour JF. Angiogenesis and hepatocellular carcinoma. *J Hepatol.* 2004, 41, 864-880.

[29] Moon WS, Rhyu KH, Kang MJ, Lee DG, Yu HC, Yeum JH, Koh GY, Tarnawski AS. Overexpression of VEGF and angiopoietin 2: a key to high vascularity of hepatocellular carcinoma? *Mod Pathol.* 2003, 16, 552-557.

[30] Huang GW, Yang LY, Lu WQ. Expression of hypoxia-inducible factor 1alpha and vascular endothelial growth factor in hepatocellular carcinoma: Impact on neovascularization and survival. *World J Gastroenterol.* 2005, 11,1705-1708.

[31] Kubo F, Ueno S, Hiwatashi K, Sakoda M, Kawaida K, Nuruki K, Aikou T. Interleukin 8 in human hepatocellular carcinoma correlates with cancer cell invasion of vessels but not with tumor angiogenesis. *Ann Surg Oncol.* 2005, 12, 800-807.

[32] Ren Y, Poon RT, Tsui HT, Chen WH, Li Z, Lau C, Yu WC, Fan ST. Interleukin-8 serum levels in patients with hepatocellular carcinoma: correlations with clinicopathological features and prognosis. *Clin Cancer Res.* 2003, 9, 5996-6001.

[33] Takeda A, Stoeltzing O, Ahmad SA, Reinmuth N, Liu W, Parikh A, Fan F, Akagi M, Ellis LM. Role of angiogenesis in the development and growth of liver metastasis. *Ann Surg Oncol.* 2002, 9, 610-616.

[34] Song BC, Chung YH, Kim JA, Choi WB, Suh DD, Pyo SI, Shin JW, Lee HC, Lee YS, Suh DJ. Transforming growth factor-beta1 as a useful serologic marker of small hepatocellular carcinoma. *Cancer* 2002, 94, 175-180.

[35] Schulte-Hermann R, Bursch W, Low-Baselli A, Wagner A, Grasl-Kraupp B. Apoptosis in the liver and its role in hepatocarcinogenesis. *Cell Biol Toxicol.* 1997, 13, 339-348.

[36] Liang YR, Wan DS, Chen G, Lu ZH, Li YJ, Lin YH, Chi PD. Detection of serum tumor supplied group of factors and its clinical significance. *Ai Zheng.* 2002, 21, 1251-1253.

[37] Ding X, Yang LY, Huang GW, Yang JQ, Liu HL, Wang W, Peng JX, Yang JQ, Tao YM, Chang ZG, Ling XS. Role of AFP mRNA expression in peripheral blood as a predictor for postsurgical recurrence of hepatocellular carcinoma: a systematic review and meta-analysis. *World J Gastroenterol.* 2005, 11, 2656-2661.

[38] Matsumura M, Niwa Y, Kato N, Komatsu Y, Shiina S, Kawabe T, Kawase T, Toyoshima H, Ihori M, Shiratori Y. Detection of alpha-fetoprotein mRNA, an indicator of hematogenous spreading hepatocellular carcinoma, in the circulation: a possible predictor of metastatic hepatocellular carcinoma. *Hepatology* 1994, 20, 1418-1425.

[39] Sheen IS, Jeng KS, Tsai YC. Is the expression of gamma-glutamyl transpeptidase messenger RNA an indicator of biological behavior in recurrent hepatocellular carcinoma? *World J Gastroenterol.* 2003, 9, 468-473.

[40] Fu XM, Yang QX, Shao CK, Feng ZY. Expressions of h-TERT, c-myc, PCNA and cell apoptosis in liver carcinogenesis. *Nan Fang Yi Ke Da Xue Xue Bao.* 2006, 26:821-823.

[41] Oh BK, Kim YJ, Park YN, Choi J, Kim KS, Park C. Quantitative assessment of hTERT mRNA expression in dysplastic nodules of HBV-related hepatocarcinogenesis. *World J Gastroenterol.* 2005, 11, 2656-2661.

[42] Parish CR. Cancer immunotherapy: the past, the present and the future. *Immunol. Cell Biol* 2003, 81, 106-113.

[43] Burnet FM. Immunological aspects of malignant disease *Lancet* 1967, 1, 1171-1174.

[44] Lewis JD, Reilly BD, Bright RK. Tumor-associated antigens: from discovery to immunity. *Int Rev Immunol* 2003, 22, 81-111.

[45] van der Bruggen P, Traversari C, Chomez P, Lurquin C, De Plaen E, Van den Eynde B, Knuth A, Boon T. A gene encoding an antigen recognized by cytolytic T lymphocytes on a human melanoma. *Science* 1991, 254, 1643-1647.

[46] Rosenberg, SA *Principles and Practice of the Biologic Therapy of Cancer*. Philadelphia: Lippincott, 2000.

[47] Parker KC, Shields M, DiBrino M, Brooks A, Coligan JE. Peptide binding to MHC class I molecules: implications for antigenic peptide prediction. *Immunol Res* 1995, 14, 34-57.

[48] van Bleek G, Nathenson S. Isolation of an endogenously processed immunodominant viral peptide from the class I H-2Kb molecule. *Nature* 1990, 348, 213-216.

[49] Liang P, Pardee AB. Differential display of eukaryotic messenger RNA by means of the polymerase chain reaction. *Science* 1992, 257, 967-971.

[50] Scanlan MJ, Gure AO, Jungbluth AA, Old LJ, Chen YT. Cancer/testis antigens: an expanding family of targets for cancer immunotherapy. *Immun Rev.* 2002, 188, 22-32.

[51] Scanlan MJ, Simpson AJG, Old LJ. The cancer/testis genes: review, standardization, and commentary. *Cancer Immunity* 2004, 4, 1.

[52] Zhao L, Mou DC, Leng XS, Peng JR, Wang WX, Huang L, Li S, Zhu JY. Expression of cancer-testis antigens in hepatocellular carcinoma. *World J Gastroenterol.* 2004, 10, 2034-2038.

[53] Wu LQ, Lu Y, Wang XF, Lv ZH, Zhang B, Yang JY. Expression of cancer-testis antigen (CTA) in tumor tissues and peripheral blood of Chinese patients with hepatocellular carcinoma. *Life Sci.* 2006, 79, 744-748.

[54] Peng JR, Chen HS, Mou DC, Cao J, Cong X, Qin LL, Wei L, Leng XS, Wang Y, Chen WF. Expression of cancer/testis (CT) antigens in Chinese hepatocellular carcinoma and its correlation with clinical parameters. *Cancer Lett.* 2005, 219, 223-232.

[55] Yin YH, Li YY, Qiao H, Wang HC, Yang XA, Zhang HG, Pang XW, Zhang Y, Chen WF. TSPY is a cancer testis antigen expressed in human hepatocellular carcinoma. *Br J Cancer.* 2005, 93, 458-463.

[56] Zhang WM, Xiao G, Zhang M, Guo AL, Dong Y, Wen JM. Expression of NY-ESO-1 and LAGE-1 cancer-testis antigens in hepatocellular carcinoma. *Zhonghua Bing Li Xue Za Zhi.* 2005, 34, 202-205.

[57] Zhang WM, Xiao G, Xie D, Zhang M, Guo AL, Wen JM. Correlation of NY-ESO-1 gene and protein expression to metastasis and clinicopathologic features of hepatocellular carcinoma. *Ai Zheng.* 2005, 24, 622-626.

[58] Shi YY, Wang HC, Yin YH, Sun WS, Li Y, Zhang CQ, Wang Y, Wang S, Chen WF. Identification and analysis of tumour-associated antigens in hepatocellular carcinoma. *Br J Cancer.* 2005, 92, 929-934.

[59] Li B, Qian XP, Pang XW, Zou WZ, Wang YP, Wu HY, Chen WF. HCA587 antigen expression in normal tissues and cancers: correlation with tumor differentiation in hepatocellular carcinoma. *Lab Invest.* 2003, 83, 1185-1192.

[60] Luo G, Huang S, Xie X, Stockert E, Chen YT, Kubuschok B, Pfreundschuh M. Expression of cancer-testis genes in human hepatocellular carcinomas. *Cancer Immun.* 2002, 2, 11.

[61] Bast RC Jr, Lilja H, Urban N, Rimm DL, Fritsche H, Gray J, Veltri R, Klee G, Allen A, Kim N, Gutman S, Rubin MA, Hruszkewycz A. Translational crossroads for biomarkers. *Clin Cancer Res.* 2005, 11, 6103-6108.

[62] Basil CF, Zhao Y, Zavaglia K, Jin P, Panelli MC, Voiculescu S, Mandruzzato S, Lee HM, Seliger B, Freedman RS, Taylor PR, Hu N, Zanovello P, Marincola FM, Wang E. Common cancer biomarkers. *Cancer Res.* 2006, 66, 2953-2961.

[63] Wilson JF. Liver cancer on the rise. *Ann Intern Med.* 2005, 142, 1029-1032.

[64] Grizzi F, Chiriva-Internati M. The complexity of anatomical systems. *Theor Biol Med Model.* 2005, 2, 26.

[65] Szathmary E, Jordan F, Pal C. Molecular biology and evolution. Can genes explain biological complexity? *Science*, 2001, 292, 1315-1316.

[66] Nurse, P. Reductionism. The ends of understanding. *Nature* 1997, 387, 657.

[67] Chiriva-Internati M, Grizzi F, Bright RK, Martin Kast W. Cancer immunotherapy: avoiding the road to perdition. *J Transl Med.* 2004, 2, 26.

[68] Juretic, A., Spagnoli, G.C., Schultz-Thater, E., Sarcevic, B. Cancer/testis tumour-associated antigens: immunohistochemical detection with monoclonal antibodies. *Lancet Oncol* 2003, 4, 104-109.

In: Tumor Markers Research Focus
Editor: Deborah H. Chang, pp. 159-162
ISBN: 978-1-60021-544-5


*Chapter IX*

# Urine Pregancy Test as a Tumor Marker in Male Patients

***Viroj Wiwanitkit***
Department of Laboratory Medicine, Faculty of Medicine, Chulalongkorn University, Bangkok Thailand 10330

## Abstract

Urine pregnancy test is a basic laboratory investigation at present. It is widely used for detection of pregnancy in suspected female cases. Basically, this test used the immunological reaction for detection of human choriogonadotropin (hCG). The hCG is a hormone that is used as a tumor marker. Here, the author reports the application of urine pregnancy test as a tumor marker for male from a tertiary hospital laboratory. It was found that there are some applications of urine pregnancy test as a tumor marker in lung cancer. This application can be an alternative and inexpensive tool in diagnosis and following up the patient with lung cancer.

## Introduction

### A. Pregnancy Test

Urine Pregnancy is an easily available diagnostic test in the present day. Due to the simple basic of immunological principle [1 – 3], many urine pregnancy diagnostic tests were produced [4]. Due to the easily using steps and inexpensive cost per test, it is widely used nowadays. Generally, urine pregnancy is a monitoring of human chorionic gonadotropin (hCG), which is secreted by the trophoblastic cells of the placenta soon after implantation of the fertilized egg into the uterine wall [5 - 6].

Urinary-based ovulation prediction and pregnancy detection tests available for use by nonprofessionals enable women and couples to take an active role in the family planning process [7]. Numerous products are available at reasonable costs to the consumer [7]. hCG from the implanting blastocyst first appears in maternal blood around 6-8 days following fertilization; the levels rise rapidly to reach a peak at 7-10 weeks [8]. With most current pregnancy test kits (sensitivity 25 units per litre) urine may reveal positive results 3-4 days after implantation; by 7 days (the time of the expected period) 98% will be positive [8]. A negative result 1 week after the missed period virtually guarantees that the woman is not pregnant [8].

Pregnancy tests are widely used both by the public and by healthcare professionals. Other pregnancy-specific materials have been proposed as pregnancy tests but none can better the sensitivity and convenience offered by immunoassay of hCG [8]. Ultrasound detection is also not as sensitive as hCG measurement [8]. The current generation of tests is based on monoclonal antibodies to the beta-subunit of hCG; these virtually eliminate the possibility of cross-reaction with pituitary luteinizing hormone (LH) and it is this feature which permits the high sensitivity [8].

As a result both the new knowledge of hCG biochemistry and the production of monoclonal antibodies a number of various tests were developed [9]. Both work consuming and sensitivity are used for estimation of pregnancy tests [9]. In some settings there has been increased testing for hCG by radioreceptor assays based on the binding of hCG to plasma membrane receptor sites and qualitative radioimmunoassay utilizing classic competitive binding techniques [10].

### B. Beta hCG as Tumor Marker

In the human blood and urine there are different antigen forms of choriogonadotropin including nonnicked hCG, nicked hCG, free subunit, free subunit, nicked free, core fragment hCG, hyperglycosylated hCG, nicked hCG missing the subunit C-terminal peptide, asialo hCG, residues 92-145, alternatively nicked hCG--cleaved at 43-44 or 44-45 and others [11]. The value of hCG measurements in the diagnosis of normal pregnancy, pathological pregnancy, Down syndrome screening and oncology: gestational trophoblastic disease, testicular, bladder, digestive tract and other cancers is documented [11].

The International Germ Cell Consensus Classification (IGCCC) of testicular germ cell tumors (TGCT) in 1997 included three serum tumor markers, serum lactate dehydrogenase catalytic concentration (S-LD), serum alpha fetoprotein concentration (S-AFP), and serum -hCG [12]. The hCG is found mainly in nonseminomatous germ cell tumors and they related to the histologic differentiation of the tumors [12]. In various types of cancer, concentrations of hCG as well as its beta-subunit may be elevated, allowing the clinical use of these substances as a tumor marker. The relation between laboratory outcome and clinical status is assessed, with emphasis on the beta-hCG in gynecological malignancies [13]. Presently, it is accepted the hCG is the first reliable tumor marker for gestational trophoblastic disease [14].

## Application of Urine Pregnancy Test as a Tumor Marker

### A. Report on Using Urine Pregnancy Test as a Tumor Marker

Information on epitope forming sequences of hCG and its subunits alpha and beta has significant impact on the examination of intra- and extracellular metabolism and the standardization of diagnostic assay systems [15]. Variants of hCG appear in biological fluids with variable modifications on different parts of the molecule [15]. The urine pregnancy test based on hCG determination is the most widely used non-serum hCG test. In addition to its main purpose for diagnosis of pregnancy, it is also used for other purposes. It is used in patients suspected of having an ectopic pregnancy [16]. It is also applied for screening for gestational trophoblastic disease although the result is not favorable [17].

## B. Experience in Using Urine Pregnancy Test as Tumor Marker in Male Patients

Here, the author reports the application of urine pregnancy test as a tumor marker for male from a tertiary hospital laboratory. This study is performed as a retrospective study. The data from medical records of all cases who got diagnostic urine pregnancy test at a division of Laboratory Medicine in Bangkok Thailand during year 2005 were reviewed. The urine pregnancy test mentioned in this study a one step pregnancy test, rapid one-step membrane test for detection of HCG in urine (One Step hCG Pregnancy Test, Search Tech Co. Ltd Thailand). The accuracy of the test is about 99%. In this work, any cases with undetermined results, presenting with weakly positive result, are re-analyzed using the second urine samples collected at 2 – 4 weeks after the first samples. Results in medical records were reviewed and collected. Records that had no complete data were excluded.

According to this review, there are upto 2,000 urine pregnancy test. Of interest, there are some requests for male subjects. These tests were verified for the correct patient identification to the physician in charge and got confirmation. The details of the 5 detected tests were studied. All of the 5 requests are from the pulmonary clinic. All patients are the suspected cases of germ cell lung cancer.

The results of a urine pregnancy test were positive in 2 cases. Further examination showed that the beta-human chorionic gonadotropin level was markedly elevated both in the serum and the urine of these 2 patients. Subsequently, testing of a bronchoscopic biopsy specimen proved these tumors to be gern cell cancer.

Generally, germ cell lung cancer in male is a rare cancer and is usually a secondary metastasis from testes [18]. A grossly elevated serum hCG concentration can be seen in the patient with this cancer [19].

Here, it can be seen that the high urine hCG can also be seen and detectable by simple urine pregnancy test. It was found that there are some applications of urine pregnancy test as a tumor marker in lung cancer. This application can be an alternative and inexpensive tool in diagnosis and following up the patient with lung cancer. This finding is concordant with a previous report of Tsai et al that that the urine pregnancy test, a simple and convenient method, would be very useful in the rapid diagnosis of primary pulmonary choriocarcinoma in men [20].

# References

[1] Cunningham FG, MacDonald PC, Gant NF, Levon KJ, Gilstrap III LC. *Pregnancy*. In: Cunningham FG, MacDonald PC, Gant NF, Levon KJ, Gilstrap III LC. William *Obstetrics*. 19th ed. Norwalk: CT Appleton Large, 1993: 11 – 56.

[2] Vattanaviboon P. Pregnancy test. *J Med Tech Assoc Thai* 1997 Jun; 25(1): 19 – 25.

[3] Dunnihoo DR. Test for pregancy. In: Dunnihoo DR. *Fundamentals of Gynecology and Obstetrics.* 1st ed. Philadelphia: Lippinncott, 1990: 262 – 3.

[4] Kin PT, Wee A, Dan L, Guo J. Diagnostic test – O & G / Pregnancy. In: Kin PT, Wee A, Dan L, Guo J. MIMS Medex 97. 1st ed. Bangkok: *Medi & Media*, 1997: 145 – 6.

[5] Chard T. Pregnancy tests: a review. *Hum Reprod.*1992;7:701-10.

[6] Morita H, Maruo T. Human chorionic gonadotropin (hCG) and subunits. *Nippon Rinsho*. 2005 Aug;63 Suppl 8:464-8

[7] Eichner SF, Timpe EM. Urinary-based ovulation and pregnancy: point-of-care testing. *Ann Pharmacother*. 2004 Feb;38(2):325-31.

[8] Chard T. Pregnancy tests: a review. *Hum Reprod.* 1992 May;7(5):701-10.

[9] Kunkel S. Pregnancy tests. *Zentralbl Gynakol.* 1988;110(12):750-6.

[10] Rippey JH. Pregnancy tests: evaluation of current status. *Crit Rev Clin Lab Sci.* 1984;19(4):353-9.

[11] Skalba P, Gajewska K, Bednarska-Czerwinska A. Choriogonadotropin measurements--critical assessment of new diagnostic possibilities. *Ginekol Pol.* 2004 Mar;75(3):221-7.

[12] von Eyben FE. Laboratory markers and germ cell tumors. *Crit Rev Clin Lab Sci.* 2003 Aug;40(4):377-427.

[13] Schutter EM, Mulder C, van Kamp GJ, Kenemans P. The beta-core fragment of human chorionic gonadotropin: biochemical background and clinical application. *Anticancer Res*. 1997 Mar-Apr;17(2B):1255-72.

[14] Lewis JL Jr. Diagnosis and management of gestational trophoblastic disease. *Cancer.* 1993 Feb 15;71(4 Suppl):1639-47.

[15] Lechner O, Dirnhofer S, Gerth R, Merz WE, Wick G, Berger P. Fragments of human chorionic gonadotropin (hCG): diagnosis of pregnancy and tumors. *Wien Klin Wochenschr*. 1995;107(1):15-9.

[16] Cartwright PS, Victory DF, Moore RA, Anderson JR, Brown DH. Performance of a new enzyme-linked immunoassay urine pregnancy test for the detection of ectopic gestation. *Ann Emerg Med.* 1986 Oct;15(10):1198-9.

[17] Civantos F, Rywlin AM. Carcinomas with trophoblastic differentiation and secretion of chorionic gonadotrophins. *Cancer*. 1972 Mar;29(3):789-98.

[18] Al-Ghamdi AM, Flint JD, Muller NL, Stewart KC. Hilar pulmonary granular cell tumor: a case report and review of the literature. *Ann Diagn Pathol.* 2000 Aug;4(4):245-51.

[19] Tilbrook LK, Slater J, Blainey AD. Testicular germ cell tumour presenting as thyrotoxicosis. *Ann Clin Biochem*. 2004 May;41(Pt 3):248-9.

[20] Tsai JR, Chong IW, Hung JY, Tsai KB. Use of urine pregnancy test for rapid diagnosis of primary pulmonary choriocarcinoma in a man. *Chest*. 2002 Mar;121(3):996-8.

In: Tumor Markers Research Focus
Editor: Deborah H. Chang, pp. 163-176

ISBN: 978-1-60021-544-5


*Chapter X*

# Epidermal Growth Factor-Like Motifs in Proteins Associated with Embryonic Development and Tumor Growth: Possible Markers for Common Functions

*A.A. Terentiev* and N.T. Moldogazieva*
Department of Biochemistry, Russian State Medical University,
Ostrovityanova Street, 1, Moscow, Russia

## Abstract

In this chapter we demonstrate that short seven-amino acid residue motifs with high degree of similarity to the sequence LDKYACN (residues 26-32) of human epidermal growth factor (EGF) are characteristic for a number of tumor-associated fetal proteins including alpha-fetoprotein (AFP) and growth factors of EGF family and transforming growth factor (TGF-β) superfamily. Besides, the EGF motifs were found in proteins involved cell adhesion and migration. In multi-modular proteins such motifs are localized within their EGF-like modules. An EGF-like motif LDSYQCT of human AFP (residues 14-20) has been obtained as isolated peptidic fragment using solid phase chemistry and tested for biological activity. Ability of this peptide to regulate cell proliferation and apoptosis has been experimentally demonstrated. Here we suppose that the short EGF-like motifs are responsible for common functions of the proteins and may be considered as a signature of their participation in regulation of embryonic and tumor cell proliferation, differentiation, migration and survival.

* E-mail address: aaterent@mtu-net.ru(Corresponding author)

# Introduction

It has been long established that growth factors and their cognate receptors are involved in regulation of proliferation, differentiation, migration and apoptosis of embryonic and tumor cells [1-4]. Among these growth factors are the members of epidermal growth factor (EGF) family and transforming growth factor (TGF-β) superfamily which have emerged as regulators of a variety of developmental processes. Expression of the growth factors and their receptors has been demonstrated to occur with high frequency in a majority of human carcinomas. Important role of the growth factors during embryonic development and tumor growth allows considering them as oncofetal proteins. They display properties similar to that of tumor-associated fetal proteins such as alpha-fetoprotein (AFP). In this chapter we demonstrate that the non-homologous and non-related proteins possessing the ability to regulate embryonic and tumor cell proliferation and survival contain short seven-residue EGF-like motifs which include highly conserved amino acids.

Earlier long epidermal growth factor (EGF)-like modules of 25-40 amino acid residues have been shown for different mosaic multi-modular proteins possessing numerous biological functions. A suggestion has been made that these modules may play a role of signals for proliferation and differentiation. In our laboratory the short seven-amino acid residue EGF-like motifs were revealed in the proteins in direct as well as in inverted form. Interestingly, in human EGF a direct motif LDKYACN (residues 26-32) and inverted motif RCQYRDL (residues 41-47) contain amino acids important for receptor binding. This may indicate that the CO- and NH- groups of human EGF main chain are not involved in binding with the receptor; direction of the polypeptide chain seems to have no significance in receptor binding.

# Epidermal Growth Factor and Its Family

Epidermal growth factor belongs to EGF family of structurally and functionally related polypeptides which includes transforming growth factor-α (TGF-α), amphiregulin, heparin-binding EGF-like growth factor, betacellulin, epiregulin, tomoregulin and isoforms of neuregulin (NRG-1, NGR-2, NRG-3 and NRG-4) [5]. More recently an EGF-CFC subfamily of EGF-related growth factors has also been described [6, 7]. Most of these growth factors are synthesized as cell membrane associated precursors that are biologically active and can function as regulators of cell adhesion and migration [8]. Such cell-anchored precursors can contribute to spreading of embryonic and tumor cells and participate in tumor invasion and metastasis.

All members of the EGF family is a single chain polypeptides which consist of approximately 50-60 amino acids in mature form and are characterized by specifically spaced six disulphide-bonded cysteine residues (Fig. 1). The disulphide bonds form three loops: loop A (residues 6-20), loop B (residues 14-31) and loop C (residues 33-42) [9, 10]. The hinge region formed by a single amino acid (N32) is located between the loops B and C. Two structurally well-defined domains are identified in human EGF by NMR spectroscopy: N-terminus domain containing major three stranded anti-parallel β-sheet and C-terminus domains with minor β-sheet.

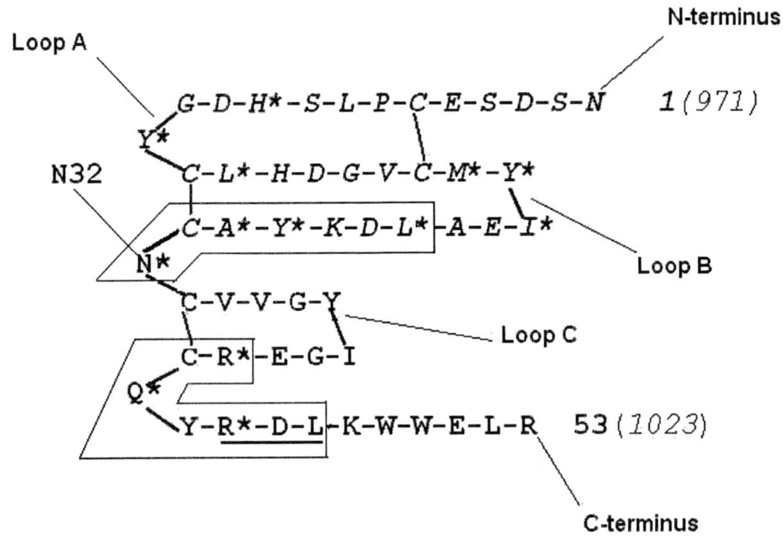


Figure 1. Primary structure of human epidermal growth factor .The direct and inverted motifs LDKYACN (residues 26-32) and RCQYRDL (residues 41-47) are indicated. Asterisks (*) mark amino acids important for receptor binding. A single amino acid N32 represents a hinge region.

Most of the EGF family growth factors can function by binding to and activating the specific transmembrane receptor tyrosine kinases (RTK) which belong to ErbB family of receptors. This family consists of four receptors (ErbB-1 or EGFR, ErbB-2, ErbB-3 and ErbB-4) which share most of the intracellular effectors activated by binding of growth factors to the extracellular domain of the receptors [11]. It has been demonstrated that the extracellular domain of EGFR may be divided into four sub-domains designated as I, II, III and IV [12]. Activating of the intracellular effectors induces RAS/RAF/MEK/MAPK signaling pathway [13].

The highly conserved half-cystine and glycine residues in EGF-related growth factors may be essential for binding to their receptors. Several other residues have been also demonstrated to be involved in receptor binding. Crystal structure of a complex of human EGFR and its ligand showed that there are three ligand-binding sites in the receptor molecule: site 1 is located in subdomain I; sites 2 and 3 are located in subdomain III of the receptor [14]. The crystal structure analysis as well as site-directed mutagenesis studies showed that the amino acid residues M21, I23 L26, A30 and N32 in the loop B participate in hydrophobic and hydrogen bonding with the site 1 [15-17]. A residue K28 is involved in electrostatic interactions with the same site. Amino acid residues H10, Y13 and L15 in the loop A interact with site 2 of EGFR [18, 19]. Amino acids located in the C-terminus of the growth factor, namely, R41, Q43, R45 and L47 participate in hydrophobic and hydrogen bonding with the site 3 of the receptor [20].

Most of the precursors of ErbB ligands contain EGF-like modules in their transmembrane region [21]. These modules consist of approximately 25-40 residues in length and contain very few conserved residues. For example an EGF precursor of 1207 amino acids in length contains not only the sequence of EGF itself but also eight EGF-like repeats [9]. The EGF-like domains that can occur as modular units can also be found in some proteins which are not considered as ErbB ligands. Such modules are characteristic for vertebrates and invertebrates and have been found in many multi-domains, mosaic proteins with various biological functions, such as regulation of cell proliferation and differentiation, cell migration and adhesion as well as blood coagulation and fibrinolysis [22-24]. Among the proteins possessing EGF-like modules are the members of EGF-CFC subfamily, extracellular matrix proteins, mouse mosaic polydom protein and others [25-27]. On the basis of revealing of EGF-like modules in proteins that exhibit growth promoting activity a suggestion has been made that these EGF-like modules may play a role of signals for proliferation and differentiation [27].

## Alpha-Fetoprotein as a Protein with EGF-like Motif

In our laboratory a short EGF-like motif consisting of seven amino acid residues has been revealed in human alpha-fetoprotein (AFP) [28, 29]. Alpha-fetoprotein is a major mammalian tumor associated fetal protein which possesses various biological activities including binding of different hydrophobic ligands, stimulation of embryonic and tumor cell proliferation, induction of apoptosis and regulation of immune cell functions [30-32]. Thus, it may be considered as a multi-functional protein.

AFP is a member of an albuminoid gene family, which currently consists of four proteins: albumin (ALB), vitamin D-binding protein (VTDB), AFP, and alpha-albumin (αALB), termed afamin in humans [33, 34]. This family is characterized by three-domain structure (domains I, II and III) which has been demonstrated by X-ray crystallography [35-37]. The family proteins also demonstrate considerable degree of primary structure similarity: up to 40% identity between human AFP and ALB. Alpha-fetoprotein is cysteine-rich protein that contains 32 highly conserved cysteine residues including double-cysteines. The cysteine residues form 15 regular spaced disulfide bonds with exception of two first ones which do not participate in disulfide bridging. Four disulfide bonds are localized in domain I, five – in domain II and six – in domain III.

To date, primary structures of AFP for eleven species have been identified including human, gorilla, chimpanzee, horse, bovine, dog, pig, woodchuck, mouse and rat (Swiss-Prot/TrEMBL and GenBank databases). The primary structure of human AFP consists of 609 amino acids including signal peptide which are removed during processing; as a consequence a mature polypeptide chain containing 591 amino acid residues arises [38, 39]. Comparison of primary structure of AFP with structures of other physiologically active proteins has shown that it is a mosaic and multi-modular protein. Overall, more than 20 distinct functionally important sites with predicted and experimentally confirmed biological activity have been revealed in human AFP [40, 41]. Localization of these sites has allowed constructing structural and functional map of alpha-fetoprotein [42]. Among these functionally important sites is the peptide LDSYQCT (residues 14-20) which represent an EGF-like motif of human AFP (figure 2). This motif has been revealed in the AFP region with low similarity to human albumin. There is up to 57% identity and 86% of total similarity between the sequences LDSYQCT of human AFP and LDKYACN (residues 26-32) of human EGF (table 1).

This EGF-like motif of human AFP has been obtained as an isolated peptide fragment using solid phase chemistry. The biological activity of this synthetic peptide has been tested experimentally. Study of this peptide in our laboratory showed that it can regulate *in vitro* cell proliferation and apoptosis as well as immune system functioning [43-45].

**Table 1. EGF-like motifs in proteins associated with development and tumor growth**

| Name of protein and position of EGF-like motif | Sequence of EGF-like motif | Identity | Conserved substitu-tions | Total similari-ty, % | Swiss-Prot/ TrEMBL database accession numbers |
|---|---|---|---|---|---|
| Hum. EGF (res. 26-32) | L D K Y A C N | 7/7 (100%) | 0/7 (0%) | 100 | P01133 |
| Mouse EGF (res. 26-32) | L D S Y T C N | 5/7 (71%) | 1/7 (14%) | 85 | P01132 |
| Hum. AFP (res.14-20) | L D S Y Q C T | 5/7 (71%) | 1/7 (14%) | 85 | P02771 |
| Hum. TGF-α (res. 27-33) | E D K P A C V | 4/7(57%) | 1/7 (14%) | 71 | P01135 |
| Hum. betacellulin (res. 57-63) | E Q T P S C V | 1/7 (14%) | 3/7 (43%) | 57 | P35070 |
| Rat HB-EFG (res. 88-94) | L R I P S C H | 2/7 (28%) | 3/7(43%) | 71 | Q06175 |
| Rab. prostaglandin G/H synthase 1 (res. 28-34) | L D R Y Q C D | 4/7(57%) | 2/7 (28%) | 85 | 097554 |
| Vaccinia growth factor (res. 45- 51) | I D G M Y C R | 2/7 (28%) | 3/7 (43%) | 71 | P20494 |
| Hum. epigen (res. 48-54) | L E K A I C R | 3/7 (43%) | 2/7 (28%) | 71 | Q6UW88 |
| Neurogenic Notch (res. 720-726) | I N G Y N C S | 27 (28%) | 4/7 (57%) | 86 | P07207 |
| Hum. lactadherin (res. 27-33 ) | F P S Y T C T | 2/7 (28%) | 4/7 (57%) | 86 | Q08431 |
| Hum.cadherin-related TSH (res. 3989-3996) | L D G A V C Q | 3/7 (43%) | 2/7 (28%) | 71 | Q14517 |
| Hum. matrilin-2 (res. 357-363) | D D S Y T C E | 4/7(57%) | 2/7 (28%) | 86 | 000339 |
| Hum. coagulation factor VII (res. 65-71) | L Q S Y I C F | 3/7 (43%) | 3/7 (43%) | 86 | P08709 |
| Hum. tomoregulin (res. 68-74) | G E S Y Q N E | 1/7 (14%) | 4/7(57%) | 71 | Q9UK5 |
| Hum. VEGF (res. 18-24) | M D V Y Q R S | 2/7 (28%) | 3/7(43%) | 71 | P15692 |
| EGF-modules of mouse polydom: | | | | | |
| a) EGF-Ca (res. 1726-1732) | L D V D E C A | 3/7 (43%) | 1/7 (14%) | 57 | Q9ES77 |
| b) EGF-Ca x6 (res.1270-1276) | L A S Y R C T | 3/7 (43%) | 2/7 (28%) | 71 | Q9ES77 |
| c) EGF-Ca x6 (res. 1384-1390) | L N S Y S C K | 3/7 (43%) | 3/7 (43%) | 86 | Q9ES77 |

Abbreviations: AFP – alpha-fetoprotein, EGF – epidermal growth factor, TGF-α – transforming growth factor-α, HB-EFG – heparin-binding EGF-like growth factor, VEGF – vascular endothelial cell growth factor, TSH – tumor suppressor homolog, EGF-Ca – EGF domain with Ca $^{2+}$-binding activity (x6 и x3 means number of repeats).

Numeration of amino acid residues is given for mature polypeptide chains.

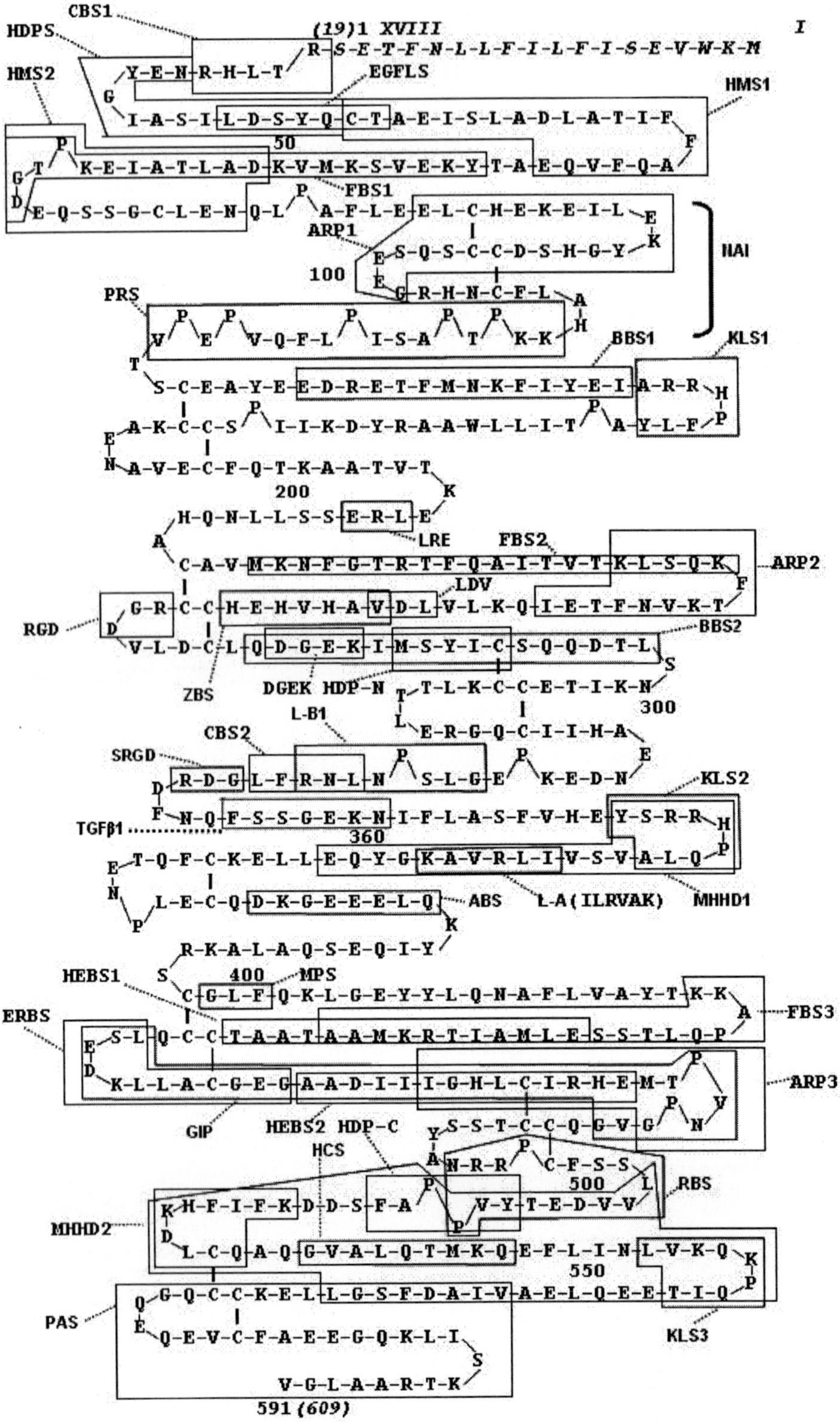


Figure 2. Structural and functional map of human alpha-fetoprotein.

I-XVIII – signal peptide;
EGFLS – epidermal growth factor like segment (residues 14-20);
TGFβ1 – segment of transforming growth factor β1 (residues 324-330);
GIP – growth inhibitory peptide (residues 446-479);
FBS – fatty acid-binding sites: FBS1 (residues 42-62), FBS2 (residues 209-228), FBS3 (residues 419-438);
HEBS1 – major estrogen-binding site (residues 428-449);
HEBS2 – additional estrogen-binding site (residues 458-471);
HDPS – homeodomain protein segment (residues 6-18); HDP-N – N-terminus segment, HDP-C – C-terminus segment (residues 267-271 and 501-508, consequently);
ERBS – estrogen-receptor-binding site (residues 446-457);
CBS1 and CBS2 – cycline-binding segments 1 and 2 (residues 1-5 and 312-316);
BBS1 and BBS2 – bilirubin-binding sites 1 and 2 (residues 135-148 and 261-277);
ABS – actin-binding site (residues 377-384);
HMS1 and HMS2 –heavy metal-binding sites 1 and 2 (residues 19-39 и 51-71);
NAI – non albumin identity site (residues 30-120);
PRS – proline rich segment (residues 111-129);
KLS1, KLS2 and KLS3 –kinetensin-like segments 1, 2 and 3 (residues 148-156, 340-348 and 538-546);
LRE, LDV, RGD, DGEK, ILRVAK – cell adhesion motifs (residues 195-197, 242-244, 253-255, 262-265 and 352-357);
SRGD – segment reverse to RGD (residues 318-320);
MHHD1 and MHHD2 –hetero- and homodimerization motifs (residues 340-361 and 497-560);
HCS – histocompatability class II segment (residues 524-532);
MPS – milk peptide segment (residues 399-401);
PAS – plasminogen activator segment (residues 553-591);
ZBS – zink-binding site (II) (residues 244-250);
RBS – receptor-binding site (residues 489-504);
L-B1 – laminin B1 segment (residues 307-314);
L-A – laminin A segment (residues 352-357);
ARP1, ARP2, ARP3 – apoptosis related peptides 1, 2, 3) (residues 79-102, 224-237 and 463-478).

# Searching the EGF-like Motifs

## Direct EGF-like Motifs

As described above, initially the short EGF-like motif displaying high similarity with the sequence LDKYACN of human EGF was found in human AFP. Then the amino acid sequence of the segment LDKYACN was compared with the protein sequences derived from Swiss-Prot/TrEMBL database using FASTA program [53, 54].

Matches were found largely with proteins associated with embryonic development and tumor growth. Short EGF-like motifs were revealed in transforming growth factors-β: TGF-β1 and TGF- β3 (table 2). These motifs represent the amino acid sequences LDTNYCF (residues 2-8) in both growth factors and LDTQYSK (residues 54-60) in TGF-β1 [42]. The role of TGF-βs and their receptors in regulation of embryonic development and tumor growth has been well established [1, 2]. All the TGF-βs (TGF-β1, TGF-β2 and TGF- β3) function through the same signaling pathway which involves binding the growth factors to and activating the type I and type II receptors. The only well-characterized intracellular effectors activated by TGF-β receptors are structurally related proteins named Smads [46-48]. However, evidence is accumulated that TGF-βs can function through effectors of other pathways [49, 50]. Recruitment of additional co-activators and co-repressors allows crosstalk with other signaling pathways. Such a crosstalk exists between the Smad-mediated and RAS/RAF/MEK/MAPK signaling pathways. In other words, there is an interaction between EGF- and TGF-β-activated pathways through their intracellular effectors.

**Table 2. EGF-like motifs in human transforming growth factors TGF-β**

| Name of protein and position of EGF-like motif | Sequence of EGF-like motif | Identity | Conservative substitutions | Total similari-ty,% | Swiss-Prot/ TrEMBL database accession number |
|---|---|---|---|---|---|
| EGF (res. 26-32) | L D K Y A C N | 7/7 (100%) | 0/7 (0%) | 100 | P01133 |
| TGF-β1 (res. 2-8) | L D T N Y C F | 3/7 (43%) | 2/7 (28%) | 71 | P01137 |
| TGF-β1 (res. 54-60) | L D T Q Y S K | 2/7 (29%) | 4/7 (57%) | 86 | P61812 |
| TGF-β3 (res.2-8) | L D T N Y C F | 3/7 (43%) | 2/7 (28%) | 71 | P10600 |

Abbreviations: EGF – epidermal growth factor, TGFβ1 – transforming growth factor β1, TGFβ3 – transforming growth factor β3.
Numeration of amino acid residues is given for mature polypeptide chains

Amino acid sequences with high similarity to EGF-like motif of human AFP were found in other members of EGF family, such as tomoregulin, betacellulin etc. EGF-like motifs were found also in other proteins which are not ErbB ligands, such as vascular endothelium growth factor (VEGF) (table 1). VEGF stimulates angiogenesis and vasculogenesis during embryonic development and tumor growth and functions through receptor tyrosine kinase-mediated signaling [51, 52]. The specific receptor of VEGF is expressed by endothelial cells and requires integrin-mediated cell adhesion to the extracellular matrix.

FASTA sequence comparison revealed matches with some proteins that play important role in cell to cell or cell to extracellular matrix communication. These interactions are necessary for cell spreading and migration during embrio- and cancerogenesis. For example, matches were fond with lactadherin, or milk fat globule EGF factor 8, (MFG-8) which can bind integrins and targets endothelial cells to integrin-dependent angiogenesis [55]. It also can bind to apoptotic cell and promotes their phagocytosis.

EGF-like motifs and their repeats of were found within the EGF-like modules of mosaic multi-domain proteins that play a role in a variety of developmental processes by regulation of cell fate. Among them: mammalian homolog of Drosophila delta-like proteins, neurogenic locus of Notch protein, and the newly described protein matrilin-2 (table 1). FASTA matches were found also with mouse polydom protein, encoded by cloning DNA in murine bone-marrow stromal cell line MS-5 [26]. The particular multi-domain structure of the polydom protein suggested its important role in cell adhesion and immune system function.

## Inverted EGF-like Motifs

The EGF-like motifs not only in direct but also in inverted form are presented in proteins associated with development and tumor growth (table 3). Largely, these proteins are the EGF-family growth factors: TGF-α, betacellulin, NRG-3, EGF itself and also the proteins involved in cell adhesion and migration. A consensus sequence CXXGY/FXGX was revealed between the direct and inverted EGF-like motifs in the most proteins. It is characteristic for EGF, TGF-α, betacellulin, vaccinia growth factor, epigen (epithelial mitogen), heparin-binding EGF-like growth factor, neurogenic locus of Notch protein, lactadherin (MFG-8), prostaglandin G/H synthase 1, cadherin-related tumor suppressor homolog, etc.

**Table 3. Inverted EGF-like motifs in proteins associated with development and tumor growth**

| Name of protein and position of EGF-like motif | Sequence of EGF-like motif | Identity | Conservative substitutions | Total similari-ty, % | Swiss-Prot/ TrEMBL database accession number |
|---|---|---|---|---|---|
| Hum. EGF (res. 41-47) | R C Q Y R D L | 7/7(100%) | 0/7(0%) | 100 | P01133 |
| Hum. TGF-α (res. 42-48) | R C E H A D L | 4/7 (57%) | 2/7 (29%) | 86 | P01135 |
| Hum. betacellulin (res. 71-77) | R C E R V D L | 4/7 (57%) | 2/7 (29%) | 86 | P35070 |
| Hum. NRG-3 (res. 5-11) | P C R D K D L | 3/7 (43%) | 2/7 (28%) | 71 | P56975 |
| Hum. delta-like protein 4 (res. 470-476) | A T C Y T D L | 3/7 (43%) | 3/7 (43%) | 86 | Q9NR61 |
| Hum. epigen (res. 63-69 ) | R C E H L T L | 3/7 (43%) | 3/7 (43%) | 86 | Q6UW88 |
| Neurogenic Notch (res. 735-341 | N C Q Y K L N | 3/7 (43%) | 2/7 (28%) | 71 | P07207 |
| Hum. lactadherin (res. 32-38) | H C E T K C V | 1/7(14%) | 6/7(86%) | 100 | Q08431 |
| Vaccinia growth factor (res. 58-64) | R C Q H V V L | 4/7 (57%) | 1/7(14%) | 71 | P20494 |
| Rat HB-EFG (res. 103-109) | R C H G L T L | 3/7 (43%) | 2/7 (28%) | 71 | Q06175 |
| Rab. prostaglandin G/H synthase 1 (res. 44-60) | N C T V P D L | 3/7 (43%) | 2/7 (28%) | 71 | 097554 |
| Hum. cadherin-related TSH (res. 4012-4018 | R C Q S D I D | 3/7 (43%) | 2/7 (28%) | 71 | Q14517 |

Abbreviations: EGF – epidermal growth factor, TGF-α – transforming growth factor-α, NRG – neuregulin, HB-EFG – heparin-binding EGF-like growth factor, TSH – tumor suppressor homolog.
Numeration of amino acid residues is given for mature polypeptide chains.

As described bellow the inverted motif of human EGF contains amino acid residues participating in receptor binding. On this basis we suggest that the inverted motifs are also important for the proteins functioning during embrio- and cancerogenesis.

## Functional Importance of Direct and Inverted EGF-like Motifs

As mentioned above the sequence LDKYACN (residues 26-32) is a part of loop B of human EGF and contains amino acid residues participating in interaction with EGFR. These residues include L26, A30 and N32 which participate in hydrophobic and hydrogen bonding with the site 1 of the receptor [14-18]. The inverted motif RCQYRDL (residues 41-47) is located near the C-terminus of human EGF and also contains amino acids which interact with the receptor. Four of the seven residues, namely R41, Q43, R45 and L47, participate in hydrophobic and hydrogen bonding with the site 3 of the receptor (figure 1). Consequently, these two sequences, the direct and inverted EGF-like motifs, are involved in very important functional property of the growth factor and provide the insight to molecular basis of receptor binding and signaling. As for inverted motif, it seems that a direction of the EGF polypeptide chain has no significance in receptor binding; CO- and NH- groups of the main chain are not involved in binding with the receptor.

Similarly, the EGF-like motifs of other growth factors and AFP might be involved in their functioning through participation in receptor binding and signal transduction. To date little is known about structure of AFP receptor and there is no experimental data on molecular basis of receptor binding and signaling.

Comparison of two sequences: LDKYACN in human EGF and LDSYQCT in human AFP, allows suggesting that the motif in human AFP might also be a part of its receptor-binding site. In these sequences the following amino acid residues correspond to each other. Residues L14 and Q18 in AFP correspond to L26 and A30 in EGF. As mentioned above the latter two residues participate in binding with the site 1 of the receptor, so it may be suggested that L14 and Q18 in AFP also can participate in hydrophobic interactions with its receptor. Residue T20 in human AFP corresponds to N32 in human EGF, which participates in hydrogen bonding. Consequently, hydroxyl group of T20 may be able to interact with the receptor of AFP in similar manner.

## Conclusion

Alpha-fetoprotein, growth factors and some other proteins which participate in regulation of embryonic development and tumor growth contain short EGF-like motifs which are proposed to be responsible for their common functions. These motifs may be considered as possible structural and functional markers of proteins for their involving in cell proliferation, survival, migration and adhesion.

In case of multi-modular and multi-functional proteins, such as AFP, other functions may be provided by other, specific, biologically important sites and may be mediated by different signaling pathways.

# References


[1] Favoni, R. E., & De Cupis, A. (2000). The role of polypeptide growth factors in human carcinomas: new targets for a novel pharmacological approach. *Pharmacol. Rev.*, 52(2), 179-206.

[2] Derynck, R., Akrhurt, R. J., & Balmain, A. (2001). TGF-β signaling in tumor suppression and cancer progression. *Nature Gen.*, *29*, 117-129.

[3] Normanno, N., Bianco, C., De Luca, A., Maiello, M.R., & Salomon, D.S. (2003). Target-based agents against ErbB receptor and their ligands: a novel approach to cancer treatment. *Endocr.-Rel. Cancer,* 10, 1-21.

[4] Chang, H., Brown, C.W., & Matzuk, M. (2002). Genetic analysis of the mammalian transforming growth factor superfamily. *Endocr. Rev.*, 23(6), 787-823.

[5] Normanno, N., Bianco, C., De Luca A, & Salomon, D.S. (2001). The role of EFG-related peptides in tumor growth. *Frontiers in Bioscience,* 6, d685-d707.

[6] Salomon, D.S., Bianco, C., Ebert, A.D., Khan, N.I., Santis, M.D., Normanno, N., Wechselberger, C., Seno, M.,Williams, K., Sanicola, M., Foley, S., Gullick, W.J., & Persico, G. (2000). The EGF-CFC family: novel epidermal growth factor-related proteins in development and cancer. *Endocr.-Rel. Cancer,* 7, 199-226.

[7] Adamson, E.D., Minchiotti, G., P., & Salomon, D.S. (2002). Cripto: a tumor growth factor and more. *J. Cell. Physiol.*, 190, 267-278.

[8] Massague, J., & Padiella, A. (1993). Membrane-anchored growth factors. *Ann. Rev. Biochem.* 62, 515-541.

[9] Bell, G.I., Fong, N.M., Stempien, M. M., Wormsted M. A., Caput , D., Ku L.L., Urdea, M. S., Rall, L.B., & Sanchez-Pescador, R. (1986). Human epidermal growth factor precursor: cDNA sequence, expression in vitro and gene organization. *Nucleic Acids Res.* 14, 8427-8446.

[10] Groenen, L.C., Nice, E.C., & Burgess A.W. (1994) Structure-function relationships for the EGF/TGF-alpha-family of mitogens. *Growth Factors,* 11(4), 235-257.

[11] Olayioye M.E., Neve R.M., Lane H. A., & Hynes N.E. (2000). The ErbB signaling network: receptor dimerization in development and cancer. *EMBO J.*, 19, 3159-3167.

[12] Ward, C.W., Hoyne, P.I., & Flegg, R.H. (1995). Insulin and epidermal growth factor receptors contain the cysteine repeat motif found in the tumor necrosis factor receptor. *Proteins,* 22, 141-153.

[13] Wellbrock, C., Karasarides, M., & Maraus, M. (2004). The RAF proteins take centre stage. *Nature Rev. Mol. Cell Biol.*, 5, 875-885.

[14] Ogiso, H., Ishitani, R., Nureki, O., Fukai, S., Yamanaka, M., Kim, J-H., Saito, K., Sakamoto, A., Inoue, M., Shirouzu, M., & Yokoyama, S. (2002). Crystal structure of the complex of human epidermal growth factor and receptor extracellular domains. *Cell,* 110, 775-787.

[15] Campion, S.R., Matsunami, R.K., Engler, D.A., & Niyogi, S.K. (1990). Biochemical properties of site-directed mutants of human epidermal growth factor: importance of solvent exposed hydrophobic residues of the amino-terminal domain in receptor binding. *Biochemistry,* 29, 9988-9993.

[16] Koide, H., Muto, Y., Kasai, H., Kohri, K., Hoshi, K., Takahashi, S., H., Tsukumo, K., Sasaki, T., Oka, T., & Miyake, T. (1992. A site-directed mutagenesis study on the role

of isoleucyne-23 of human epidermal growth factor in receptor binding. *Biochim. Biophys. Acta.,* 1120, 257-261.

[17] Koide, H., Muto, Y., Kasai, H., Hoshi, K., Takusari, H., Kohri, K., Takahashi, S., Sasaki, T., Tsukumo, K., & Miyake, T. (1992). Recognition of antiparallel beta-sheet structure of human epidermal growth factor by its receptor. Site-directed mutagenesis studies of Ala-30 and Asn-32. *FEBS Lett.,* 302, 39-42.

[18] Tadaki, D.K., & Niyogi, S.K. (1993). The functional importance of hydrophobicity of the tyrosine at position 13 of human epidermal growth factor in receptor binding. *J. Biol.Chem.,* 268, 10114-10119.

[19] Murray, M.B., Tadaki, D.K., Campion, S.R., Lamerdin, J.A., Srepersu, E.H., Bradrick, T.D., & Niyogi, S.K. (1998). Structure-function analysis of a conserved aromatic cluster in the N-terminal domain of human epidermal growth factor. *Protein engineering,* 11(11), 1041-1050.

[20] Engler, D.A., Campion, R.S., Hauser, M.R., Cook, J.S., & Nioyagi S.K. (1992). Critical functional requirement for the guanidinium group of the arginine 41 side chain of human epidermal growth factor as revealed my mutagenic inactivation and chemical reactivation. *J. Biol. Chem.,* 267, 2271-2281.

[21] Davis, G.G. (1990). The many faces of epidermal growth factor repeats. *New Biol.,* 2, 410-419.

[22] Doolitlte F.R., (1995). The multiplicity of domains in proteins. *Annu. Rev. Biochem.,* 64, 287-314.

[23] Bork P., Downing A.K., Kieffer B., & Campbell I.D. (1996). Structure and function of modules in extracellular proteins. *Q. Rev. Biophys.,* 29, 119-167.

[24] Wouters, M.A., Rigoutsos, I., Chu, C.K., Feng, L.L., Sparrow, D.B., & Dunwoodie, S.L. Evolution of distinct EGF domains with specific functions. (2005). *Protein Sci.,* 14, 1091-1103.

[25] Bianco, C., Strizzi, L., Normanno, N., Khan, N., & Salomon, D.S. (2005). Cripto-1: an oncofetal gene with many faces. *Curr. Top. Dev. Biol.,* 67, 85-133.

[26] Gilges, D., Vinit, M-A., Callebut, I., Cuolombel, L., Cacheaux, V., Romeo, P-H., & Vigon, I. (2000). Polydom: a secreted protein with pentraxin, complement control protein, epidermal growth factor and von Willebrand factor A domains. *Biochem. J.,* 352, 49-59.

[27] Engel, J. EGF-like domains in extracellular matrix proteins: localized signals for growth and differentiation? (1989). *FEBS Lett.,* 251 *(*1,2*)*, 1-7.

[28] Terentiev, A.A., & Tatarinov, Yu.S. (1997). Display strong homology of the peptide regions: 13-18 of AFP and 26-31 of Epidermal Growth Factor (EGF). *Tumor Biol.* 18, *Suppl.* 2, 42.

[29] Terentiev, A.A., & Tatarinov, Yu.S. (1999). Homology of oligopeptide sequences in primary structures of glycodelin, AFP, insulin alpha-chain and EGF. *Tumor Biol.,* 20, Suppl. 2, 44.

[30] Abelev, G.I. (1983). Alpha-fetoprotein: the genesis. *Oncodev. Biol. Med.,* 4, 371-381.

[31] Tatarinov, Yu.S. (1994). *Human alpha-fetoprotein. 30 years from basic research to clinical application.* Moscow. 90p.

[32] Mizejewski G.J. (1997). Alpha-fetoprotein as a biologic response modifier: relevance to domain and subdomain structure. *Proc. Soc. Exp. Biol. Med..* 215, 333-362.

[33] McLeod, J.F, & Cooke, N.E. (1989). The vitamin D-binding protein, alpha-fetoprotein, albumin multigene family: Detection of transcripts in multiple tissues. *J. Biol. Chem.* 264, 21760–21769.

[34] Lichenstein, H.S, Lyons, D.E, Wurfel, M.M, Johnson, D.A, McGinley, M.D, Leidle, J.C, Trollinger, D.B, Mayer, J.P, Wright, S.D, & Zukowski, M.M. (1994). Afamin is a new member of the albumin, alpha-fetoprotein and vitamin D-binding protein gene family. *J. Biol. Chem.*, 269, 18149–18154.

[35] Luft, A.J., & Loscheider, F.L. (1983). *Biochemistry,* 22, 5971–5978.

[36] Zizkovsky, V., Strop, P., Korcakova, J., Havranova, M., & Mikes, F. (1983). Fluorescence spectroscopy, fluorescence polarization and circular dichroism in studies of pH-dependent changes in the alpha-fetoprotein molecule. *Ann. N.Y. Acad. Sci.,* 417, 49–56.

[37] He, X-M., & Carter, D. (1992). Atomic structure and chemistry of human serum albumin. *Nature,* 358, 209-215.

[38] Morinaga, T., Sakai, M., Wegmann, T.G., & Namaoki, T. (1983). Primary structure of human alpha-fetoprotein and its mRNA. *Proc. Natl. Acad. Sci. USA,* 80, 4604-4608.

[39] Pucci, P., Siliciano, R., Malorni, A., Marino, G., Tecce, M.F., Ceccarini, C., & Terrana, B. (1991). Human alpha-fetoprotein primary structure: a mass spectrometric study. *Biochemistry,* 30, 5061-5066.

[40] Mizejewski, G.J. (2001). Alpha-fetoprotein structure and function: relevance to isoforms, epitopes and conformational variants. *Exp. Biol. Med.*, 226, 377-408.

[41] Mizejewski, G.J. & Butterstein, G. (2006). Survey of functional activities alpha-fetoprotein-derived growth inhibitory peptides: review and prospects. *Curr. Prot. Pept. Sci.,* 7, 73-100.

[42] Terentiev, A.A., & Moldogazieva, N.T. (2006). Structural and functional mapping of alpha-fetoprotein. *Biochemistry (Mosc),* 71(2), 120-132. Review.

[43] Terentiev, A.A., Simonova, A.V., Arshinova, S.S., Kulakov, V.V., Bahus, G.O., Kudryavtseva, E.V., Bespalova, J.D., Ovchinnikov, M.V., & Tatarinov, Yu.S. (2003). Influence of peptide LDSYQCT (sequence 14-20 of human AFP) on proliferative activity of human lymphocytes. *Tumor Biol.,* 24, Suppl.1, 54.

[44] Kazimirsky, A.N., Terentiev, A.A., Salmasi , J.M., & Poryadin, G.V. (2001). Restoration of FAS-mediated apoptosis of lymphocytes in patients with myocarditis by specific peptide sequence of human alpha-fetoprotein ($AFP_{13\text{-}19}$). *Russ. J. Immunol.,* 6 (12), 394–398.

[45] Terentiev, A.A., Simonova, A.V., Arshinova, S.S., Kulakov, V.V., Bahus, G.O., Pavlichenkov, A.V., Kudryavtseva, E.V., Bespalova, J.D., Ovchinnikov, M.V., Moldogazieva, N.T., & Tagirova, A.K. (2004). Influence of the human alpha-fetoprotein-derived peptide LDSYQC(ACM)T ($AFP_{14\text{-}20}$) on proliferative and cytotoxic activity of human peripheral blood lymphocytes. *Immunologia (in Russian),* 5,279–281.

[46] Chang, H., Brown, C.W., & Matzuk, M. (2002). Genetic analisys of the mammalian transforming growth factor superfamily. *Endocr. Rev.,* 23(6), 787-823.

[47] Shi, Y., & Massague, J. (2003). Mechanisms of TGF-β signaling from cell membrane to the nucleus *Cell,* 113, 685-700.

[48] Massague, J., Seoane, J. &, Wotton, D. (2005). Smad transcription factors. *Genes Dev.,* 19(23), 2783-2810.

[49] Moustakas, A., &, Heldin, C-H. (2005). Non-Smad TGF-β signals. *J. Cell Sci.,* 118, 3573-3584.

[50] Derynck, R., &, Zhang, Y.E. (2003). Smad-dependent and Smad-independent pathways in TGF-β signaling. *Nature,* 425, 577- 584.

[51] Schlessinger, J., & Ullrich, A. (1992). Growth factor signaling by receptor tyrosine kinases. *Neuron,* 9, 383-391.

[52] Schlessinger, J. (2000). Cell signaling by receptor tyrosine kinases. *Cell,* 103, 211-225.

[53] Smith, T.F., & Waterman, M.S. (1981).Identification of common molecular subsequences. *J. Mol. Biol.,* 147, 195-197.

[54] Pearson, W.R. (1991). Searching protein sequence libraries: comparison of the sensitivity and selectivity of the Smith-Waterman and FASTA algorithms. *Genomics,* 11, 635-650.

[55] Andersen, M.H., Graversen, H., Fedosov, S.N., Petersen, T.E.. & Rasmussen, J.T. (2000) Functional analisys of two cellular binding domains of bovine lactadherin. *Biochemistry,* 39, 6200-6206.

In: Tumor Markers Research Focus
Editor: Deborah H. Chang, pp. 177-184
ISBN: 978-1-60021-544-5


*Chapter X A*

# Specific Gene Methylation as a Gastrointestinal Tumor Marker

***Juan Carlos Roa*** [*] ***and Miguel Villaseca***
Department of Pathology. Universidad de La Frontera, Temuco, Chile
Supported by Fondecyt GRANT N°1050603

## Draft Abstract. Specific Gene Methylation as a Gastrointestinal Tumor Marker

A biological marker is a substance, a structure or a process that entails a cellular, biochemical, molecular or genetic alteration, measurable qualitatively or quantitatively in biological samples from tissue, cells or bodily fluids and that can determine or predict the current status or outcome of a disease.

The detection of tumor-specific DNA changes, such as promoter gene hypermethylation, seems to be a more advantageous strategy than the techniques based on protein or RNA detection because DNA is more stable than RNA and, in contrast to proteins, DNA is amplifiable, which results in a heightened sensitivity to protein detection.

Aberrant methylation of the promoter gene regions has been identified early in the tumor genesis process, with it being presented in preneoplastic lesions and in preinvasive carcinomas. This enables the detection of these changes in DNA isolated in bodily fluids or from gastrointestinal washings. Recently, it has been reported that patients with infiltrating tumors present free-circulating DNA in the plasma that originates predominantly from necrotic or apoptotic tumor cells. This facilitates the development of diagnostic or plasmatic screening methods by means of the identification of typical genetic patterns for each tumor or group of tumors.

[*] E-mail address: Jcroa@ufro.cl. Correspondence to Dr. Juan Carlos Roa. Department of Pathology. Faculty of Medicine. Universidad de la Frontera. Manuel Montt 112, Zip code 478-1176 Temuco, Chile, 56-45-216273; 56-45-264909

The frequency of these alterations, the earliness of their appearance and the development of decision sensitive and efficient mechanisms for the detection of DNA methylation by means of methylation-specific PCR techniques convert into hypermethylation of the gene promoter areas in a biological marker of risk states that could enable the development of a screening method for the early diagnosis of neoplasias.

**Keywords:** Promoter hypermethylation; gastrointestinal tumor, tumor markers

It is well known and accepted that malignant tumors in human beings present significant changes in DNA methylation and the change in histone patterns produce a significant alteration in gene function without causing a change in the nucleotide sequence -- a condition known as epigenetics. (1)

In vertebrates, the DNA methylation pattern is established early on in embryogenesis, and in general, it is maintained throughout the life of the organism (2, 3). Inactivation is produced by the interaction of the methylated cytosine (methylcytosine) and other proteins and chromatin structural components (4), which probably makes the DNA inaccessible to transcription factors due to chromatin structural changes and histone deacetylation (5, 6). These differentially methylated regions are key elements, as for example in the transcriptional regulation of genes whose expression depends on the gender of the parent they were inherited from ("imprinted genes") (7). In this same way, the initiation and maintenance of the inactivation of the X chromosome (8) very early in development (9) is a consequence of the differential methylation of various genes.

The importance of the loss of epigenetically mediated gene function in cancer has been highlighted recently by the recognition that this process precedes and seems to be essential to various genetic events that control the initiation and progression of the tumor process. This link may be indirect and is associated with the hypermethylation of important promoter genes in the appearance and early progression of tumors and genes related to the DNA repair system. To measure the importance of hypermethylation, it must be pointed out that approximately half of the known tumor suppressor genes can be inactivated by promoter hypermethylation.

There are essentially five types of clinical application studies that can use the aberrant DNA methylation pattern in cancer (10-13).

**1. Identification of tumor cells from biological samples.** If the aberrant gene methylation of some gastrointestinal cancers is specifically present in the tumor cells, this can be used to detect the neoplastic cells in samples from biopsies or from free-circulating DNA in plasma or other bodily fluids. Since methylation occurs early on the carcinogenetic process, both early and advanced cancers can be detected. This would be of particular importance in patient groups with a family history of cancer who are at greatest risk of developing specific neoplasias. In prostate cancer, detecting methylation in only one gene (*GSTP1*) is informative in 80-90% of the cases (14, 15); and the determination of methylation in gene groups can be informative in 100 % of cases (16).

**2. Prognostic marker through individual gene methylation or methylation profiles for groups of specific genes.**

The study of single or combined genes that are inactivated by promoter hypermethylation, such as p16, can be used as to predict survival, time free of disease and tumor phenotype.

**3. Markers to predict the response to chemotherapy and/or hormone therapy.** The products of the genes that are silenced by DNA methylation can be used as biomarkers to predict the response to chemotherapy or radiotherapy.

**4. Reactivation of genes inactivated by methylation through the use of demethylating drugs** with the aim of reversing the neoplastic phenotype.

**5. Markers of preneoplastic lesions.** If the aberrant methylation is found to be linked to conditions that most frequently develop into some type of gastrointestinal cancer, this can be used as a marker to select patients with the greatest risk of developing a neoplasia.

This review will center mainly on DNA methylation detection used as a tumor marker in the diagnosis of gastrointestinal cancer.

## Detection of Free-Circulating Tumor DNA in Plasma/Serum

It has been described that under normal conditions, very little free DNA circulates in the plasma of healthy individuals. However, patients with cancer have on average an amount of DNA fragments circulating in the plasma four times greater than normal controls. This DNA would not have come from blood cells but rather from necrotic or apoptotic cells, presumably from neoplastic cells and some non-neoplastic cells close to the tumor (17-19). The first report on the detection of extracellular nucleic acids in blood circulation was published by Mandel and Métais in 1948, where they demonstrated the presence of DNA and RNA in the plasma of healthy and ill individuals. (29). Research on this topic was taken up again in the 1960s with the discovery of DNA circulating in patients with systemic lupus eritematoso (21). Only around 1977 was an increase in the DNA serum concentrations in cancer patients described, proving that the circulating DNA concentrations were greater in patients with metastasic disease and that these concentrations decreased after successful treatments (22). In 1989, Stroun et al. (23) suggested that the circulating DNA in cancer patients shows certain tumor DNA characteristics. This observation was reinforced in 1994 when two groups proved the presence of tumor-associated oncogene mutations in the plasma of patients with myelodysplastic syndrome or acute myelogenous leukemia (24) and pancreatic cancer (25).

The detection of free-circulating nucleic acids in cancer patients allows the development of molecular markers useful in the diagnosis, prognostic evaluation and follow-up of these patients. The cancer-associated molecular changes that can be detected include genetic mutations, chromosomal rearrangements, loss of heterozygocity (LOH), microsatellite instability, presence of viral sequences and hypermethylation of the gene-promoter region (26). Since 1996, several studies have described various genetic and epigenetic changes in the plasma and serum of patients with malignant neoplastic diseases (27-31).

The detection of tumor-specific DNA changes, as with gene hypermethylation, is a more profitable strategy than those techniques based on protein or RNA detection because DNA is more stable than RNA and, furthermore, in contrast to proteins, DNA is amplifiable, which means a more heightened sensitivity than protein detection (17). Methylated DNA detection also offers comparative advantages in relation to the early detection of neoplastic lesions owing to its high degree of specificity, to the fact that it constitutes a test which detects a positive signal and not the loss of a signal (as with loss of heterozygocity (LOH) determinations), and to the sensitivity of the method even in the presence of a marker for an excess of unmethylated DNA (17).

## Gene Hypermethylation in Free-Circulating Tumor DNA in Plasma/Serum in Patients with Gastrointestinal Tumors

In gastrointestinal tumors, aberrant methylation in free-circulating DNA in serum or plasma has been proven through methylation-specific PCR (MSP) in esophageal (32), gastric (33-36), hepatic (30, 31, 37) and colorectal (29, 38-41) carcinomas. The changes in methylation detected at the circulating DNA level show the correlation to the DNA methylation isolated from the tumor tissue extracted from the primary tumor. Due to the similarity in the changes observed in serum and tumor DNA, it is possible to use this tool as a prognostic indicator in order to allow an assessment of the risk of local recurrence or recurrence with distant spread and to show the correlation to survival, which is useful in patient follow-up and in the evaluation of response to treatment.

### Esophageal Cancer

In epidermoid carcinomas as well as in esophageal adenocarcinomas, hypermethylation of the p16 and APC promoter genes has been proven. The aberrant methylation of the p16 promoter gene has been detected in up to 82% of esophageal epidermoid carcinomas and, in 23% of those patients, hypermethylation of this gene in free-circulating serum DNA was concomitantly proven (42). On the other hand, hypermethylation of the promoter gene for adenomatous polyposis coli (APC), located in chromosome 5q21-22, has been proven in more than 90% of esophageal adenocarcinomas. 27% of these cases also showed hypermethylation of this gene in free-circulating plasma DNA. The plasma hypermethylation of this gene is largely associated with a lower survival rate ($p = .016$) (32).

### Gastric Cancer

In a significant proportion of patients with gastric cancer, aberrant methylation of various promoter genes such as DAP-quinase (70.3%), E-cadherin (75.9%), GSTP1 (18.5%), p15 (68.5%) and p16 (66.7%) has been proven. More than two thirds of the patients with aberrant methylation in the primary tumor showed this change in the serum samples with correlations that fluctuated between 68% and 81% (33). One series proved 28% of aberrant p16 and E-cadherin methylation in the serum of patients with early gastric cancer (34). Other hypermethylated genes have also been detected in the serum of patients with gastric cancer: APC (17%), hMLH1 (41%), TIMP3 (17%) and retinoic acid receptor, beta (RARbeta) (25%) (35, 36). The isolated or combined use of detecting aberrant APC and E-cadherin methylation has enabled the identification of subgroups of patients with the worst prognosis (35, 36). In accordance with Leung et al, with the combined analysis of aberrant APC and E-cadherin methylation, significant differences can be seen in the survival rate average of each subgroup (3.3 months vs. 16.1 months, $p = 0.006$) (35).

### Hepatocellular Carcinoma

The aberrant methylation of the p16 and p15 promoter genes is frequent in hepatocellular carcinoma, being observed in 73% and 64% of primary tumors, respectively (30, 37). The correlation of hypermethylation in tumor tissue and in free-circulating plasma or serum DNA was greater for p16 (81%) than for p15 (25%), with aberrant plasma or serum methylation being detected for p16 or p15 in 92% of the cases (30). With real-time quantitative studies of methylation-specific PCR (RTQ-MSP), a significant drop in the plasma methylation indices was proven after surgery (37), which demonstrates its clinical usefulness in the detection of recurrences and in post-treatment monitoring.

### Colorectal Cancer

In tumor tissue from patients with colorectal carcinoma, hypermethylation of promoter genes hMLH1 (21-47%), MGMT (40%), p16 (32-53%), p14 (38%), APC (32%), DAP-quinase (55%) and E-cadherin (40%) has been described (29, 38-40, 43, 44). Aberrant methylation of some of these genes has been detected in free-circulating plasma or serum DNA. One-third of the patients that presented hypermethylation of the hMLH1 gene in the primary tumor showed the same change in the free-circulating serum DNA (29). Of the colorectal carcinomas that present aberrant methylation of the p16 promoter gene, 68% present this change in free-circulating plasma DNA (38). The presence of p16 hypermethylation in serum shows a significant association to the most advanced Dukes stages ($p = 0.03$) (43). Only in 21% of the tumors that showed hypermethylation of the DAP-quinase promoter gene was the change proven at the serum level (44). In contrast to what was reported regarding tumors of other origins (45, 46), a correlation has not been proven between aberrant DAP-quinase methylation expression and survival rate or other prognosis variables.

## Conclusion

The presence of free-circulating DNA in plasma and serum, in healthy individuals as well as cancer patients, is a phenomenon that has been under observation for many years. Recently, practical applications have been described for the detection of aberrant DNA methylation in cancer patients that could be converted into powerful diagnostic instruments, biological markers to evaluate the clinical response to treatment, prognostic markers or useful tools for following up on the disease in these patients.

# References


[1] Esteller M. The necessity of a human epigenome project. Carcinogenesis. 2006;27:1121-5. Epub 2006 May 13.

[2] Razin A, Cedar H. DNA methylation and gene expression. *Microbiol Rev* 1991;55: 451-8.

[3] Razin A, Cedar H. DNA methylation and genomic imprinting. *Cell* 1994;77:473-6.

[4] Chen B, Kung HF, Bates RR. Effects of methylation of the beta-galactosidase genome upon in vitro synthesis of beta-galactosidase. *Chem Biol Interact* 1976;14:101-11.

[5] Bestor TH. The DNA methyltransferases of mammals. *Hum Mol Genet* 2000;9: 2395-402.

[6] Rice JC, Futscher BW. Transcriptional repression of BRCA1 by aberrant cytosine methylation, histone hypoacetylation and chromatin condensation of the BRCA1 promoter. *Nucleic Acids Res* 2000;28:3233-9.

[7] Li E, Beard C, Jaenisch R. Role for DNA methylation in genomic imprinting. *Nature* 1993;366:362-5.

[8] Panning B, Jaenisch R. RNA and the epigenetic regulation of X chromosome inactivation. *Cell* 1998;93:305-8.

[9] Li E, Bestor TH, Jaenisch R. Targeted mutation of the DNA methyltransferase gene results in embryonic lethality. *Cell* 1992;69:915-26.

[10] Esteller M. Relevance of DNA methylation in the management of cancer. *Lancet Oncol.* 2003;4:351-8.

[11] Esteller M. DNA methylation and cancer therapy: new developments and. *Curr Opin Oncol.* 2005;17:55-60.

[12] Esteller M. Profiling aberrant DNA methylation in hematologic neoplasms: a view from the tip of the iceberg. *Clin Immunol* 2003;109:80-8.

[13] Roa JC. [Genetic methylation in carcinogenesis and its application in oncology]. *Med Clin (Barc).* 2006;126:455-6.

[14] Lee WH, Morton RA, Epstein JI, Brooks JD, Campbell PA, Bova GS, et al. Cytidine methylation of regulatory sequences near the pi-class S-transferase gene accompanies human prostatic carcinogenesis. *Proc Natl Acad Sci U S A.* 1994;91:11733-7.

[15] Jeronimo C, Usadel H, Henrique R, Oliveira J, Lopes C, Nelson WG, et al. Quantitation of GSTP1 methylation in non-neoplastic prostatic organ-confined prostate adenocarcinoma. *J Natl Cancer Inst.* 2001;93:1747-52.

[16] Esteller M, Corn PG, Baylin SB, Herman JG. A gene hypermethylation profile of human cancer. Cancer Res 2001;61:3225-9.

[17] Widschwendter M, Jones PA. The potential prognostic, predictive, and therapeutic values of DNA methylation in cancer. Commentary re: J. Kwong et al., Promoter hypermethylation of multiple genes in nasopharyngeal carcinoma. *Clin. Cancer Res.*, 8: 131-137, 2002, and H-Z. Zou et al., Detection of p16 methylation in the serum of colorectal cancer patients. Clin. Res., 8: 188-191, 2002. Clin Cancer Res. 2002;8:17-21.

[18] Jahr S, Hentze H, Englisch S, Hardt D, Fackelmayer FO, Hesch RD, et al. DNA fragments in the blood plasma of cancer patients: quantitations and evidence for their origin from apoptotic and necrotic cells. *Cancer Res.* 2001;61:1659-65.

[19] Anker P, Stroun M. Circulating DNA in plasma or serum. *Medicina (B Aires).* 2000;60:699-702.
[20] Mandel P, Metais P. Les acides nucléiques du plasma sanguin chez l'homme. *Acad. Sci. Paris* 1948;142:241-243.
[21] Tan EM, Schur PH, Carr RI, Kunkel HG. Deoxybonucleic acid (DNA) and antibodies to DNA in the serum of with systemic lupus erythematosus. *J Clin Invest.* 1966;45: 1732-40.
[22] Leon SA, Shapiro B, Sklaroff DM, Yaros MJ. Free DNA in the serum of cancer patients and the effect of therapy. *Cancer Res.* 1977;37:646-50.
[23] Stroun M, Anker P, Maurice P, Lyautey J, Lederrey C, Beljanski M. Neoplastic characteristics of the DNA found in the plasma of cancer patients. *Oncology.* 1989;46:318-22.
[24] Vasioukhin V, Anker P, Maurice P, Lyautey J, Lederrey C, Stroun M. Point mutations of the N-ras gene in the blood plasma DNA of patients myelodysplastic syndrome or acute myelogenous leukaemia. *Br J Haematol.* 1994;86:774-9.
[25] Sorenson GD, Pribish DM, Valone FH, Memoli VA, Bzik DJ, Yao SL. Soluble normal and mutated DNA sequences from single-copy genes in blood. *Cancer Epidemiol Biomarkers Prev.* 1994;3:67-71.
[26] Taback B, Hoon DS. Circulating nucleic acids in plasma and serum: past, present and. *Curr Opin Mol Ther.* 2004;6:273-8.
[27] Chen XQ, Stroun M, Magnenat JL, Nicod LP, Kurt AM, Lyautey J, et al. Microsatellite alterations in plasma DNA of small cell lung cancer patients. *Nat Med.* 1996;2:1033-5.
[28] Anker P, Lefort F, Vasioukhin V, Lyautey J, Lederrey C, Chen XQ, et al. K-ras mutations are found in DNA extracted from the plasma of patients with colorectal cancer. *Gastroenterology.* 1997;112:1114-20.
[29] Grady WM, Rajput A, Lutterbaugh JD, Markowitz SD. Detection of aberrantly methylated hMLH1 promoter DNA in the serum of patients with microsatellite unstable colon cancer. *Cancer Res.* 2001;61:900-2.
[30] Wong IH, Lo YM, Yeo W, Lau WY, Johnson PJ. Frequent p15 promoter methylation in tumor and peripheral blood from hepatocellular carcinoma patients. *Clin Cancer Res.* 2000;6:3516-21.
[31] Wong IH, Lo YM, Zhang J, Liew CT, Ng MH, Wong N, et al. Detection of aberrant p16 methylation in the plasma and serum of liver cancer patients. *Cancer Res.* 1999;59:71-3.
[32] Kawakami K, Brabender J, Lord RV, Groshen S, Greenwald BD, Krasna MJ, et al. Hypermethylated APC DNA in plasma and prognosis of patients with esophageal adenocarcinoma. *J Natl Cancer Inst* 2000;92:1805-11.
[33] Lee T-L, Leung WK, Chan MWY, Ng EKW, Tong JHM, Lo K-W, et al. Detection of Gene Promoter Hypermethylation in the Tumor and Serum of Patients with Gastric Carcinoma. *Clin Cancer Res* 2002;8:1761-1766.
[34] Ichikawa D, Koike H, Ikoma H, Ikoma D, Tani N, Otsuji E, et al. Detection of aberrant methylation as a tumor marker in serum of with gastric cancer. *Anticancer Res.* 2004;24:2477-81.
[35] Leung WK, To KF, Chu ES, Chan MW, Bai AH, Ng EK, et al. Potential diagnostic and prognostic values of detecting promoter hypermethylation in the serum of patients with gastric cancer. *Br J Cancer.* 2005;92:2190-4.

[36] Ikoma H, Ichikawa D, Koike H, Ikoma D, Tani N, Okamoto K, et al. Correlation between serum DNA methylation and prognosis in gastric patients. *Anticancer Res.* 2006;26:2313-6.

[37] Wong IH, Zhang J, Lai PB, Lau WY, Lo YM. Quantitative analysis of tumor-derived methylated p16INK4a sequences in plasma, serum, and blood cells of hepatocellular carcinoma patients. *Clin Cancer Res*. 2003;9:1047-52.

[38] Lecomte T, Berger A, Zinzindohoue F, Micard S, Landi B, Blons H, et al. Detection of free-circulating tumor-associated DNA in plasma of cancer patients and its association with prognosis. *Int J Cancer*. 2002;100:542-8.

[39] Nakayama H, Hibi K, Taguchi M, Takase T, Yamazaki T, Kasai Y, et al. Molecular detection of p16 promoter methylation in the serum of cancer patients. *Cancer Lett.* 2002;188:115-9.

[40] Nakayama H, Hibi K, Takase T, Yamazaki T, Kasai Y, Ito K, et al. Molecular detection of p16 promoter methylation in the serum of colorectal cancer patients. *Int J Cancer*. 2003;105:491-3.

[41] Sanchez-Cespedes M, Esteller M, Wu L, Nawroz-Danish H, Yoo GH, Koch WM, et al. Gene promoter hypermethylation in tumors and serum of head and patients. *Cancer Res*. 2000;60:892-5.

[42] Hibi K, Taguchi M, Nakayama H, Takase T, Kasai Y, Ito K, et al. Molecular detection of p16 promoter methylation in the serum of with esophageal squamous cell carcinoma. Clin Cancer Res. 2001;7:3135-8.

[43] Zou HZ, Yu BM, Wang ZW, Sun JY, Cang H, Gao F, et al. Detection of aberrant p16 methylation in the serum of colorectal cancer patients. *Clin Cancer Res.* 2002;8:188-91.

[44] Yamaguchi S, Asao T, Nakamura J, Ide M, Kuwano H. High frequency of DAP-kinase gene promoter methylation in colorectal cancer specimens and its identification in serum. *Cancer Lett*. 2003;194:99-105.

[45] Sanchez-Cespedes M, Esteller M, Wu L, Nawroz-Danish H, Yoo GH, Koch WM, et al. Gene promoter hypermethylation in tumors and serum of head and neck cancer patients. *Cancer Res* 2000;60:892-5.

[46] Tozawa T, Tamura G, Honda T, Nawata S, Kimura W, Makino N, et al. Promoter hypermethylation of DAP-kinase is associated with poor in primary biliary tract carcinoma patients. *Cancer Sci*. 2004;95:736-40.

In: Tumor Markers Research Focus
Editor: Deborah H. Chang, pp. 185-191

ISBN: 978-1-60021-544-5


*Chapter X B*

# Potential Tumor Marker for Cholangiocarcinoma

***Viroj Wiwanitkit***
Department of Laboratory Medicine, Faculty of Medicine, Chulalongkorn University, Bangkok Thailand

## Abstract

Cholangiocarcinoma, a malignancy of the biliary duct system, tends to grow slowly and to infiltrate the walls of the ducts, dissecting along tissue planes and leading to biliary tract obstruction. Surgery remains the only curative treatment option for cholangiocarcinoma. Currently, the diagnosis is still hard and the specific tumor marker for cholangiocarcinoma is not available. Several serum and bile markers for the diagnosis of cholangiocarcinoma have been mentioned including fast liver alkaline phosphatase, carbohydrate antigen (CA) 19-9, interleukin-6, lactate, trypsinogen-2, pancreatic polypeptide, p53 mutations, p16 (INK4a), p14 (ARF) promoter hypermethylation. In this article, these new potential tumor markers for cholangiocarcinoma will be reviewed.

## Introduction

Cholangiocarcinoma is the cancer of the bile duct. This malignancy arising from biliary tract epithelia, or cholangiocarcinoma, is a tumor that has a poor prognosis [1]. They are broadly classified into intrahepatic tumors, (extrahepatic) hilar tumors and (extrahepatic) distal bile duct tumors. Considering the natural history of this cancer, it tends to grow slowly and to infiltrate the walls of the ducts, dissecting along tissue planes and leading to biliary tract obstruction [2]. At present, the incidence of this cancer is gradually increasing in many countries, with the peak incidence in Southeast Asia, especially for Thailand and Laos. Recent advances have been made in identifying some of the risk factors, and the need for appropriate classification is emerging [1]. The major risk factor for this cancer in Thailand is believed to be exposure to liver fluke in insufficiently cooked traditional foods [2]. As it is still endemic in Thailand, continuous prevention and surveillance of this public health problem are necessary [2]. Surgery remains the only curative treatment option for cholangiocarcinoma.

Currently, the diagnosis is still hard and the specific tumor marker for cholangiocarcinoma is not available. The diagnosis of cholangiocarcinoma is often difficult and requires multiple complementary studies [1]. Most of the patients usually visit the physician with the late manifestation, severe obstructive jaundice [2]. The high fatality of this cancer is generally due to the late diagnosis. Uttaravichien et al found that the results of surgery according to pathological staging showed that survival time in early stage was extremely better than that in late stage [3]. Patients with unresectable cholangiocarcinoma or pre-existing primary sclerosing cholangitis should be considered for liver transplantation with neoadjuvant chemoirradiation, in specialized centers [4]. Early diagnosis of this cancer can become an effective tool in lowering the high mortality. Non-jaundiced cases have the potential for curative resection [5]. In suspected cases, the diagnosis can be established with non-invasive imaging studies [4]. Early diagnosis of bile duct carcinomas not associated with jaundice, detailed ultrasonographic examination is useful, and subtle changes indicate a need for direct cholangiography [5]. Tumor markers for early diagnosis of cholangiocarcinoma become a new hope in management of this problematic cancer [6].

# Possible Tumor Marker for Cholangiocarcinoma

Several serum and bile markers for the diagnosis of cholangiocarcinoma have been mentioned including fast liver alkaline phosphatase, carbohydrate antigen (CA) 19-9, interleukin-6 (IL-6), lactate, trypsinogen-2, pancreatic polypeptide, p53 mutations, p16 (INK4a), p14 (ARF) promoter hypermethylation. In this article, these new potential tumor markers for cholangiocarcinoma will be reviewed.

## A. Fast Liver Alkaline Phosphatase

Fast liver alkaline phosphatase is an isoenzyme of alkaline phosphatase (ALP). Basically, ALP is an important enzyme mainly derived from the liver, bones and in lesser amounts from intestines, placenta, kidneys and leukocytes [7]. An increase in ALP levels in the serum is frequently associated with a variety of diseases [7]. High serum ALP levels in hospitalized patients were commonly found in three major groups having obstructive biliary diseases, infiltrative liver disease and sepsis [7]. Cholangiocarcionoma and some tropical diseases unique to tropical setting were also detected in these cases, where there was a marked elevation of serum ALP [7]. In laboratory medicine, fast liver ALP isoenzyme was measured by cellulose acetate electrophoresis in the sera obtained from the suspected patients. Ricci et al showed that the presence of fast liver isoenzyme, besides being highly specific, was also an early marker for cholestasis [8].According to a recent study by Paritpokee et al, concluded that the fast liver isoenzyme could be a useful marker in diagnosis of malignant extrahepatic obstruction [9].

## B. CA19-9

CA19-9 is an important tumor marker widely used in gastrointestinal cancer [10]. Almost all of these studies show that CA19-9 determination has a good sensitivity in the diagnosis of advanced pancreatic cancer and that its diagnostic accuracy is superior to that of the other serum tumor markers currently available [11]. Various immunoassay kits including CLEIA, FEIA, LPIA and RIA are available for CA19-9 determination. However, it is well known that serious method-related differences exist in results of serum CA19-9, and the necessity of standardization has been pointed out [12]. It is suggested that the obtained CA19-9 values could be approximated by recalculation with the assumed standard material would be able to correct between-method and between-laboratory discrepancies in particular systematic errors [12].

For cholangiocarcinoma, there are many reports on using CA19-9 as tumor marker. In 2005, Levy et al performed an interesting study aiming to characterize the test properties of CA 19-9 and of a change in CA 19-9 over time in predicting cholangiocarcinoma [13]. According to this work, the positive predictive value of an elevated CA 19-9 was 56.6%; only advanced cases were detected by this method [13]. In 2006, Chen et al performed a similar study to assess the value of CA19-9 in diagnosing hepatocellular carcinoma and intrahepatic cholangiocarcinoma [14]. A similar result to the study of Levy et al's work [13 - 14]. The diagnostic property of CA19-9 for diagnosis of cholangiocarcinoma is still questionable.

## C. IL-6

IL-6 is reported to be altered in the patients with cholangiocarcinoma. It has recently identified a critical role for the p44/p42 mitogen-activated protein kinase (MAPK) pathway in interleukin 6 (IL-6)-stimulated growth of human cholangiocytes [15]. According to a recent study by Park et al, both p38 and p44/p42 MAPKs were constitutively present and active in malignant cholangiocytes, and increased activity of both was observed within 15 minutes of stimulation with IL-6 [15]. Selective inhibition of either the p44/p42 MAPK pathway, by PD098059, or of the p38 MAPK pathway, by SB203580, blocked proliferation in response to IL-6 [15]. Thus, IL-6 can contribute to the autocrine and/or paracrine growth stimulation of malignant cholangiocytes via activation of either p38 or p44/p42 MAPK signaling pathways [15]. Enhanced telomerase activity in response to IL-6 stimulation can prevent cellular senescence and thereby contribute to cholangiocarcinoma growth [16]. Inhibition of telomerase activity may therefore be therapeutically useful in biliary tract malignancies [16].

In 1998, Goydos et al performed a study to determine if the serum level of interleukin-6 (IL-6) was elevated in patients with hepatic malignancies or correlated with radiologic tumor burden [17]. According to this study, in selected patients, a high serum level of IL-6 marks patients with cholangiocarcinoma and correlates with tumor burden both before and after resection [17]. IL-6 levels are elevated in patients with other liver neoplasms and may distinguish patients with hepatic malignancies from those with benign disease [17]. In 2004, Tangkijvanich performed another work toinvestigate the accuracy of CA 19-9 and IL-6 in the diagnosis of cholangiocarcinoma [18]. Tangkijvanich et al noted that the combined assays of both serum CA 19-9 and IL-6 could be useful in diagnosing cholangiocarcinoma, particularly in populations where this cancer was prevalent [18].

## D. Lactate

Lactate is a tumor marker that can be measured both in serum and bile [19]. Nishijima et al said that the measurement of lactate levels in serum and bile using proton nuclear magnetic resonance (1H-NMR) might be useful for the detection of hepatobiliary malignancies [20]. They found thatbiochemical enzymatic measurement of serum lactate levels revealed no such difference among patients with, without malignancy and healthy volunteer [20]. They also found that the spectrum of lactate in bile was observed in all of the studied patients with malignant diseases, but in none of healthy volunteers and the patients with non-malignant diseases [20].

## E. Trypsinogen-2

Trypsinogen-2 pancreatic polypeptide is a marker for acute pancreatitis. Application of this serum marker for diagnosis of cholangiocarcinoma has been performed for a few years [19]. In 1996, Hedstrom found that high trypsinogen-2 and trypsin-2-AAT concentrations were found most often in patients with biliary and pancreatic cancer, but also in benign obstructive biliary disease [22]. They suggested that trypsinogen-2 and trypsin-2-AAT were new potential markers for cholangiocarcinoma [22].

## F. Pancreatic Polypeptide

Pancreatic polypeptide can be classified as a gastrointestinal hormone controlling appetite [23]. In contrast to trypsinogen-2 polypeptide, pancreatic polypeptide is a serum marker for chronic pancreatitis [24 - 25]. Application of this serum marker for diagnosis of cholangiocarcinoma has been performed for a few years [19].

## G. p53 Mutation

Inactivation of the tumor suppressor gene p53, is the commonest genetic abnormality in human cancer and has been implicated in the genesis of cholangiocarcinoma in various immunohistochemical and molecular epidemiological investigations, including gene sequencing studies [26]. The majority of serum anti-p53 antibodies detected in cholangiocarcinoma are specifically associated with the accumulation of p53 protein in tumor tissues [27]. However, antibody generation against the p53 protein is a relatively uncommon event in cholangiocarcinoma [27]. According to a recent study of Tangkijvanich et al, anti-p53 antibodies could be detected in only 7.3% of the cases tested [28].They also found that anti-p53 antibodies were rapidly detected more frequently among patients with peripheral tumors than those with central tumors [28].

## H. p16 Promoter Hypermethylation

p16(INK4a) inactivation has been implicated in cholangiocarcinoma for a few years. It is suggested that suggest that inactivation of the p16 gene was a frequent event in cholangiocarcinoma [29]. The most common somatic alteration is promotor methylation of the p16 gene which is closely associated with K-ras mutations [29]. Taniai et al showed that functional point mutations in the p16(INK4a) promoter region likely contributed to the initiation/progression of cholangiocarcinoma in primary sclerosing cholangitis [30]. Promoter mutations in CpG islands may function as a methylation equivalent phenomenon resulting in gene inactivation [30].

## I. p14 Promoter Hypermethylation

Similar to p16, p14(ARF) inactivation has been implicated in cholangiocarcinoma for a few years. Klump et al performed an interesting study to evaluate the potential diagnostic role of p16(INK4a) and p14(ARF) promoter methylation in biliary disease [31].This study demonstrates: (a) a high frequency and specificity of INK4a/ARF methylation in malignant biliary disease compared with mere cholangitis; and (b) the capability to detect these alterations reliably in endoscopically obtained bile [14]. Thus, INK4a/ARF's promoter methylation status represents a candidate marker for the endoscopic diagnosis of biliary disease [31].

**Table 1. Summary on the new possible tumor markers for cholangiocarcinoma.**

| Markers | Specimen | Comments |
|---|---|---|
| fast liver ALP | Serum | Enzyme electrophoresis is required. |
| CA 19-9 | Serum | The clinical usefulness is questionable. |
| IL-6 | Serum | The clinical usefulness is questionable. |
| Lactate | Serum, Bile | Bile determination is more reliable. |
| trypsinogen-2 | Serum | This test is more proper for pancreatitis |
| pancreatic polypeptide p53 | Serum | This test is more proper for pancreatitis |
| mutations | Serum | Low detection rate is derived. |
| p16 (INK4a) | Bile | Endoscopic bile collection is required. |
| p14 (ARF) | Bile | Endoscopic bile collection is required. |

# References


[1] Reddy SB, Patel T. Current approaches to the diagnosis and treatment of cholangiocarcinoma. *Curr Gastroenterol Rep*. 2006 Feb;8(1):30-7.

[2] Wiwanitkit V. Clinical findings among 62 Thais with cholangiocarcinoma. *Trop Med Int Health*. 2003 Mar;8(3):228-30.

[3] Uttaravichien T, Bhudhisawasdi V, Pairojkul C, Pugkhem A. Intrahepatic cholangiocarcinoma in Thailand. *J Hepatobiliary Pancreat Surg*. 1999;6(2):128-35.

[4] Malhi H, Gores GJ. Review article: the modern diagnosis and therapy of cholangiocarcinoma. *Aliment Pharmacol Ther*. 2006 May 1;23(9):1287-96.

[5] Sugiyama M, Atomi Y, Kuroda A, Muto T. Bile duct carcinoma without jaundice: clues to early diagnosis. *Hepatogastroenterology*. 1997 Sep-Oct;44(17):1477-83.

[6] Sirisinha S. Tumor markers for early diagnosis of cholangiocarcinoma. *Asian Pac J Allergy Immunol.* 1989 Jun;7(1):1-3.
[7] Wiwanitkit V. High serum alkaline phosphatase levels, a study in 181 Thai adult hospitalized patients. *BMC Fam Pract.* 2001;2:2.
[8] Ricci OE, Tozzi P, Caldini M, Pasquinelli IT, Orsini B, Ventura L, Borsotti M, Surrenti C. Serum alkaline phosphatase isoenzymes: the fast liver fraction in the diagnosis of hepatobiliary disease with or without cholestasis. *Boll Soc Ital Biol Sper.* 1984 Jul 31;60(7):1363-8.
[9] Paritpokee N, Tangkijvanich P, Teerasaksilp S, Wiwanitkit V, Lertmaharit S, Tosukhowong P. Fast liver alkaline phosphatase isoenzyme in diagnosis of malignant biliary obstruction. *J Med Assoc Thai.* 1999 Dec;82(12):1241-6.
[10] Odagiri E. CA19-9. *Nippon Rinsho.* 2005 Aug;63 Suppl 8:642-4.
[11] Gullo L. CA19-9: the Italian experience. *Pancreas.* 1994 Nov;9(6):717-9.
[12] Hayashi K, Hoshino T, Yanai M, Tsuchiya T, Kumasaka K, Kawano K. An attempt for standardization of serum CA19-9 levels, in order to dissolve the gap between three different methods. *Rinsho Byori.* 2004 Jun;52(6):500-5.
[13] Levy C, Lymp J, Angulo P, Gores GJ, Larusso N, Lindor KD. The value of serum CA 19-9 in predicting cholangiocarcinomas in patients with primary sclerosing cholangitis. *Dig Dis Sci.* 2005 Sep;50(9):1734-40.
[14] Chen Y, Wang ZM, Ren ZG, LE F, Zhang BH, Xia JL, Ye SL, Tang ZY. The value of CA19-9 in diagnosing hepatocellular carcinoma and intrahepatic cholangiocarcinoma. *Zhonghua Gan Zang Bing Za Zhi.* 2006 Apr 20;14(4):299-300.
[15] Park J, Tadlock L, Gores GJ, Patel T. Inhibition of interleukin 6-mediated mitogen-activated protein kinase activation attenuates growth of a cholangiocarcinoma cell line. *Hepatology.* 1999 Nov;30(5):1128-33.
[16] Yamagiwa Y, Meng F, Patel T. Interleukin-6 decreases senescence and increases telomerase activity in malignant human cholangiocytes. *Life Sci.* 2006 Apr 18;78(21):2494-502.
[17] Goydos JS, Brumfield AM, Frezza E, Booth A, Lotze MT, Carty SE. Marked elevation of serum interleukin-6 in patients with cholangiocarcinoma: validation of utility as a clinical marker. *Ann Surg.* 1998 Mar;227(3):398-404.
[18] Tangkijvanich P, Thong-ngam D, Theamboonlers A, Hanvivatvong O, Kullavanijaya P, Poovorawan Y. Diagnostic role of serum interleukin 6 and CA 19-9 in patients with cholangiocarcinoma. *Hepatogastroenterology.* 2004 Jan-Feb;51(55):15-9.
[19] Nehls O, Gregor M, Klump B. Serum and bile markers for cholangiocarcinoma. *Semin Liver Dis.* 2004 May;24(2):139-54.
[20] Nishijima T, Nishina M, Fujiwara K. Measurement of lactate levels in serum and bile using proton nuclear magnetic resonance in patients with hepatobiliary diseases: its utility in detection of malignancies. *Jpn J Clin Oncol.* 1997 Feb;27(1):13-7.
[21] Matull WR, Pereira SP, O'Donohue JW. Biochemical markers of acute pancreatitis. *J Clin Pathol.* 2006 Apr;59(4):340-4.
[22] Hedstrom J, Haglund C, Haapiainen R, Stenman UH. Serum trypsinogen-2 and trypsin-2-alpha(1)-antitrypsin complex in malignant and benign digestive-tract diseases. Preferential elevation in patients with cholangiocarcinomas. *Int J Cancer.* 1996 May 3;66(3):326-31.

[23] Fukuda K, Inagaki N, Seino Y. Pancreatic polypeptide. *Nippon Rinsho.* 2005 Aug;63 Suppl 8:521-3.

[24] Seino Y. Plasma pancreatic polypeptide assay and the clinical significance. *Nippon Rinsho.* 1990 Feb;48 Suppl:40-2.

[25] Yamamura T, Mori K, Tatsumi M, Kotoura Y, Yoshiya K, Itoh N, Seino Y. Availability of plasma pancreatic polypeptide measurement in diagnosis of chronic pancreatitis. *Scand J Gastroenterol.* 1981;16(6):757-61.

[26] Khan SA, Thomas HC, Toledano MB, Cox IJ, Taylor-Robinson SD. p53 Mutations in human cholangiocarcinoma: a review. *Liver Int.* 2005 Aug;25(4): 704-16.

[27] Limpaiboon T, Sripa B, Wongkham S, Bhudhisawasdi V, Chau-in S, Teerajetgul Y. Anti-p53 antibodies and p53 protein expression in cholangiocarcinoma. *Hepatogastroenterology.* 2004 Jan-Feb;51(55):25-8.

[28] Tangkijvanich P, Kasemsupatana K, Janchai A, Kullavanijaya P, Theamboonlers A, Poovorawan Y. Prevalence and clinical relevance of serum anti-p53 antibodies in patients with cholangiocarcinoma. Asian Pac J Allergy Immunol. 2000 Sep;18(3):173-6.

[29] Tannapfel A, Benicke M, Katalinic A, Uhlmann D, Kockerling F, Hauss J, Wittekind C. Frequency of p16(INK4A) alterations and K-ras mutations in intrahepatic cholangiocarcinoma of the liver. *Gut.* 2000 Nov;47(5):721-7.

[30] Taniai M, Higuchi H, Burgart LJ, Gores GJ. p16INK4a promoter mutations are frequent in primary sclerosing cholangitis (PSC) and PSC-associated cholangiocarcinoma. *Gastroenterology.* 2002 Oct;123(4):1090-8.

[31] Klump B, Hsieh CJ, Dette S, Holzmann K, Kiebetalich R, Jung M, Sinn U, Ortner M, Porschen R, Gregor M. Promoter methylation of INK4a/ARF as detected in bile-significance for the differential diagnosis in biliary disease. *Clin Cancer Res.* 2003 May;9(5):1773-8.

In: Tumor Markers Research Focus
Editor: Deborah H. Chang, pp. 193-196

ISBN: 978-1-60021-544-5


*Chapter XI*

# Alpha Fetoprotein as a Tumor Marker for Hepatoma in Populations with High Incidence of Viral Hepatitis

***Viroj Wiwanitkit***
Department of Laboratory Medicine, Faculty of Medicine, Chulalongkorn University, Bangkok Thailand 10330

## Abstract

Hepatoma is a common gastrointestinal malignancy in viral hepatitis cases which is difficult to detect in early stages. The two important viral hepatitis associated with hepatoma are hepatitis B and hepatitis C viruses. Alpha fetoprotein (AFP) is a tumor marker which has been introduced for screening but in the settings where the rate of hepatitis B and hepatitis C seropositivity is very high, the diagnostic benefit is still doubtful. Here, a metanalysis on the previous reports is conducted and the conclusion that serum AFP can not be recommended for viral hepatitis carriers over standard tests is set.

## Introduction

Hepatoma is a common gastrointestinal malignancy in viral hepatitis cases which is difficult to detect in early stages. Hepatoma is the most common hepatic malignancy worldwide [1]. The primary risk factor for the development of hepatoma is cirrhosis [1]. Even patients without cirrhosis who develop hepatoma are typically found to have some underlying hepatic abnormality, such as steatohepatitis or chronic viral hepatitis [1]. Although cirrhosis of any cause increases the risk of developing HCC, cirrhosis associated with viral hepatitis carries the greatest risk. The two important viral hepatitis associated with hepatoma are hepatitis B and hepatitis C viruses.

Chronic hepatitis B is the most common cause of hepatoma in tropical Asia. Integration of hepatitis B virus genome is likely an early event of carcinogenesis [2]. The integrated hepatitis B virus genome may activate neighboring cellular genes directly to offer a selective growth advantage to the liver cells [2]. It has been proposed that the insertion of hepatitis B virus DNA into the human genome results in chromosomal instability and inactivation of tumor suppressor genes [3]. Transactivation of oncogenes, inactivation of tumor suppressor genes, and alteration of the cell cycle by hepatitis B virus proteins are also involved in the progression of hepatocellular carcinogenesis [3]. Production of hepatitis B X protein can act as a transactivator on various cellular genes for tumor development. Hepatic inflammation and cirrhosis also favors the process of carcinogenesis [2]. For hepatitis C, Chronic hepatitis C is highly heterogeneous in clinical presentation and outcomes [4]. This heterogeneity is largely related to host factors that have been clearly proven to affect the severity and rapidity of disease progression [4]. Of those exposed to hepatitis C virus, 80% become chronically infected, and at least 30% of carriers develop chronic liver disease, including cirrhosis and hepatocellular carcinoma [5].

Screening for hepatoma offers the best hope for early detection, eligibility for treatment, and improved survival [6]. Most physicians routinely screen at-risk patients with chronic viral hepatitis and cirrhosis for hepatoma, despite the lack of official guidelines [6]. The current consensus recommendations are to screen healthy hepatitis B virus carriers with annual or semiannual serum alpha-fetoprotein (AFP); carriers with chronic hepatitis or cirrhosis and patients with cirrhosis of any etiology are surveyed with twice yearly serum AFP and liver ultrasound [6]. Alpha fetoprotein (AFP) is a tumor marker which has been introduced for HCC screening in recent years [7 – 8] and in some countries it has become routinely employed [9]. However, use for screening in developing Asian countries is limited and the marker is not specific, being elevated in various liver diseases [7].

# Screening for Hepatocellular Cancer in Populations with Viral Hepatitis B and C: an Appraisal in Thailand

Alpha fetoprotein (AFP) is a tumor marker which has been introduced for screening but in the settings where the rate of hepatitis B and hepatitis C seropositivity is very high, the diagnostic benefit is still doubtful. Here, a metanalysis on the previous Thai reports is conducted and the conclusion that serum AFP can not be recommended for viral hepatitis carriers over standard tests is set.

## A. AFP, Hepatitis B and Hepatoma

Wiwanitkit recently performed a study to appraise the use of serum AFP in screening for hepatocellular cancer in Thai cases with hepatitis B [10]. In this study, a literature review of three Thai reports [11 - 13] was conducted, covering 4,295 cases. The overall diagnostic activity showed sensitivity, specificity, false positives and false negatives of 73.5 %, 98.9 %,

26.5 % and 1.1 %, respectively [10]. Thus the sensitivity is insufficient for screening purposes and serum AFP can not be recommended for hepatitis B carriers over standard tests [10].

**Table 1. Reports of using serum AFP measurement comparing to standard histopathological study in screening for hepatocellular cancer due to hepatitis B in Thailand.**

| References | Number of screenees | Positive rate (%) | Sensitivity (%) | Specificity (%) |
|---|---|---|---|---|
| 11 | 2,006 | 0 | 100 | 98.6 |
| 12 | 2,50 | 43.2 | 75.5 | 88.7 |
| 13 | 2,039 | 1.4 | 67.6 | 100 |

## B. AFP, Hepatitis C and Hepatoma

Here, the author performed a similar metanalysis to study the situation for hepatits C. A literature review was conducted of previous reports of serum AFP measurement in comparison with standard histopathological studies for hepatoma screening in patients with hepatitis C in Thailand was performed with the electronic search engine PubMed (www.pubmed.com). Published work in all 256 local Thai journals, which are not included in the international citation index by the database Thai Index Medicus were also considered. Reports that did not present diagnostic properties (sensitivity, specificity, false positives and false negatives) analysis were excluded. With the three reports satisfying the selection criteria, the sensitivity, specificity, false positives and false negatives were calculated. SPSS 11.0 for Windows was used for statistical analysis.

According to the literature review, 2 reports [11, 14] were recruited for further analysis (Table 2), covering 2,078 cases. The overall prevalence of hepatoma was 3.5 % (72/2,078). The overall diagnostic activity showed sensitivity, specificity, false positives and false negatives to be 88.9 %, 98.6 %,11.1 % and 1.4 %, respectively (Table 2).

**Table 2. Reports of using serum AFP measurement comparing to standard histopathological study in screening for hepatocellular cancer due to hepatitis C in Thailand.**

| References | Number of screenees | Positive rate (%) | Sensitivity (%) | Specificity (%) |
|---|---|---|---|---|
| 11 | 2,006 | 0 | 100 | 98.6 |
| 14 | 72 | 88.9 | 88.9 | 100 |

It can indicate that the overall sensitivity with AFP is not good, disproving the hypothesis that this marker would be appropriate for screening for hepatoma among hepatitis B or C carriers. Comparing to hepatitis B, screening in hepatitis C giving better sensitivity. The results are not concordant with an earlier report that the monitoring of serum AFP level in high-risk patients with viral hepatitis infection is valuable [14].

# References

[1] Nissen NN, Martin P. Hepatocellular carcinoma: the high-risk patient. *J Clin Gastroenterol.* 2002 Nov-Dec;35(5 Suppl 2):S79-85.

[2] Chan HL, Sung JJ. Hepatocellular carcinoma and hepatitis B virus. *Semin Liver Dis.* 2006 May;26(2):153-61.

[3] Wong CH, Chan SK, Chan HL, Tsui SK, Feitelson M. The molecular diagnosis of hepatitis B virus-associated hepatocellular carcinoma. *Crit Rev Clin Lab Sci.* 2006 Jan;43(1):69-101.

[4] Alberti A, Vario A, Ferrari A, Pistis R. Review article: chronic hepatitis C--natural history and cofactors. *Aliment* 2005 Nov;22 Suppl 2:74-8.

[5] Thomson BJ, Finch RG. Hepatitis C virus infection. *Clin Microbiol Infect.* 2005 Feb;11(2):86-94.

[6] Nguyen MH, Keeffe EB.Screening for hepatocellular carcinoma. *J Clin Gastroenterol.* 2002 Nov-Dec;35(5 Suppl 2):S86-91.

[7] Lee HY, Jung JH, Kang YS, et al. Clinical significance of transiently elevated serum AFP level in developing hepatocellular carcinoma in HBsAg positive-liver cirrhosis. *Korean J Gastroenterol* 2004; 43: 252-9.

[8] Daniele B, Bencivenga A, Megna AS, Tinessa V (2004). Alphafetoprotein and ultrasonography screening for hepatocellular carcinoma. *Gastroenterology.* 2004; 127(5 Suppl 1): S108-12.

[9] Di Bisceglie AM (2004). Issues in screening and surveillance for hepatocellular carcinoma. *Gastroenterology.* 2004; 127(5 Suppl 1): S104-7.

[10] Wiwanitkit V. Alpha fetoprotein for screening for hepatocellular cancer in populations with viral hepatitis B: an appraisal of Thai reports. *Asian Pac J Cancer Prev.* 2005;6:535-6.

[11] Srivatanakul P, Sriplung H, Deerasamee S. Epidemiology of liver cancer: an overview. *Asian Pac J Cancer Prev.* 2004; 5: 118-25.

[12] Chudhabuddhi C, Srivatanakul P, Boonyapisit S, Anukarahanonta T. Diagnostic value of alpha-fetoprotein and gammaglutamyl transpeptidase in hepatocellular carcinoma. *Intern Med* 1985;1: 21-4.

[13] Rinsurongkawong S. Search for hepatocellular carcinoma in the Thai population with viral B hepatitis by using ultrasonography and alpha-fetoprotein level. *Thai Cancer J.* 1993;19: 14-18.

[14] Songsivilai S, Dharakul T, Senawong S. Hepatitis B- and hepatitis C-associated hepatocellular carcinoma: evaluation of alpha-fetoprotein as a diagnostic marker. *Asian Pac J Allergy Immunol.* 1995; 13: 167-71.

In: Tumor Markers Research Focus
Editor: Deborah H. Chang, pp. 197-219

ISBN: 978-1-60021-544-5


*Chapter XII*

# Tumor Biomarkers for Early Detection of Hepatocellular Carcinoma

*Nikki P.Y. Lee and John M. Luk*
Department of Surgery and Center for Cancer Research, the University of Hong Kong, Pokfulam, Hong Kong

## Abstract

Hepatocellular carcinoma (HCC) is one of the most common and aggressive malignant tumor and recently ranked the third leading cause of cancer death worldwide. The incidence of HCC has been steadily increasing; and the major etiologic factors such as alcoholism and chronic hepatitis virus infection are the causative agents. Currently, there is no definite cure available and surgery is the primary treatment modality. Regardless of the advanced surgical technique, the prognosis is still poor, owing to the high rate of cancer recurrence and late diagnosis when the tumor becomes practically unresectable. Today, the liver cancer surveillance program relies on the detection of serum alfa-fetoprotein (AFP) and ultrasound imaging, which however, has limited sensitivity and specificity, and often operator dependent, respectively. Thus, identification of new biomarkers for better diagnosis of HCC is of great interest and high clinical priorities. Recent efforts on genomic and proteomic research have led to the discovery of panel diagnostic and prognostic markers for HCC. These include fucosylated fraction of AFP, heat shock proteins, glypican-3, and other biomarkers. Some of these markers are being evaluated in multi-center trials under the auspice of Early Detection Research Network. Besides, there have been significant efforts on unearthing a handful of biomarkers that are correlated with different clinical situations of liver diseases as in the cases of cirrhosis and tumor metastasis. In the foreseeable future, at-risk patients (viral hepatitis and cirrhosis) would benefit from earlier intervention and better treatment options for liver cancer that is made possible as a result of cancer biomarker discovery.

## Liver Cancer

Hepatocellular carcinoma (HCC) is a global liver hepatoma accounting for approximately 598 000 deaths each year and ranks as the third most common cause of cancer-related mortality [1]. The incidence of HCC is rising in both western and Asian countries, despite the endemic etiologies are quite distracted due to the spatial and racial differences. In westerns, the major risk factors attributable for HCC are hepatitis C virus (HCV) infection (~60%) and alcoholism (~45%), whereas hepatitis B virus (HBV) infection (~60-80%) is the main cause for the prevalence in Asian regions [2, 3]. Having these determinants, the mortal rates vary between them with Asians have a better survival rate [4]. In general, the overall 5-year survival rate of patients after HCC diagnosis remains at ~5% [1, 5]. The principal reason leading to this dismal is the late diagnosis of HCC in high-risk populations due to the late presentation and unawareness of the symptoms. Given the opportunity of detecting HCC before advancing to an aggressive stage, more treatment options are available and patients will have better curative chances with favorable improvements in post-operative outcomes [6]. To address this issue and lower the mortality of patients, improvement in clinical management of patients is necessary. The core procedures for early detection of HCC include regular screening of nodular lesions in livers and periodic testing of biomarkers in at-risk groups. As such, the discovery and utilization of biomarkers for early HCC detection bears a paramount role for better patient care and prolongs the long-term survival of patients.

## Molecular and Cellular Pathogenesis of HCC

HCC is a common liver malignance resulting from liver function failure. Etiologically, the causative agents include, but not limited to, viral hepatitis infection and alcoholism, and to a lesser extent the consumption of tobacco and exposure to aflatoxin B1 [3, 7]. In addition, HCC is also triggered by some other metabolic abnormalities as in steatosis, type 2 diabetes, and obesity [8, 9]. Rapid aggravation of the situations are noted when more than one risk factor synergistically pressurize on the livers, deteriorating the conditions [10]. Histologically, HCC development accompanies with the appearance of nodular lesions in the inflamed livers, which can be detected using imaging technologies as mentioned below [11, 12]. For the cellular progression, HCC incidence is preceded with liver cirrhosis, which is the one of the end-stages of fibrosis. Liver fibrosis is goaded by the procarcinogenic stimulants mentioned, which trigger a serial of inflammatory mechanism and chronic hepatic injury simultaneously. From that, HCC is the ultimate event of long-term inflammation and fibrosis. Hepatic fibrosis involves the modifications of extracellular matrix to become fibrous-like by abnormal deposition of matrix proteins, distorting the normal architecture of the livers [13-15].

Cirrhosis, in contrary to fibrosis, is an irreversible process. In the course of HCC development, it undergoes several phases, such as preneoplasia, dysplasia, and neoplasia [16]. Subsequently, these occurrences accompany with multifactorial events in the liver lesions. Most notable is the involvement of massive chronic inflammation [17, 18]. In fact, inflammations involving the participations of immune cells in the circulations are frequently associated with tumor development in other organs as well [19]. Besides, direct cell killing and apoptotic events are frequently observed in dysplastic livers [20]. Within the cellular compartment, opinions diverge regarding the origins of HCC. Along the hepatic lineage, four levels of cells are known as the precursors of tumor cells due to their susceptibilities to carcinogenic stimuli: the hepatocytes, the bile duct cells, the bipolar ductal progenitor cells, and the periductular oval cells [21, 22]. Beneath these physiological abnormalities, the genetic composition differs throughout the period of HCC development [16, 23, 24]. Common genetic and epigenetic changes encompass chromosomal aberration, appearance of genetic variants, microsatellite instability, and erratic methylation patterns [16, 24]. These genetic transformations eventually modify the genetic and protein profilings and the morphology in the neoplastic livers when compared to healthy livers.

# Clinical Diagnosis and Treatments of HCC

Two broad categories of diagnostic screening procedures are adopted nowadays for the detection of HCC in patients with histories of previous hepatitis infections, fibrosis, and/or cirrhosis [12, 25, 26]. These are part of the practices employed for the clinical management of patients, aiming to uncover the possible HCC incidence in high-risk populations. Since the symptoms of HCC usually present late and HCC becomes incurable when discovered because of the limited treatment options and poor prognosis for the advanced stage of this incidence. Even after surgery, the post-operative morbidity remains high in HCC patients in aggressive stage [26]. On the contrary, early detection of HCC means better curative plan and better prognosis. For better patient care, imaging technologies for spotting hepatic nodular lesions including the magnetic resonance imaging, ultrasound screening, angiography, and computed tomography scan are developed for early diagnosis [12, 27]. In parallel, existence and quantity of tumor biomarkers, such as the serum α-fetoprotein level, are detected in patient serum and recorded for tracking the HCC occurrence [12]. It is documented that serological materials reflect liver conditions, since plasma proteins are largely synthesized in livers. As such, plasma compositions act as clinical relevance, which is subjected to alterations in response to liver situations, for the overall status of liver diseases. These precautious schemes put a step forward in facilitating the early diagnosis and detection of HCC and directly benefit the healing opportunity of patients.

Varieties of treatment modalities are established to meet clinical criteria based on different HCC situations. Guidelines for applying treatment options depend on the number and size of hepatic tumors, the tumor locations, the associated hepatic dysfunctions, and the patient conditions, since no one absolute strategy is widely applicable to all status of HCC [25, 28-30]. Four main categories of remedies are broadly grouped as follows: (1) surgical approaches: surgical resection and liver transplantation [25, 31]; (2) percutaneous treatments: radiofrequency ablation [32, 33]; (3) transarterial interventions: embolization and chemoembolization [28]; (4) therapies: gene therapy, tagged antibody application, and drug medication [25, 34, 35]. Despite all the targeted approaches to treat this liver malignancy, there is no promise of complete recovery, further implicating the need for finding early HCC biomarkers to halt HCC progression at the first instance. Knowledge originated from these studies definitely advances the diagnostic and therapeutic of HCC.

# Approaches for the Discovery of Biomarkers

For the espial of HCC biomarkers, two technological platforms have been successfully capitalized to delineate the genomic and proteomic profiles of serum, liver tissue, and urine sample from patients [36, 37]. These samples should be the matched counterpart and are selected based on representative criteria as to reveal the gene and protein patterns among different clinicopathological features of HCC patients. After pair-wise matching and comparison, differential expressions of genes/proteins are displayed. Based on these analyses, biomarkers correlated with clinical situations can be distinguished for further validation and characterization, as sketched in Fig.1. For this purpose, we have also established a surgical tissue banking repository to facilitate biomarker identification and characterization by genomic and proteomic approaches as well as to contribute to a better understanding of human diseases resulting in improvements in diagnostics and therapies (Fig 2)

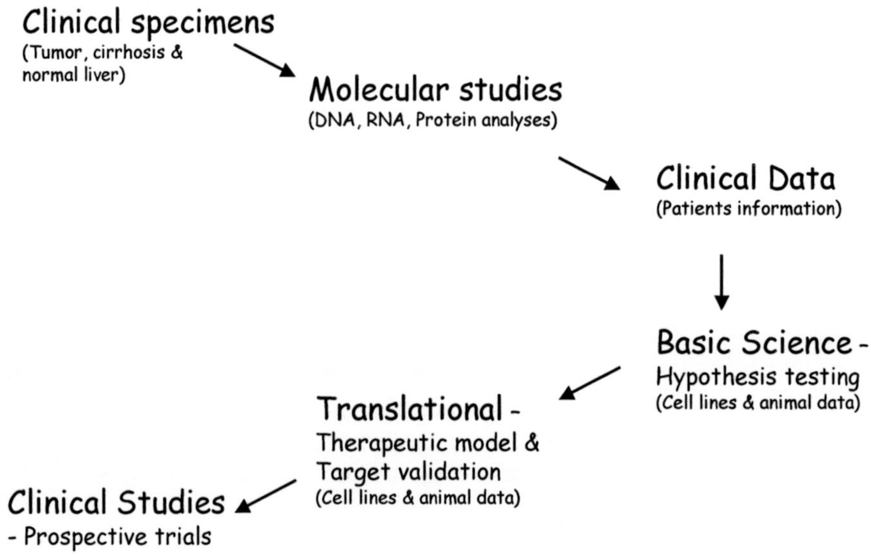


Figure 1. Biomarkers discovery program. Experimental approaches to identify and validate cancer biomarkers

(1) *Genomic platform.* Traditional methodology for identifying HCC biomarkers in genomics is mainly array- or chip-based [38, 39]. This not only depicts the genomic profiling, but also assesses the copy number of a target gene [40]. Later, this platform is further extended to study the gene polymorphism. One of the outstanding applications is to study single nucleotide polymorphism via mapping the allelic deletion or substitution [41, 42]. The investigation of the non-coding genes and its relationship with HCC can also be revealed. Although genomics can virtually address all the questions regarding the gene expression alteration and is imperative at the gene level, the conclusion generated is sometimes ambiguous due to its deficiency in revealing the functional end products. To this end, functional genomics, as a bridge to correlate gene and protein, is devoted to supplement the shortcomings [23, 40]. In general, genomics is still important in delineating the genetic background and information of HCC.

(2) *Proteomic platform.* The study of proteins is made feasible with the advancement of 2-dimensional (2D) gel electrophoresis, which segregates a pool of proteins according to the distinct pI value and molecular weight of each component [36, 37]. Data derived is in the format of gel spot intensity and gel spot profiles. Unlike the gene array platform with

identified gene name, each protein spot is anonymous, which requires further identification using mass spectrometry (MS) [36]. MS is a device for reading the mass-to-charge ratio of the ionized analytes after enzymatic digestion, which provides information for differentiating individual peptide. Electrospray ionization (ESI) and matrix-assisted laser desorption/ionization (MALDI) are two basic technologies for ionizing the peptides [43, 44]. The accuracy of MS is further enhanced with the implementation of tandem MS (MS/MS) machine that directly outputs the amino acid sequences. So far, the innovation of liquid chromatography (LC) MS/MS with enhanced resolving abilities further ameliorates the discriminative powers [45]. The analytic capability of the MS is greatly improved and scarce amount of digested peptides derived from intact proteins can be detected and identified [44]. In view of the complexity of proteome in intact cells, liquid phase isoelectric focusing, sub-cellular compartment fractionation, and high capacity chromatography are used as supplements [46, 47]. In addition, quantitative proteomics is integrated to analyze differential expressions of distinct proteomes in a comparative way [48-50]. With all those innovations and improvements, the efficiency and accuracy of biomarker discovery is drastically facilitated [37, 51].

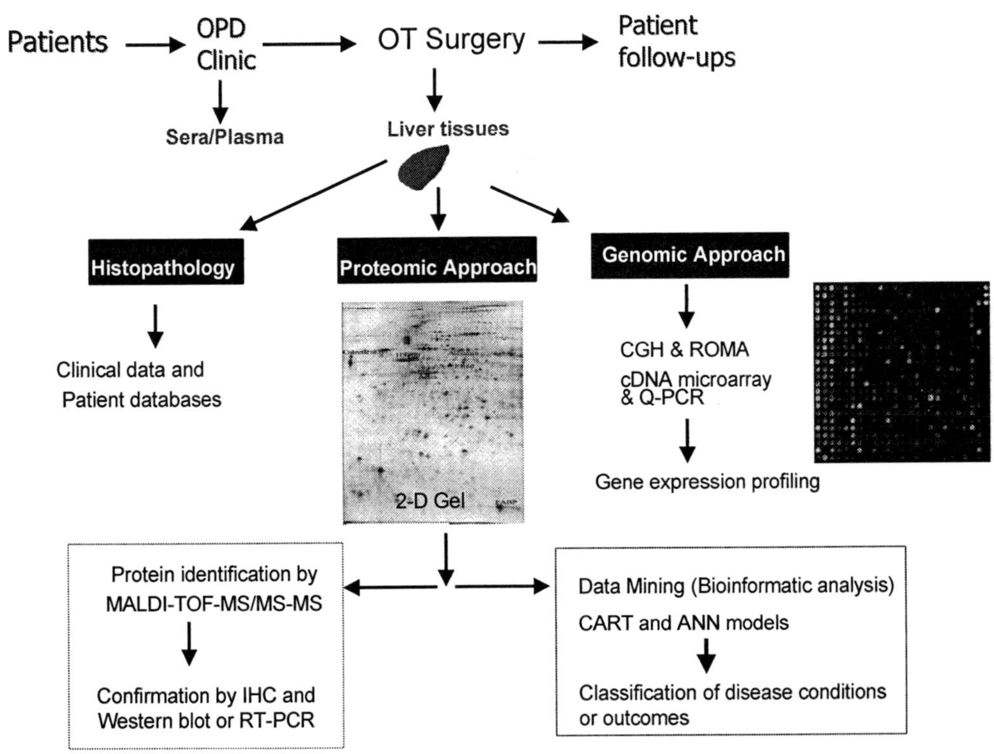


Figure 2. Workflow in genomic and proteomic expression profiling analyses on clinical tissues.

(3) *Animal models.* In addition for the early diagnosis of HCC, biomarkers identified could form the basis for HCC intervention. However, the suitability of these HCC biomarkers as candidates needs further validation in animal models developed with HCC, which is a prerequisite step before proceeding to human clinical trials. HCC in animals can be provoked by several means, such as exposure to carcinogenic stimuli or substances, such as HBV and

aflatoxin B1. Both woodchuck and tree shrews are widely used models for the study of human HCC, due to their vulnerability in HCC as a way similar to those exhibited in human [52-56]. Woodchuck shares coherent glycosylation patterns of liver proteins, as those viewed in human HCC [57]. This is clearly exemplified by using Golgi Protein 73, illustrating consistent glycosylation patterns in accordance to those in human HCC patients [57]. However, woodchuck does not display total reflection to the human HCC conditions due to the lack of p53 mutation [58]. This makes an urge to search for other animal models with consistency. In light of that, tree shrew, a non-human primate, turns as an alternate model [59-61]. It is well susceptible to HCC and manifests p53 mutation in the same manner as in human HCC [62][63, 64]. Using this model, signaling pathways known to exist in human HCC can be found and novel pathways can be mapped using this model, which may partially represent the scenario in human.

## Biomarkers for the Early Detection of HCC

Using the strategies described, several proteins having expression alterations in HCC, termed as HCC biomarkers, are discovered. After validation, they could serve as the diagnostic references for HCC incidence. In addition to the biomarkers with descriptions below, panels of biomarkers with different physiological functions are gradually uncovered using genomic or proteomic approaches [65-67] (Table 1). However, not all of them are practically used in routine clinical screenings and they require individual detailed validation. Indeed, the combined effects of quantifying more than one type of tumor markers significantly increase the sensitivity, accuracy, and specificity, the three principal criteria determining the efficacy of biomarkers, of HCC prediction [68-70]. In brief, the concurrent applications of multiple biomarkers benefit the early detection of HCC tremendously (Table 1). Thereafter, evaluations and examinations are performed following the guidelines set forth by the Early Detection Research Network of the National Cancer Institute [71] (Fig. 1). Through all these procedures, the biomarkers are ready for clinical diagnosis of HCC.

*α-Fetoprotein (AFP) and Lens culinaris agglutinin A-reaction fraction of AFP (AFP-L3).* AFP is a classic and most established serological HCC indicator, working in conjunction with ultrasonography, for routine use in early detection of HCC in patients [72, 73]. In addition, it is implemented in patient surveillance program for routine screening of HCC incidence in high-risk groups. Despite its prevalent use, it is criticized for its low sensitivity in HCC detection and high false positive rate. In order to overcome this deficiency, other biomarkers, such as des-γ-carboxy-prothrombin, are used in parallel to provide more trustworthy clinical conclusions [72] (Table 1). AFP-L3 is a fraction of AFP pool and is rated as a decisive biomarkers for HCC with high specificity and accuracy [72, 74, 75]. It is practically useful for screening small HCC. When compared with AFP-L3 seronegative patients, AFP-L3 positive patients have worsen liver functions and the possessions of larger tumor [76]. In addition, the mean AFP-L3 value is significantly elevated in moderately- or poorly-differentiated HCC than in well-differentiated HCC [75]. As such, AFP-L3 can be worked as a complement biomarker for HCC prediction.

**Table 1. Selected HCC Biomarkers and their Characteristics in HCC Prediction***

| Biomarkers | Correlation with clinicopathological features of HCC | Source | Cut-off level | Diagnostic accuracy | Sensitivity | Specificity | Combinations with other biomarkers <Cut-off level> (accuracy/sensitivity/specificity) | Selected references |
|---|---|---|---|---|---|---|---|---|
| α-Fetoprotein (AFP) | Tumor size | Serum | 20 ng/ml | - | 55% | 90% | Refer below for joint use with other biomarkers (AFP-L3, DCP, GPC3, IGF-II, AFU, SCCA-IgM IC, TGF-β1) | [84, 93, 140] |
| Lens culinaris agglutinin A-reaction fraction of AFP (AFP-L3) | AFP level; nodule diameter; tumor differentiation; liver function; metastasis | Serum | 15% relative to total AFP | 95.5% | 96.9% | 92% | AFP-L3 <10%> + AFP <20 ng/ml> + DCP <40 mAU/ml> (82.2%/82.1%/82.4%) | [70, 75, 76] |
| Cancer antigen 125 (CA 125) | Child-Pugh scores | Serum | 200 ng/ml | - | 92% | - | - | [83, 84, 141] |
| Des-γ carboxy-prothrombin (DCP) | Tumor differentiation, vascular invasion, metastasis, TNM staging, tumor size; prognosis; hepatitis infection | Serum | 125 mAU/ml | - | 89% | 95% | DCP <40 mAU/ml> + AFP-L3 <10%> (84.1%/-/97.8%) | [87, 142-144] |
| Glucose-regulated protein 78 (GRP78) | Tumor venous infiltration | Tissue | - | - | - | - | - | [104] |

**Table 1. (Continued)**

| Biomarkers | Correlation with clinicopathological features of HCC | Source | Cut-off level | Diagnostic accuracy | Sensitivity | Specificity | Combinations with other biomarkers <Cut-off level> (accuracy/sensitivity/specificity) | Selected references |
|---|---|---|---|---|---|---|---|---|
| Soluble glypican-3 (GPC3) | - | Serum | 2 ng/ml | - | 51% | 90% | GPC3 <2 ng/ml> + AFP <20 ng/ml> (-/72%/-) | [93] |
| Golgi protein-73 (GP73) | - | Serum | 10 relative intensity units | - | 69% | 86% | - | [98] |
| Heat shock protein 27 (HSP27) | Hepatitis B infection; tumor stage; AFP level | Tissue | - | - | - | - | - | [100, 104, 106] |
| Heat shock protein 70 (HSP70) | Tumor size; portal vein invasion; tumor stage | Tissue | - | - | - | - | - | [100] |
| Human telomerase reverse transciptase (hTERT) | Tumor stage; tumor size; tumor differentiation | Serum, tissue | 12500 copies/0.2 ml | - | 88.2% | 68.7% | - | [107, 109, 111] |
| Insulin-like growth factor-II (IGF-II) | AFP | Serum | 4.5 mg/g prealbumin | 69% | 42% | 96% | IGF-II <4.5 mg/g prealbumin>+ AFP <100 ng/ml> (96.5%/97.9%/95.1%) | [114] |
| Soluble interleukin-2 receptor (IL-2R) | Child-Pugh scores; tumor size; tumor differentiation | Serum | 850 U/ml | - | 99% | 95.6% | - | [117, 145] |

**Table 1. (Continued)**

| Biomarkers | Correlation with clinicopathological features of HCC | Source | Cut-off level | Diagnostic accuracy | Sensitivity | Specificity | Combinations with other biomarkers <Cut-off level> (accuracy/sensitivity/specificity) | Selected references |
|---|---|---|---|---|---|---|---|---|
| α-L-fucosidase (AFU) | Tumor size; hepatitis infection | Serum | 443 nmol/ml/h | - | 76% | 90.9% | AFU <870 nmol/ml/h> + AFP <400 ng/ml> (-/82.6%/-) | [119, 120, 126] |
| Nitrite/nitrate plasma ratio | Tumor size; tumor volume | Plasma | 36.8 nmol/ml | 75.3% | 79.5% | 72% | - | [127, 128] |
| Squamous cell carcinoma antigen-immunoglobulin M immune complexes (SCCA-IgM IC) | - | Serum | 120 AU/ml | - | 70% | 100% | SCCA-IgM IC <120 AU/ml> + AFP <20 ng/ml> (-/96%/100%) | [129] |
| Transforming growth factor-β1 (TGF-β1) | AFP level; Child-Pugh scores; tumor size; tumor differentiation | Plasma, urine | 50 μg/g creatinine | - | 53.1% | 99% | TGF-β1 <50 μg/g creatinine> + AFP <100 ng/ml> (90.1%/84%/98%) | [133, 136, 146] |

* Information in this table does not mean to be inclusive for all works and just represents selected studies specified. The diagnostic accuracy, sensitivity, and specificity are based on the cut-off values tabulated in the studies.

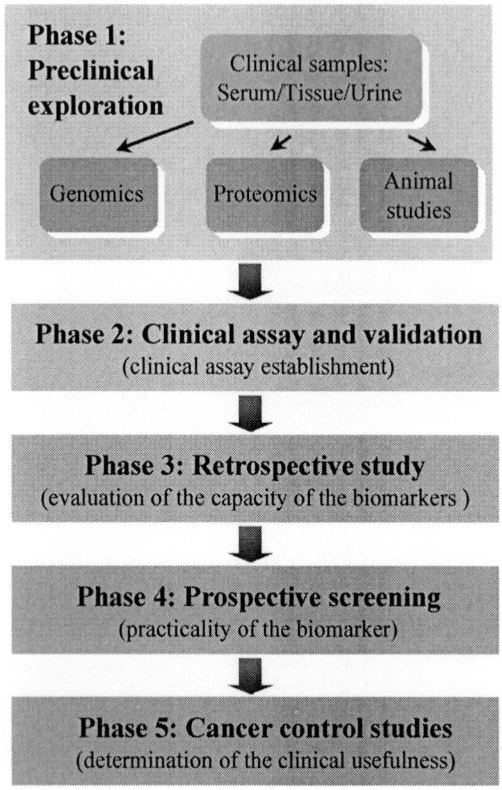


Figure 3. Flow-chart depicts the sequential processes in the Early Detection Research Network leading to the discovery of clinical HCC biomarkers. With patient serum, tissue, and urine sample as the starting materials in Phase 1 of the Early Detection Research Network, putative HCC biomarkers are discovered using genomic and proteomic approaches and detailed analyses of these markers can be performed in HCC animal models. Thereafter, the procedure will move forwards from Phase 2 to Phase 5, during which consists of serial steps involving the clinical assay and validation, retrospective study, prospective screening, and cancer control studies with different aims and purposes.

*Albumin-γ-glutamyltransferase isoenzyme (Albumin-GGT isoenzyme).* GGT is a glycoenzyme catalyzing the synthesis and metabolism of glutathione [77]. Different isoforms of GGT are found in circulation and are named according to their associated serum proteins. Albumin-GGT is one of the isoenzymes with a diagnostic value in HCC [78]. Presence of albumin-GGT is not specific to HCC only and is also implicated for the development of cirrhosis and metastasis. Despite that, it also serves as an accurate marker for HCC prediction in cooperation with AFP [72, 78]. Apart from albumin-GGT, other GGT in complex with low-density lipoprotein plus very low-density lipoprotein is examined to have clinical correlations with HCC [79], making GGT isoenzyme as a distinct group of HCC biomarkers.

*Cancer antigen 125 (CA 125).* CA 125 is a HCC biomarker associated with general liver abnormalities [80]. However, its level is elevated in both benign and malignant liver disorders [80-82]. Despite its limited specificity, it is still a explicit marker when used jointly with AFP, since the double negative of both markers almost excludes the possibility of having HCC [83, 84].

*Des-γ carboxy-prothrombin (DCP).* DCP is an abnormal prothrombin protein with induced serum levels in HCC patients [85, 86]. It is a specific tumor marker that enables the unequivocal discrimination of HCC from other nonmalignant liver lesions, such as chronic hepatitis and cirrhosis [87]. The predictive application of DCP is further extended to depict the clinicopathological features of HCC in the aspects of tumor size and liver histology [88, 89]. In addition, DCP-seropositive patients are usually found to associate with a more severe HCC status when compared to patients who are seronegative [90], making DCP as a good indicator for HCC severity. Still, it should be used in conjunction with AFP to generate the optimal conclusions.

*Glypican-3 (GPC3).* GPC3 is a plasma membrane-anchoring heparan sulfate proteoglycan [91, 92]. It is appraised to be a novel serological marker for early stage of HCC [93]. The levels of GPC3 are induced in HCC tissues [94, 95]. Elevated levels of GPC3 are also detected in human HCC cell lines and secreted GPC3 is measured in the culture medium of HCC cell lines [96, 97]. Significantly, HCC patients have enhanced levels of soluble GPC3, a cleaved product of GPC3, in the circulation [93]. Patients with chronic hepatitis and cirrhosis are seronegative for this marker, implying its usefulness in diagnosis of HCC among various benign liver disorders [93, 94]. The simultaneous use of soluble GPC3 and AFP as a HCC predictive reference improves the overall sensitivity of both markers [93].

*Golgi protein-73 (GP73).* GP73 is a serum Golgi glycoprotein being up-regulated in HCC [98]. The level of GP73 is augmented in serum from HCC patients. Its utilization as a predictive HCC biomarker is recently authenticated [98]. On the advantage side, it is a more precise marker than the conventional AFP for early detection of HCC [98]. GP73 is used as a clinical diagnostic marker in concord with SELDI-TOF profiling to monitor HCC incidence in high-risk patients with HCV infection [99].

*Heat shock proteins (HSP).* HSP is a family of stress-induced proteins and is recently known to function as the HCC biomarker for early diagnosis. Among the family members, HSP27, HSP70, and glucose-regulated protein 78 (GRP78) demonstrate incremental expression in HCC conditions [100-105]. For HSP70, it can specifically differentiate early HCC from noncancerous and precancerous tissues [103]. In addition, HSP70 coincides with several clinical matters, such as tumor size, portal vein invasion, and aggravated tumor staging in HCC [100]. On the other hand, HSP27 significantly relates with HBV infection and histological stages in HCC [100, 106]. For GRP78, its expression is linked with tumor venous infiltration in HCC [104].

*Human telomerase reverse transciptase (hTERT).* The level of hTERT reflects the course of HCC development with induced RNA expression [107-110]. It demonstrates preferential elevation in poorly-differentiated HCC when compared to highly- or moderately-differentiated HCC [111]. Besides HCC, hTERT is implicated to be a cancer marker in bladder carcinoma [112]. .

*Insulin-like growth factor-II (IGF-II).* Serological IGF-II is valuated to be a rather sensitive marker for the detection of small HCC [113]. In combined use with AFP, the specificity, sensitivity, and accuracy is further enhanced [113, 114]. Despite that, abnormal level of IGF-II is observed in tumors with non-hepatic origins, such as prostate cancers [115] and endometrial cancer [116].

*Interleukin-2 receptor (IL-2R).* Circulating level of soluble IL-2R is raised in HCC conditions and is regarded as a more sensitive marker than AFP [117]. It is used as an index to envision the incidence of HCC in a retrospective fashion [117]. However, it is also known as biomarker for other neoplasms, such as those happened in ovaries [118].

*α-L-fucosidase (AFU).* AFU is a specific marker for early conjecture of HCC development among other liver malignances. Up-regulation in its level prognosticates the onset of HCC, since patients with hepatitis infection and cirrhosis have non-significant AFU level [119-121]. This characteristic makes AFU a useful marker for continuous monitoring for HCC incidence in high-risk populations by periodic quantification of serum AFU levels and activities. An increase in AFU level and activity in cirrhotic patients during follow-up period indicates the high possibility of progression from cirrhosis to HCC and this procedure facilitates the early detection of HCC [122, 123]. However, enhanced level of AFU has restricted interpretation due to its association with the development of other tumors, such as the head and neck squamous cell carcinoma [124] and the colorectal tumor [125], in addition to HCC. This situation leads to the use of AFU activity in conjunction with AFP and ultrasonography for the accurate detection of HCC [126].

*Nitrite/nitrate plasma ratio.* Nitrite and nitrate are two of the indicators for the nitric oxide levels and activities and are quantified using Griess reaction [72]. Abnormal nitrite/nitrate ratio signifies HCC incidence [127]. In the clinicopathological aspects, high nitrite/nitrate ratio shows positive correlations with tumor size and tumor volume [127]. The sensitivity and specificity of using nitrite/nitrate ratio is further enhanced with the complementary use of AFP [128].

*Squamous cell carcinoma antigen-immunoglobulin M immune complexes (SCCA-IgM IC).* SCCA-IgM IC is an immune complex, composed of SCCA and IgM. Augmented SCCA-IgM IC level in circulation is observed in HCC conditions [129]. However, moderate and low levels of this IC are detected, in certain cases, in cirrhotic and hepatitis-infected patients, respectively [129]. Its concurrent use with other markers, such as AFP, is preferable for yielding optimal results in differentiating HCC from other benign hepatic dysfunctions [130].

*Transforming growth factor-β1 (TGF-β1).* Elevation in the level of TGF-β1 in plasma and urine serves as an indicator for HCC incidence [131, 132]. Combined use of TGF-β1 and AFP as the predictive markers for HCC can successfully differentiate HCC from cirrhosis [133]. On the other hand, the usefulness of TGF-β1 as a HCC marker can be illustrated in its accuracy of HCC diagnosis in patients having serological insignificant AFP level [134, 135], complementing the clinical use of conventional AFP. In addition, plasma TGF-β1 can selectively detect the incidence of small HCC development, for which the detection is not absolutely accurate using AFP as a sole predictor [136]. Besides, its level accords with the extent of tumor vascularity, implicating the phenomenon of tumor angiogenesis in HCC [137]. Due to the fact that elevation in TGF-β1 level is also documented in other non-hepatic tumors, such as colorectal tumor [138] and renal cell carcinoma [139], the use of TGF-β1 is usually accompanied with other markers.

## Conclusion

HCC is one of the most common tumors nowadays and ranks third in causing cancer-related mortality. Liver cirrhosis is preceding HCC, in some instances, and is the general consequences of long-term inflammation and liver function failure that is goaded by hepatitis virus infection and alcoholism as part of the stimulants. Different fields of modalities for HCC are established, however, the overall survival of HCC patients is grim. It is grossly due to the late presentation of the symptoms, resulting in poor prognostic outcomes. One of the main tasks is to have the applicable patient surveillance program for high-risk groups to facilitate the early detection of HCC. These include the ultrasonography to reveal tumor nodules in a periodic screening and the serological testing of the presence of HCC biomarkers on a routine basis. In the context of biomarker utilization, the insensitivity and non-specificity of current clinical biomarkers, such as AFP, poses a serious problem in its accuracy in predicting HCC occurrence. This leads to the large-scale mapping of HCC biomarkers to supplement the deficiency. Two promising disciplines of HCC biomarker discovery rely on genomics and proteomics and these approaches largely solve the problems of the complexity of cellular genomes and proteomes and the presence of low-copy number genes and low abundant proteins. After targeting the putative biomarkers, the evaluation and development of these biomarkers in clinical applications follow part of the 5-phase scheme in the Early Detection Research Network. Resultant biomarkers can then be used to prognosticate HCC incidence and progression. In the midst of exponential emergence of a huge number of HCC biomarkers, validations of their clinical practicality are the major theme of future study. Apart from being diagnostic biomarkers, the established biomarkers can provide starting ground in the investigation of their putative roles in HCC treatment. Along the paths of HCC progression, signals that destine the precancerous cells to evolve into benign or malignant hepatocellular tumors are not totally disclosed. It is not yet dissected whether silencing the actions or removal of the tumor associated genes or proteins would intervene further HCC progression or reverse the tumorigenic conditions. The optimal curable time frames for treating HCC still need subsequent exploration. These are some of the unanswered questions that worth the merit of further intense focus.

## Acknowledgements

The study was supported by CRCG Seed Grant of University Research Committee and the Research Grants Council of Hong Kong (N_HKU718/03; HKU7320/02M).

## References

[1] Parkin, DM; Bray, F; Ferlay, J& Pisani, P. Global cancer statistics, 2002. CA *Cancer J Clin*, 2005, 55, 74-108.

[2] Bosch, FX; Ribes, J; Cleries, R& Diaz, M. Epidemiology of hepatocellular carcinoma. *Clin Liver Dis*, 2005, 9, 191-211, v.

[3] Bosch, FX; Ribes, J; Diaz, M& Cleries, R. Primary liver cancer: worldwide incidence and trends. *Gastroenterology*, 2004, 127, S5-S16.

[4] Davila, JA& El-Serag, HB. Racial differences in survival of hepatocellular carcinoma in the United States: a population-based study. *Clin Gastroenterol Hepatol*, 2006, 4, 104-110; quiz 104-105.

[5] El-Serag, HB; Mason, AC& Key, C. Trends in survival of patients with hepatocellular carcinoma between 1977 and 1996 in the United States. *Hepatology*, 2001, 33, 62-65.

[6] Kudo, M. Early detection and curative treatment of early-stage hepatocellular carcinoma. *Clin Gastroenterol Hepatol*, 2005, 10 Suppl 2, S144-S148.

[7] Bruix, J; Boix, L; Sala, M& Llovet, JM. Focus on hepatocellular carcinoma. *Cancer Cell*, 2004, 5, 215-219.

[8] Powell, EE; Jonsson, JR& Clouston, AD. Steatosis: co-factor in other liver diseases. *Hepatology*, 2005, 42, 5-13.

[9] Caldwell, SH; Crespo, DM; Kang, HS& Al-Osaimi, AM. Obesity and hepatocellular carcinoma. *Gastroenterology*, 2004, 127, S97-103.

[10] Marrero, JA; Fontana, RJ; Fu, S; Conjeevaram, HS; Su, GL& Lok, AS. Alcohol, tobacco and obesity are synergistic risk factors for hepatocellular carcinoma. *J Hepatol*, 2005, 42, 218-224.

[11] Frazer, C. Imaging of hepatocellular carcinoma. *J Gastroenterol Hepatol*, 1999, 14, 750-756.

[12] Kudo, M. Early detection and characterization of hepatocellular carcinoma: value of imaging multistep human hepatocarcinogenesis. *Intervirology*, 2006, 49, 64-69.

[13] Lotersztajn, S; Julien, B; Teixeira-Clerc, F; Grenard, P& Mallat, A. Hepatic fibrosis: molecular mechanisms and drug targets. *Annu Rev Pharmacol Toxicol*, 2005, 45, 605-628.

[14] Hui, AY& Friedman, SL. Molecular basis of hepatic fibrosis. *Expert Rev Mol Med*, 2003, 2003, 1-23.

[15] Bataller, R& Brenner, DA. Liver fibrosis. *J Clin Invest*, 2005, 115, 209-218.

[16] Thorgeirsson, SS& Grisham, JW. Molecular pathogenesis of human hepatocellular carcinoma. *Nat Genet*, 2002, 31, 339-346.

[17] Umeda, T& Hino, O. Molecular aspects of human hepatocarcinogenesis mediated by inflammation: from hypercarcinogenic state to normo- or hypocarcinogenic state. *Oncology*, 2002, 62 Suppl 1, 38-42.

[18] Moss, SF& Blaser, MJ. Mechanisms of disease: Inflammation and the origins of cancer. *Nat Clin Pract Oncol*, 2005, 2, 90-97; quiz 91 p following 113.

[19] Mantovani, A. Cancer: inflammation by remote control. *Nature*, 2005, 435, 752-753.

[20] Ghavami, S; Hashemi, M; Kadkhoda, K; Alavian, SM; Bay, GH& Los, M. Apoptosis in liver diseases--detection and therapeutic applications. *Med Sci Monit*, 2005, 11, RA337-345.

[21] Sell, S. Cellular origin of hepatocellular carcinomas. *Semin Cell Dev Biol*, 2002, 13, 419-424.

[22] Wu, XZ& Chen, D. Origin of hepatocellular carcinoma: Role of stem cells. *J Gastroenterol Hepatol*, 2006, 21, 1093-1098.

[23] Thorgeirsson, SS; Lee, JS& Grisham, JW. Functional genomics of hepatocellular carcinoma. *Hepatology*, 2006, 43, S145-150.

[24] Laurent-Puig, P& Zucman-Rossi, J. Genetics of hepatocellular tumors. *Oncogene*, 2006, 25, 3778-3786.

[25] Cormier, JN; Thomas, KT; Chari, RS& Pinson, CW. Management of hepatocellular carcinoma. *J Gastrointest Surg*, 2006, 10, 761-780.

[26] Gish, RG. Hepatocellular carcinoma: overcoming challenges in disease management. *Clin Gastroenterol Hepatol*, 2006, 4, 252-261.

[27] Digumarthy, SR; Sahani, DV& Saini, S. MRI in detection of hepatocellular carcinoma (HCC). *Cancer Imaging*, 2005, 5, 20-24.

[28] Llovet, JM. Updated treatment approach to hepatocellular carcinoma. *J Gastroenterol*, 2005, 40, 225-235.

[29] Blum, HE. Treatment of hepatocellular carcinoma. *Best Pract Res Clin Gastroenterol*, 2005, 19, 129-145.

[30] Bruix, J; Hessheimer, AJ; Forner, A; Boix, L; Vilana, R& Llovet, JM. New aspects of diagnosis and therapy of hepatocellular carcinoma. *Oncogene*, 2006, 25, 3848-3856.

[31] Llovet, JM; Schwartz, M& Mazzaferro, V. Resection and liver transplantation for hepatocellular carcinoma. *Semin Liver Dis*, 2005, 25, 181-200.

[32] Curley, SA& Izzo, F. Radiofrequency ablation of primary and metastatic hepatic malignancies. *Int J Clin Oncol*, 2002, 7, 72-81.

[33] Curley, SA; Izzo, F; Ellis, LM; Nicolas Vauthey, J& Vallone, P. Radiofrequency ablation of hepatocellular cancer in 110 patients with cirrhosis. *Ann Surg*, 2000, 232, 381-391.

[34] Mohr, L; Yeung, A; Aloman, C; Wittrup, D& Wands, JR. Antibody-directed therapy for human hepatocellular carcinoma. *Gastroenterology*, 2004, 127, S225-231.

[35] Palmer, DH; Hussain, SA& Johnson, PJ. Gene- and immunotherapy for hepatocellular carcinoma. *Expert Opin Biol Ther*, 2005, 5, 507-523.

[36] Poon, TC& Johnson, PJ. Proteome analysis and its impact on the discovery of serological tumor markers. *Clin Chim Acta*, 2001, 313, 231-239.

[37] Chignard, N& Beretta, L. Proteomics for hepatocellular carcinoma marker discovery. Gastroenterology, 2004, 127, S120-125.

[38] Kim, JW& Wang, XW. Gene expression profiling of preneoplastic liver disease and liver cancer: a new era for improved early detection and treatment of these deadly diseases? *Carcinogenesis*, 2003, 24, 363-369.

[39] Bucca, G; Carruba, G; Saetta, A; Muti, P; Castagnetta, L& Smith, CP. Gene expression profiling of human cancers. *Ann N Y Acad Sci*, 2004, 1028, 28-37.

[40] Lee, JS& Thorgeirsson, SS. Comparative and integrative functional genomics of HCC. *Oncogene*, 2006, 25, 3801-3809.

[41] Kato, N; Ji, G; Wang, Y; Baba, M; Hoshida, Y; Otsuka, M; Taniguchi, H; Moriyama, M; Dharel, N; Goto, T; Shao, RX; Matsuura, T; Ishii, K; Shiina, S; Kawabe, T; Muramatsu, M& Omata, M. Large-scale search of single nucleotide polymorphisms for hepatocellular carcinoma susceptibility genes in patients with hepatitis C. *Hepatology*, 2005, 42, 846-853.

[42] Midorikawa, Y; Yamamoto, S; Ishikawa, S; Kamimura, N; Igarashi, H; Sugimura, H; Makuuchi, M& Aburatani, H. Molecular karyotyping of human hepatocellular carcinoma using single-nucleotide polymorphism arrays. *Oncogene*, 2006,

[43] Aebersold, R& Mann, M. Mass spectrometry-based proteomics. *Nature*, 2003, 422, 198-207.

[44] Guerrera, IC& Kleiner, O. Application of mass spectrometry in proteomics. *Biosci Rep*, 2005, 25, 71-93.

[45] Wang, H& Hanash, S. Multi-dimensional liquid phase based separations in proteomics. *J Chromatogr B Analyt Technol Biomed Life Sci*, 2003, 787, 11-18.

[46] Wang, H& Hanash, S. Intact-protein based sample preparation strategies for proteome analysis in combination with mass spectrometry. *Mass Spectrom Rev*, 2005, 24, 413-426.

[47] Parent, R& Beretta, L. Proteomics in the study of liver pathology. *J Hepatol*, 2005, 43, 177-183.

[48] Ong, SE& Mann, M. Mass spectrometry-based proteomics turns quantitative. *Nat Chem Biol*, 2005, 1, 252-262.

[49] Sechi, S& Oda, Y. Quantitative proteomics using mass spectrometry. *Curr Opin Chem Biol*, 2003, 7, 70-77.

[50] Julka, S& Regnier, F. Quantification in proteomics through stable isotope coding: a review. *J Proteome Res*, 2004, 3, 350-363.

[51] Feng, JT; Shang, S& Beretta, L. Proteomics for the early detection and treatment of hepatocellular carcinoma. *Oncogene*, 2006, 25, 3810-3817.

[52] Tennant, BC. Animal models of hepadnavirus-associated hepatocellular carcinoma. *Clin Liver Dis*, 2001, 5, 43-68.

[53] Gouillat, C; Manganas, D; Zoulim, F; Vitrey, D; Saguier, G; Guillaud, M; Ain, JF; Duque-Campos, R; Jamard, C; Praves, M& Trepo, C. Woodchuck hepatitis virus-induced carcinoma as a relevant natural model for therapy of human hepatoma. *J Hepatol*, 1997, 26, 1324-1330.

[54] Yan, RQ; Su, JJ; Huang, DR; Gan, YC; Yang, C& Huang, GH. Human hepatitis B virus and hepatocellular carcinoma. I. Experimental infection of tree shrews with hepatitis B virus. *J Cancer Res Clin Oncol*, 1996, 122, 283-288.

[55] Yan, RQ; Su, JJ; Huang, DR; Gan, YC; Yang, C& Huang, GH. Human hepatitis B virus and hepatocellular carcinoma. II. Experimental induction of hepatocellular carcinoma in tree shrews exposed to hepatitis B virus and aflatoxin B1. *J Cancer Res Clin Oncol*, 1996, 122, 289-295.

[56] Li, Y; Su, JJ; Qin, LL; Yang, C; Ban, KC& Yan, RQ. Synergistic effect of hepatitis B virus and aflatoxin B1 in hepatocarcinogenesis in tree shrews. Ann Acad Med Singapore, 1999, 28, 67-71.

[57] Block, TM; Comunale, MA; Lowman, M; Steel, LF; Romano, PR; Fimmel, C; Tennant, BC; London, WT; Evans, AA; Blumberg, BS; Dwek, RA; Mattu, TS& Mehta, AS. Use of targeted glycoproteomics to identify serum glycoproteins that correlate with liver cancer in woodchucks and humans. *Proc Natl Acad Sci U S A,* 2005, 102,779-784.

[58] Rivkina, M; Cote, PJ; Robinson, WS; Tennant, BC& Marion, PL. Absence of mutations in the p53 tumor suppressor gene in woodchuck hepatocellular carcinomas associated with hepadnavirus infection and intake of aflatoxin B1. *Carcinogenesis*, 1996, 17, 2689-2694.

[59] Reddy, JK; Svoboda, DJ& Rao, MS. Induction of liver tumors by aflatoxin B1 in the tree shrew (Tupaia glis), a nonhuman primate. *Cancer Res*, 1976, 36, 151-160.

[60] Yang, EB; Cao, J; Su, JJ& Chow, P. The tree shrews: useful animal models for the viral hepatitis and hepatocellular carcinoma. *Hepatogastroenterology*, 2005, 52, 613-616.

[61] Cao, J; Yang, EB; Su, JJ; Li, Y& Chow, P. The tree shrews: adjuncts and alternatives to primates as models for biomedical research. *J Med Primatol*, 2003, 32, 123-130.

[62] Su, JJ; Li, Y; Ban, KC; Qin, LL; Wang, HY; Yang, C; Ou, C; Duan, XX; Lee Yl, Y& Yan, RQ. Alteration of the p53 gene during tree shrews' hepatocarcinogenesis. *Hepatobiliary Pancreat Dis Int*, 2003, 2, 612-616.

[63] Lunn, RM; Zhang, YJ; Wang, LY; Chen, CJ; Lee, PH; Lee, CS; Tsai, WY& Santella, RM. p53 mutations, chronic hepatitis B virus infection, and aflatoxin exposure in hepatocellular carcinoma in Taiwan. *Cancer Res,* 1997, 57, 3471-3477.

[64] Bergsland, EK. Molecular mechanisms underlying the development of hepatocellular carcinoma. *Semin Oncol*, 2001, 28, 521-531.

[65] Blanc, JF; Lalanne, C; Plomion, C; Schmitter, JM; Bathany, K; Gion, JM; Bioulac-Sage, P; Balabaud, C; Bonneu, M& Rosenbaum, J. Proteomic analysis of differentially expressed proteins in hepatocellular carcinoma developed in patients with chronic viral hepatitis C. *Proteomics*, 2005, 5, 3778-3789.

[66] Li, C; Tan, YX; Zhou, H; Ding, SJ; Li, SJ; Ma, DJ; Man, XB; Hong, Y; Zhang, L; Li, L; Xia, QC; Wu, JR; Wang, HY& Zeng, R. Proteomic analysis of hepatitis B virus-associated hepatocellular carcinoma: Identification of potential tumor markers. *Proteomics*, 2005, 5, 1125-1139.

[67] Lee, IN; Chen, CH; Sheu, JC; Lee, HS; Huang, GT; Yu, CY; Lu, FJ& Chow, LP. Identification of human hepatocellular carcinoma-related biomarkers by two-dimensional difference gel electrophoresis and mass spectrometry. *J Proteome Res,* 2005, 4, 2062-2069.

[68] Toyoda, H; Kumada, T; Kiriyama, S; Sone, Y; Tanikawa, M; Hisanaga, Y; Yamaguchi, A; Isogai, M; Kaneoka, Y& Washizu, J. Prognostic significance of simultaneous measurement of three tumor markers in patients with hepatocellular carcinoma. *Clin Gastroenterol Hepatol*, 2006, 4, 111-117.

[69] el-Houseini, ME; Mohammed, MS; Elshemey, WM; Hussein, TD; Desouky, OS& Elsayed, AA. Enhanced detection of hepatocellular carcinoma. *Cancer Control,* 2005, 12, 248-253.

[70] Shimizu, A; Shiraki, K; Ito, T; Sugimoto, K; Sakai, T; Ohmori, S; Murata, K; Takase, K; Tameda, Y& Nakano, T. Sequential fluctuation pattern of serum des-gamma-carboxy prothrombin levels detected by high-sensitive electrochemiluminescence system as an early predictive marker for hepatocellular carcinoma in patients with cirrhosis. *Int J Mol Med*, 2002, 9, 245-250.

[71] Marrero, JA& Lok, AS. Newer markers for hepatocellular carcinoma. *Gastroenterology*, 2004, 127, S113-119.

[72] Lopez, JB. Recent developments in the first detection of hepatocellular carcinoma. *Clin Biochem Rev*, 2005, 26, 65-79.

[73] Talwalkar, JA& Gores, GJ. Diagnosis and staging of hepatocellular carcinoma. *Gastroenterology*, 2004, 127, S126-132.

[74] Lamerz, R. AFP isoforms and their clinical significance (overview). *Anticancer Res,* 1997, 17, 2927-2930.

[75] Khien, VV; Mao, HV; Chinh, TT; Ha, PT; Bang, MH; Lac, BV; Hop, TV; Tuan, NA; Don, LV; Taketa, K& Satomura, S. Clinical evaluation of lentil lectin-reactive alpha-fetoprotein-L3 in histology-proven hepatocellular carcinoma. *Int J Biol Markers*, 2001, 16, 105-111.

[76] Yamashiki, N; Seki, T; Wakabayashi, M; Nakagawa, T; Imamura, M; Tamai, T; Nishimura, A; Inoue, K; Okamura, A; Arita, S& Harada, K. Usefulness of Lens culinaris agglutinin A-reactive fraction of alpha-fetoprotein (AFP-L3) as a marker of distant metastasis from hepatocellular carcinoma. *Oncol Rep*, 1999, 6, 1229-1232.

[77] Goldberg, DM. Structural, functional, and clinical aspects of gamma-glutamyltransferase. *CRC Crit Rev Clin Lab Sci*, 1980, 12, 1-58.

[78] Pompili, M; Addolorato, G; Pignataro, G; Rossi, C; Zuppi, C; Covino, M; Grieco, A; Gasbarrini, G& Rapaccini, GL. Evaluation of the albumin-gamma-glutamyltransferase isoenzyme as a diagnostic marker of hepatocellular carcinoma-complicating liver cirrhosis. *J Gastroenterol Hepatol*, 2003, 18, 288-295.

[79] Sacchetti, L; Castaldo, G; Cimino, L; Budillon, G& Salvatore, F. Diagnostic efficiency in discriminating liver malignancies from cirrhosis by serum gamma-glutamyltransferase isoforms. *Clin Chim Acta*, 1988, 177, 167-172.

[80] Devarbhavi, H; Kaese, D; Williams, AW; Rakela, J; Klee, GG& Kamath, PS. Cancer antigen 125 in patients with chronic liver disease. *Mayo Clin Proc*, 2002, 77, 538-541.

[81] Molina, R; Filella, X; Bruix, J; Mengual, P; Bosch, J; Calvet, X; Jo, J& Ballesta, AM. Cancer antigen 125 in serum and ascitic fluid of patients with liver diseases. *Clin Chem*, 1991, 37, 1379-1383.

[82] Elias, J& Kew, MC. Evaluation of CA 125 as a serum marker of hepatocellular carcinoma. *Int J Cancer*, 1990, 46, 805-807.

[83] Lopez, JB; Balasegaram, M& Thambyrajah, V. Serum CA 125 as a marker of hepatocellular carcinoma. *Int J Biol Markers*, 1996, 11, 178-182.

[84] Lopez, JB; Balasegaram, M; Timor, J& Thambyrajah, V. Comparison of alpha-fetoprotein with some other tumour markers in Malaysians with hepatocellular carcinoma. *Malays J Pathol*, 1997, 19, 53-58.

[85] Okuda, H; Nakanishi, T; Furukawa, M& Obata, H. Vitamin K-dependent proteins and hepatocellular carcinoma. *J Gastroenterol Hepatol*, 1991, 6, 392-399.

[86] Yamagata, H; Nakanishi, T; Furukawa, M; Okuda, H& Obata, H. Levels of vitamin K, immunoreactive prothrombin, des-gamma-carboxy prothrombin and gamma-glutamyl carboxylase activity in hepatocellular carcinoma tissue. *J Gastroenterol Hepatol*, 1995, 10, 8-13.

[87] Marrero, JA; Su, GL; Wei, W; Emick, D; Conjeevaram, HS; Fontana, RJ& Lok, AS. Des-gamma carboxyprothrombin can differentiate hepatocellular carcinoma from nonmalignant chronic liver disease in American patients. *Hepatology*, 2003, 37, 1114-1121.

[88] Okuda, H; Nakanishi, T; Takatsu, K; Saito, A; Hayashi, N; Takasaki, K; Takenami, K; Yamamoto, M& Nakano, M. Serum levels of des-gamma-carboxy prothrombin measured using the revised enzyme immunoassay kit with increased sensitivity in relation to clinicopathologic features of solitary hepatocellular carcinoma. *Cancer*, 2000, 88, 544-549.

[89] Nakamura, S; Nouso, K; Sakaguchi, K; Ito, YM; Ohashi, Y; Kobayashi, Y; Toshikuni, N; Tanaka, H; Miyake, Y; Matsumoto, E& Shiratori, Y. Sensitivity and specificity of

des-gamma-carboxy prothrombin for diagnosis of patients with hepatocellular carcinomas varies according to tumor size. *Am J Gastroenterol*, 2006, in press.

[90] Okuda, H; Nakanishi, T; Takatsu, K; Saito, A; Hayashi, N; Yamamoto, M; Takasaki, K& Nakano, M. Comparison of clinicopathological features of patients with hepatocellular carcinoma seropositive for alpha-fetoprotein alone and those seropositive for des-gamma-carboxy prothrombin alone. *J Gastroenterol Hepatol*, 2001, 16, 1290-1296.

[91] Nakatsura, T& Nishimura, Y. Usefulness of the novel oncofetal antigen glypican-3 for diagnosis of hepatocellular carcinoma and melanoma. *BioDrugs*, 2005, 19, 71-77.

[92] Moriguchi, H& Sato, C. The values and limitations of glypican-3 as a novel tumor marker for hepatocellular carcinoma from clinical and economic viewpoints. *Gastroenterology*, 2004, 127, 679-680.

[93] Hippo, Y; Watanabe, K; Watanabe, A; Midorikawa, Y; Yamamoto, S; Ihara, S; Tokita, S; Iwanari, H; Ito, Y; Nakano, K; Nezu, J; Tsunoda, H; Yoshino, T; Ohizumi, I; Tsuchiya, M; Ohnishi, S; Makuuchi, M; Hamakubo, T; Kodama, T& Aburatani, H. Identification of soluble NH2-terminal fragment of glypican-3 as a serological marker for early-stage hepatocellular carcinoma. *Cancer Res*, 2004, 64, 2418-2423.

[94] Nakatsura, T; Yoshitake, Y; Senju, S; Monji, M; Komori, H; Motomura, Y; Hosaka, S; Beppu, T; Ishiko, T; Kamohara, H; Ashihara, H; Katagiri, T; Furukawa, Y; Fujiyama, S; Ogawa, M; Nakamura, Y& Nishimura, Y. Glypican-3, overexpressed specifically in human hepatocellular carcinoma, is a novel tumor marker. *Biochem Biophys Res Commun*, 2003, 306, 16-25.

[95] Capurro, M; Wanless, IR; Sherman, M; Deboer, G; Shi, W; Miyoshi, E& Filmus, J. Glypican-3: a novel serum and histochemical marker for hepatocellular carcinoma. *Gastroenterology*, 2003, 125, 89-97.

[96] Midorikawa, Y; Ishikawa, S; Iwanari, H; Imamura, T; Sakamoto, H; Miyazono, K; Kodama, T; Makuuchi, M& Aburatani, H. Glypican-3, overexpressed in hepatocellular carcinoma, modulates FGF2 and BMP-7 signaling. *Int J Cancer*, 2003, 103, 455-465.

[97] Sung, YK; Hwang, SY; Park, MK; Farooq, M; Han, IS; Bae, HI; Kim, JC& Kim, M. Glypican-3 is overexpressed in human hepatocellular carcinoma. *Cancer Sci,* 2003, 94, 259-262.

[98] Marrero, JA; Romano, PR; Nikolaeva, O; Steel, L; Mehta, A; Fimmel, CJ; Comunale, MA; D'Amelio, A; Lok, AS& Block, TM. GP73, a resident Golgi glycoprotein, is a novel serum marker for hepatocellular carcinoma. *J Hepatol*, 2005, 43, 1007-1012.

[99] Schwegler, EE; Cazares, L; Steel, LF; Adam, BL; Johnson, DA; Semmes, OJ; Block, TM; Marrero, JA& Drake, RR. SELDI-TOF MS profiling of serum for detection of the progression of chronic hepatitis C to hepatocellular carcinoma. *Hepatology*, 2005, 41, 634-642.

[100] Joo, M; Chi, JG& Lee, H. Expressions of HSP70 and HSP27 in hepatocellular carcinoma. *J Korean Med Sci*, 2005, 20, 829-834.

[101] Song, HY; Liu, YK; Feng, JT; Cui, JF; Dai, Z; Zhang, LJ; Feng, JX; Shen, HL& Tang, ZY. Proteomic analysis on metastasis-associated proteins of human hepatocellular carcinoma tissues. *J Cancer Res Clin Oncol*, 2006, 132, 92-98.

[102] Feng, JT; Liu, YK; Song, HY; Dai, Z; Qin, LX; Almofti, MR; Fang, CY; Lu, HJ; Yang, PY& Tang, ZY. Heat-shock protein 27: a potential biomarker for hepatocellular carcinoma identified by serum proteome analysis. *Proteomics*, 2005, 5, 4581-4588.

[103] Chuma, M; Sakamoto, M; Yamazaki, K; Ohta, T; Ohki, M; Asaka, M& Hirohashi, S. Expression profiling in multistage hepatocarcinogenesis: identification of HSP70 as a molecular marker of early hepatocellular carcinoma. *Hepatology*, 2003, 37, 198-207.

[104] Luk, JM; Lam, CT; Siu, AF; Lam, BY; Ng, IO; Hu, MY; Che, CM& Fan, ST. Proteomic profiling of hepatocellular carcinoma in Chinese cohort reveals heat-shock proteins (Hsp27, Hsp70, GRP78) up-regulation and their associated prognostic values. *Proteomics*, 2006, 6, 1049-1057.

[105] Takashima, M; Kuramitsu, Y; Yokoyama, Y; Iizuka, N; Toda, T; Sakaida, I; Okita, K; Oka, M& Nakamura, K. Proteomic profiling of heat shock protein 70 family members as biomarkers for hepatitis C virus-related hepatocellular carcinoma. *Proteomics*, 2003, 3, 2487-2493.

[106] King, KL; Li, AF; Chau, GY; Chi, CW; Wu, CW; Huang, CL& Lui, WY. Prognostic significance of heat shock protein-27 expression in hepatocellular carcinoma and its relation to histologic grading and survival. *Cancer*, 2000, 88, 2464-2470.

[107] Miura, N; Shiota, G; Nakagawa, T; Maeda, Y; Sano, A; Marumoto, A; Kishimoto, Y; Murawaki, Y& Hasegawa, J. Sensitive detection of human telomerase reverse transcriptase mRNA in the serum of patients with hepatocellular carcinoma. *Oncology*, 2003, 64, 430-434.

[108] Nagao, K; Tomimatsu, M; Endo, H; Hisatomi, H& Hikiji, K. Telomerase reverse transcriptase mRNA expression and telomerase activity in hepatocellular carcinoma. *J Gastroenterol*, 1999, 34, 83-87.

[109] Miura, N; Maeda, Y; Kanbe, T; Yazama, H; Takeda, Y; Sato, R; Tsukamoto, T; Sato, E; Marumoto, A; Harada, T; Sano, A; Kishimoto, Y; Hirooka, Y; Murawaki, Y; Hasegawa, J& Shiota, G. Serum human telomerase reverse transcriptase messenger RNA as a novel tumor marker for hepatocellular carcinoma. *Clin Cancer Res*, 2005, 11, 3205-3209.

[110] Toshikuni, N; Nouso, K; Higashi, T; Nakatsukasa, H; Onishi, T; Kaneyoshi, T; Kobayashi, Y; Kariyama, K; Yamamoto, K& Tsuji, T. Expression of telomerase-associated protein 1 and telomerase reverse transcriptase in hepatocellular carcinoma. *Br J Cancer*, 2000, 82, 833-837.

[111] Takuma, Y; Nouso, K; Kobayashi, Y; Nakamura, S; Tanaka, H; Matsumoto, E; Fujikawa, T; Suzuki, M; Hanafusa, T& Shiratori, Y. Telomerase reverse transcriptase gene amplification in hepatocellular carcinoma. *J Gastroenterol Hepatol*, 2004, 19, 1300-1304.

[112] Bialkowska-Hobrzanska, H; Bowles, L; Bukala, B; Joseph, MG; Fletcher, R& Razvi, H. Comparison of human telomerase reverse transcriptase messenger RNA and telomerase activity as urine markers for diagnosis of bladder carcinoma. *Mol Diagn*, 2000, 5, 267-277.

[113] Tsai, JF; Jeng, JE; Chuang, LY; You, HL; Wang, LY; Hsieh, MY; Chen, SC; Chuang, WL; Lin, ZY; Yu, ML& Dai, CY. Serum insulin-like growth factor-II as a serologic marker of small hepatocellular carcinoma. *Scand J Gastroenterol*, 2005, 40, 68-75.

[114] Tsai, JF; Jeng, JE; Chuang, LY; You, HL; Ho, MS; Lai, CS; Wang, LY; Hsieh, MY; Chen, SC; Chuang, WL; Lin, ZY; Yu, ML& Dai, CY. Serum insulin-like growth factor-II and alpha-fetoprotein as tumor markers of hepatocellular carcinoma. Tumour Biol, 2003, 24, 291-298.

[115] Harman, SM; Metter, EJ; Blackman, MR; Landis, PK& Carter, HB. Serum levels of insulin-like growth factor I (IGF-I), IGF-II, IGF-binding protein-3, and prostate-specific antigen as predictors of clinical prostate cancer. *J Clin Endocrinol Metab*, 2000, 85, 4258-4265.

[116] Oh, JC; Wu, W; Tortolero-Luna, G; Broaddus, R; Gershenson, DM; Burke, TW; Schmandt, R& Lu, KH. Increased plasma levels of insulin-like growth factor 2 and insulin-like growth factor binding protein 3 are associated with endometrial cancer risk. *Cancer Epidemiol Biomarkers Prev*, 2004, 13, 748-752.

[117] Izzo, F; Cremona, F; Delrio, P; Leonardi, E; Castello, G; Pignata, S; Daniele, B& Curley, SA. Soluble interleukin-2 receptor levels in hepatocellular cancer: a more sensitive marker than alfa fetoprotein. *Ann Surg Oncol*, 1999, 6, 178-185.

[118] Hurteau, JA; Woolas, RP; Jacobs, IJ; Oram, DC; Kurman, CC; Rubin, LA; Nelson, DL; Berchuck, A; Bast, RC, Jr.& Mills, GB. Soluble interleukin-2 receptor alpha is elevated in sera of patients with benign ovarian neoplasms and epithelial ovarian cancer. *Cancer*, 1995, 76, 1615-1620.

[119] Deugnier, Y; David, V; Brissot, P; Mabo, P; Delamaire, D; Messner, M; Bourel, M& Legall, JY. Serum alpha-L-fucosidase: a new marker for the diagnosis of primary hepatic carcinoma? *Hepatology*, 1984, 4, 889-892.

[120] Giardina, MG; Matarazzo, M; Varriale, A; Morante, R; Napoli, A& Martino, R. Serum alpha-L-fucosidase. A useful marker in the diagnosis of hepatocellular carcinoma. *Cancer*, 1992, 70, 1044-1048.

[121] Hutchinson, WL; Johnson, PJ; Du, MQ& Williams, R. Serum and tissue alpha-L-fucosidase activity in the pre-clinical and clinical stages of hepatocellular carcinoma. *Clin Sci (Lond)*, 1991, 81, 177-182.

[122] Giardina, MG; Matarazzo, M; Morante, R; Lucariello, A; Varriale, A; Guardasole, V& De Marco, G. Serum alpha-L-fucosidase activity and early detection of hepatocellular carcinoma: a prospective study of patients with cirrhosis. *Cancer*, 1998, 83, 2468-2474.

[123] Ishizuka, H; Nakayama, T; Matsuoka, S; Gotoh, I; Ogawa, M; Suzuki, K; Tanaka, N; Tsubaki, K; Ohkubo, H; Arakawa, Y& Okano, T. Prediction of the development of hepato-cellular-carcinoma in patients with liver cirrhosis by the serial determinations of serum alpha-L-fucosidase activity. *Intern Med*, 1999, 38, 927-931.

[124] Ayude, D; Gacio, G; Paez de la Cadena, M; Pallas, E; Martinez-Zorzano, VS; de Carlos, A& Rodriguez-Berrocal, FJ. Combined use of established and novel tumour markers in the diagnosis of head and neck squamous cell carcinoma. *Oncol Rep*, 2003, 10, 1345-1350.

[125] Ayude, D; Fernandez-Rodriguez, J; Rodriguez-Berrocal, FJ; Martinez-Zorzano, VS; de Carlos, A; Gil, E& Paez de La Cadena, M. Value of the serum alpha-L-fucosidase activity in the diagnosis of colorectal cancer. *Oncology*, 2000, 59, 310-316.

[126] Tangkijvanich, P; Tosukhowong, P; Bunyongyod, P; Lertmaharit, S; Hanvivatvong, O; Kullavanijaya, P& Poovorawan, Y. Alpha-L-fucosidase as a serum marker of hepatocellular carcinoma in Thailand. *Southeast Asian J Trop Med Public Health*, 1999, 30, 110-114.

[127] Moriyama, A; Masumoto, A; Nanri, H; Tabaru, A; Unoki, H; Imoto, I; Ikeda, M& Otsuki, M. High plasma concentrations of nitrite/nitrate in patients with hepatocellular carcinoma. *Am J Gastroenterol*, 1997, 92, 1520-1523.

[128] Moriyama, A; Tabaru, A; Unoki, H; Abe, S; Masumoto, A& Otsuki, M. Plasma nitrite/nitrate concentrations as a tumor marker for hepatocellular carcinoma. *Clin Chim Acta*, 2000, 296, 181-191.

[129] Beneduce, L; Castaldi, F; Marino, M; Quarta, S; Ruvoletto, M; Benvegnu, L; Calabrese, F; Gatta, A; Pontisso, P& Fassina, G. Squamous cell carcinoma antigen-immunoglobulin M complexes as novel biomarkers for hepatocellular carcinoma. *Cancer*, 2005, 103, 2558-2565.

[130] Giannelli, G; Marinosci, F; Trerotoli, P; Volpe, A; Quaranta, M; Dentico, P& Antonaci, S. SCCA antigen combined with alpha-fetoprotein as serologic markers of HCC. *Int J Cancer*, 2005, 117, 506-509.

[131] Shirai, Y; Kawata, S; Tamura, S; Ito, N; Tsushima, H; Takaishi, K; Kiso, S& Matsuzawa, Y. Plasma transforming growth factor-beta 1 in patients with hepatocellular carcinoma. Comparison with chronic liver diseases. *Cancer*, 1994, 73, 2275-2279.

[132] Tsai, JF; Chuang, LY; Jeng, JE; Yang, ML; Chang, WY; Hsieh, MY; Lin, ZY& Tsai, JH. Clinical relevance of transforming growth factor-beta 1 in the urine of patients with hepatocellular carcinoma. *Medicine (Baltimore),* 1997, 76, 213-226.

[133] Tsai, JF; Jeng, JE; Chuang, LY; Yang, ML; Ho, MS; Chang, WY; Hsieh, MY; Lin, ZY& Tsai, JH. Clinical evaluation of urinary transforming growth factor-beta1 and serum alpha-fetoprotein as tumour markers of hepatocellular carcinoma. *Br J Cancer,* 1997, 75, 1460-1466.

[134] Sacco, R; Leuci, D; Tortorella, C; Fiore, G; Marinosci, F; Schiraldi, O& Antonaci, S. Transforming growth factor beta1 and soluble Fas serum levels in hepatocellular carcinoma. *Cytokine*, 2000, 12, 811-814.

[135] Tsai, JF; Jeng, JE; Chuang, LY; Chang, WY; Hsieh, MY; Lin, ZY& Tsai, JH. Urinary transforming growth factor-beta 1 in relation to serum alpha-fetoprotein in hepatocellular carcinoma. *Scand J Gastroenterol*, 1997, 32, 254-260.

[136] Song, BC; Chung, YH; Kim, JA; Choi, WB; Suh, DD; Pyo, SI; Shin, JW; Lee, HC; Lee, YS& Suh, DJ. Transforming growth factor-beta1 as a useful serologic marker of small hepatocellular carcinoma. *Cancer*, 2002, 94, 175-180.

[137] Ito, N; Kawata, S; Tamura, S; Shirai, Y; Kiso, S; Tsushima, H& Matsuzawa, Y. Positive correlation of plasma transforming growth factor-beta 1 levels with tumor vascularity in hepatocellular carcinoma. *Cancer Lett*, 1995, 89, 45-48.

[138] Narai, S; Watanabe, M; Hasegawa, H; Nishibori, H; Endo, T; Kubota, T& Kitajima, M. Significance of transforming growth factor beta1 as a new tumor marker for colorectal cancer. *Int J Cancer*, 2002, 97, 508-511.

[139] Hegele, A; Varga, Z; von Knobloch, R; Heidenreich, A; Kropf, J& Hofmann, R. TGF-beta1 in patients with renal cell carcinoma. *Urol Res*, 2002, 30, 126-129.

[140] Takahashi, H; Saibara, T; Iwamura, S; Tomita, A; Maeda, T; Onishi, S; Yamamoto, Y& Enzan, H. Serum alpha-L-fucosidase activity and tumor size in hepatocellular carcinoma. *Hepatology*, 1994, 19, 1414-1417.

[141] Xiao, WB& Liu, YL. Elevation of serum and ascites cancer antigen 125 levels in patients with liver cirrhosis. *J Gastroenterol Hepatol*, 2003, 18, 1315-1316.

[142] Grazi, GL; Mazziotti, A; Legnani, C; Jovine, E; Miniero, R; Gallucci, A; Palareti, G& Gozzetti, G. The role of tumor markers in the diagnosis of hepatocellular carcinoma,

with special reference to the des-gamma-carboxy prothrombin. *Liver Transpl Surg*, 1995, 1, 249-255.

[143] Tang, W; Miki, K; Kokudo, N; Sugawara, Y; Imamura, H; Minagawa, M; Yuan, LW; Ohnishi, S& Makuuchi, M. Des-gamma-carboxy prothrombin in cancer and non-cancer liver tissue of patients with hepatocellular carcinoma. *Int J Oncol*, 2003, 22, 969-975.

[144] Sassa, T; Kumada, T; Nakano, S& Uematsu, T. Clinical utility of simultaneous measurement of serum high-sensitivity des-gamma-carboxy prothrombin and Lens culinaris agglutinin A-reactive alpha-fetoprotein in patients with small hepatocellular carcinoma. *Eur J Gastroenterol Hepatol*, 1999, 11, 1387-1392.

[145] Parasole, R; Izzo, F; Perrone, F; Pignata, S; Galati, MG; Leonardi, E; Castiglione, F; Orlando, R; Castello, G; Esposito, G; Gallo, C& Daniele, B. Prognostic value of serum biological markers in patients with hepatocellular carcinoma. *Clin Cancer Res*, 2001, 7, 3504-3509.

[146] Tsai, JF; Jeng, JE; Chuang, LY; Yang, ML; Ho, MS; Chang, WY; Hsieh, MY; Lin, ZY& Tsai, JH. Elevated urinary transforming growth factor-beta1 level as a tumour marker and predictor of poor survival in cirrhotic hepatocellular carcinoma. *Br J Cancer*, 1997, 76, 244-250.

In: Tumor Markers Research Focus
Editor: Deborah H. Chang, pp. 221-239

ISBN: 978-1-60021-544-5


*Chapter XIII*

# Galectin-3: An Useful Tumor Marker in Thyroid and Colorectal Cancer*

***Ludviková Marie[1,4], Holubec Luboš jr[2], Topolčan Ondřej[3], Pešta Martin[3] and Reischig Josef[1]***
[1]Institute of Biology,
[2]Department of Oncology,
[3]Department of Internal Medicine Medical Faculty in Plzen, and
[4]Department of Pathology, 1st Medical Faculty in Prague,
Charles University, Czech Republic

## Abstract

Tissue tumor markers play important role in diagnosis of variety neoplasms. This review aims to summarize: 1/ diagnostic and prognostic difficulties in thyroid and colorectal cancer; 2/ currently available thyroid and colorectal tumor markers; 3/ role of galectin-3 in diagnosis and/or prognosis of these tumors. Results of our current related studies will be also presented.

Thyroid tumors of follicular cell origin represent diagnostically and prognostically difficult group of neoplasms. Namely differentiation between follicular adenoma and carcinoma or between follicular tumor and follicular variant of papillocarcinoma desires additional methods of evaluation, such as immunohistochemical examination of tumor markers (proliferative markers, thyroid peroxidase (TPO), cytokeratin 19 (CK-19), galectin-3 etc).

Colorectal carcinoma is the common cancer in the industrial countries with the high mortality. The main task at the time of pathologist's diagnosis consists in assessment of metastatic potential of colorectal cancer using tumor markers such as metalloproteinases (MMP), tissue inhibitors of metalloproteinases (TIMPS), mucins, and galectin-3 as well.

Galectin-3 (endogenous ß-galactoside-binding protein) as a member of widely distributed carbohydrate-binding proteins that have beeen implicated in the spectrum physiological and pathobiological processes including malignant transformation. Galectin-3 was proven to be expressed in variety cancer cells, mainly of thyroid and colorectal cancer. Its expression in

* Supported by Czech Foundantion League against Cancer (LPR 756) and partly by research project VZ MSM 0021620819

above mentioned tumors has been intensively studied in respects of diagnostic and prognostic role of this tumor marker.
In conclusion, plenty of prognostic and diagnostic thyroid and colorectal tumor markers has been so far studied. However, the ideal specific marker occuring solely within malignant tumor and reliably predicting its biological behavior does not exist. Galectin-3 seems to be promising diagnostic marker in malignant thyroid tumors of follicular cell origin as well as prognostic marker predicting metastases in colorectal carcinomas. Based on our research results and literary experience we recommend to add this marker to the list of significant thyroid and colorectal tissue tumor markers.

# Introduction

Pathology traditionally has been considered to be strictly descriptive morphological discipline based on gross and microscopical examination of tissues only. However, with the advent of new sophisticated laboratory technique (namely immunohistochemistry) pathology has significantly changed during past 20 years. Immunohistochemistry enabled to study a broad range of tissue antigens. Majority of these antigens plays important role of molecular markers in tumor pathology and serve for diagnostic, prognostic and/or predictive purposes. In this way pathologist takes up an important position along with gastroenterologist, surgeon and oncologist in multidisciplinary team attending oncological patient. Current pathology enables not only diagnostic procedure, but also prognostic and predictive evaluation. In this chapter we would like to inform about thyroid and colorectal tumor markers and to focus on a novel marker galectin-3.

# Tumor Markers: an Important Prognostic and Diagnostic Tool

Tumor marker is according to definition any measurable entity that can be used to evaluation of diagnostic and prognostic tumor aspects. Most tumor markers are proteins that are qualitatively abnormal or quantitatively excessive [Eissa 1995].

Tumor markers may be detected either in blood as well as in the other somatic fluids (biochemical markers) or within tumor tissues (tissue markers). The latter group of markers is subject of pathologist´s interest. The great advantages of biochemical markers seems to be possibility to quantify them and to monitore changes in level of their expression. However, they do not provide any information abour site of their expression. These biochemical markers fulfill predominantly prognostic and predictive functions, but their diagnostic role is low. On the other hand, detection of tumor tissue markers enables their accurate localisation within definite neoplasm. Function of tissue markers is not only diagnostic, but also prognostic and predictive as well. In this chapter we would like to focused on tissue tumor markers from pathologist´s point of view.

The most common method used for study of tissue biomarkers is immunohistochemistry, which applies on tissue section immunological principles of linkage between antigen (molecular marker) and specific primary antipody [Asa 2005]. Tissue tumor markers are classified according to their role in diagnostic-therapeutic process into subsequent groups:

- diagnostic molecular markers (specific markers for definite tumor or histogenetically defined group of tumors)
- prognostic molecular markers (molecules are produced by either the tumor or the host (patient) and their expression is usually associated with clinical outcome. Three types of these markers exist reflecting different aspects of tumorous process: markers of cellular growth, markers of invasion/metastaziing, and markers of angiogenesis)
- predictive molecular markers (indicate prospective response of malignant tumor to specific therapy. A typical example of application of this type of marker in routine practice is appraisal of estrogen and progesteron receptor status and HER-2 status in patients with breast cancer)[Tesech 1993].

## Galectin-3: a Novel Promising Tumor Marker

Galectins are β-galactoside binding mammalian lectins and they share characteristic carbohydrate recognition-binding domains, which are evolutionary highly conversed..To date, 14 members of galectin family have been cloned and identified under multiple names, they were re-named as galectin-1 to galectin-14 [Nakahara 2005, Wada 2001]. Galectins play a key role in diverse biological events (e.g. embryogenesis, oncogenesis, adhesion and proliferation of the cells, mRNA splicing, bacterial colonization, apoptosis and in modulation of the immune response) and have implications to clinical diagnostic and therapeutic interventions [Wada 2001]. Distribution of galectins encompasses intracellular space, cell surface as well as extracellular matrix. Each type of galectin participates in a variety of specific biological functions in a given cell type or tissue. Differential expression of the most common galectins (galectin-1 and 3) was documented in progressive colorectal cancer [Sanjuan 1997].

Galectin-3 is a 26 kDa β-galactoside-binding protein with a unique structure consisting of three different domains. Galectin-3 is normally expressed in epithelia of many organs and various inflammatory cells, dendritic cells and Kupfer cells [Brustman 2003, Hsu 1996]. Galectin-3 is distributed within cytoplasma, translocated to the nucleus and/or secreted as soluble proteins[ Nakahara 2005]. Increased galectin-3 levels are associated with various pathological conditions, such as atherosclerosis, inflammations, viral infections, and neoplastic transformation a progression [Nachtigal 1998, Pugliese 2000]. Principal functions of galectin-3 recently were described as follows [Wada 2001, Nakahara 2005, Sano 2000]:

- cell-cell and cell-matrix interaction
- cell migration regulation
- cell growth regulation
- chemoattractant for monocytes and macrophages
- inflammation (activates various type od inflammatory cells)
- modulation of immune system
- modulation of apoptosis
- tumor invasion and metastasis

## Thyroid Cancer: Diagnostic Difficulties and Significance of Tumor Markers

Well differentiated thyroid tumors of follicular cell origin constitute the most common group of thyroid lesions encountered by pathologist [Rosai 1992] (Table 1). Futhermore, oncocytic (Hurthle cell, oxyphilic) variants of above mentioned thyroid neoplasms are known as controversial tumors concerning their natural history and biological behaviour. By the World Health Organisation they are contemporary regard as variant of the existing thyroid tumors categories of follicular cell origin although possibility to consider oncocytic tumors as distinct neoplastic entities is continually discussed [Broner 1997, Carcangiu 1991, Hedinger 1988, Rosai 1992, Rosen 1985, Tallini 1998].

**Table 1. Classification of thyroid tumors of follicular cell origin**

| TUMOR DIFFERENTIATION | TYPE OF BENIGN TUMOR | TYPE OF MALIGNANT TUMOR |
|---|---|---|
| Well differentiated (low-grade) | Follicular adenoma | Follicular carcinoma<br>Papillary carcinoma |
| Poorly differentiated (intermediate-grade) | | Poorly differentiated carcinoma - insular |
| Undifferentiated (high-grade) | | Undifferentiated (anaplastic) carcinoma |

All these tumors (oncocytic and non-oncocytic) can represent a serious challenge for diagnosis owing to unusual morphological criteria of malignancy, such as capsular and/or vascular invasion and nuclear characteristics, respectively [Rosai 1992]. The histological detection of capsular and/or vascular invasion discriminating follicular carcinoma from adenoma as well as the evaluation of nuclear characteristics of papillary carcinoma may be inconclusive in some cases [Fonseca 1995, Suster 2006]. Capsular invasion should only be diagnosed when there is infiltration spreding through capsule into the surrounding thyroid parenchyma and connection between infiltrative tumor islands and the main tumor inside the capsule exists. Likewise, vascular invasion should be assessed in vessels located beyond the capsule. Nuclear characteristics include intranuclear inclusions and clearing, grooving and crowding of nuclei [Rosai 1992]. These criteria are occasionally poorly reproducible and considerably differ from conventional criteria of malignancy, e.g. cellular and nuclear size, polymorphism, hyperchromasia, mitotic activity etc. Considerable inter-observer subjectivity exists in the interpretation of the above mentioned histological features [Kakudo 2002, Williams 2000]. Distinguishing between follicular adenoma and carcinoma or between follicular tumor and follicular variant of papillocarcinoma can often be subtle and subjective and desires additional methods of evaluation, namely immunohistochemical examination of tumor markers.

Molecular markers are expected to solve the diagnostic and prognostic dilemmas [Asa 2005, Eissa 1995, Dabbs 2002, Katoh 2000]. Diagnostic thyroid markers can be divided into following categories: tissue specific markers (essential to determine the origin of sample or origin of neoplastic cells, e.g. thyroglobulin-TG; thyroid transcription factor 1-TTF1; human thyroid peroxidase-TPO) and cancer specific markers (essential to discriminate benign from malignant tumors).

**Table 2. Diagnostic and prognostic markers investigated in thyroid tumors of follicular cell origin**

| Group of tumor marker | Example of tumor marker |
|---|---|
| Differentiation markers | TSH-R, TG, TPO, TTF1, PAX-8 |
| Proliferation markers | Ki-67 (MIB-1), PCNA, topoisomerase II-α |
| Markers of cellular growth (e.g. products of oncogenes, tumor suppressor and apoptosis regulating genes) | TGF-α, VEGF, cerb2/neu, met, ret/PTC, trk, ras,G-protein,cyclins,$p27^{kip}$,telomerase,p53, bax, bcl-2 |
| Tumor-host interaction markers | galectin-3,CD44,E-cadherin,angiogenetic markers, matrix proteases, cell adhesion molecules |
| Other markers | DPPIV,CD-56(NCAM),CD-57,HBME-1 |

**Abbreviations**: TSH-R, thyroid stimulating hormone receptor; TG, thyroglobulin; TPO, thyroid peroxidase; TTF1, thyroid transcription factor 1; PAX-8, specific transcriptional factor activated promoters for TG and TPO; PCNA, proliferative cell nuclear antigen; TGF-α, transforming growth factor; VEGF, vascular endothelial growth factor; DPPIV, dipeptidylaminopeptidase IV; NCAM (CD56), neural cell adhesion molecule;CK19, cytokeratin 19; CEA, carcinoembryonic antigen.

Many tumor markers have been so far tested. However, for the routine use to differentiate among non-neoplastic, benign, and malignant nodules of follicular cell origin, the majority of these diagnostic markers are not sufficiently specific and sensitive [Raphael 2002] (Table 2). Multicenter studies were disappointing and often showed serious limitations in the diagnostic value of these markers due to lack of significant specificity, sensitivity or both [Wada 2001]. From daily practice point of view, implemetation of single tumor marker test in diagnostic process as influenced by methodologic problems as well as fundamental biologic variables. Satisfactory thyroid tumor marker has not been so far revealed, if ever. None of studied markers has been 100% specific, however using them in the panel increases specificity and predictive value and can prone to be helpful in the diagnosis [Raphael 2002]. Immunoprofil of selected thyroid tumors is demonstrated in Table 3.

**Table 3. Significant molecular marker profile of thyroid neoplasms**

| Tumor Phenotype | Tissue Molecular Marker Expression | |
|---|---|---|
| | Positivity | Negativity |
| Follicular adenoma | TG, TPO, TTF-1, CD56 | galectin-3, DPPIV |
| Follicular carcinoma | ras, DPPIV | TPO, CD56 |
| Papillary carcinoma | CK19,galectin-3,HBME-1,CD44, DPPIV, ret/PTC | TPO, CD56 |
| Anaplastic carcinoma | p53, MIB-1 index (increased) | TG,TPO,CD56, TTF-1 |
| Medullary carcinoma | calcitonin,CEA,synaptophysin | TG, TPO |

**Abbreviations**: TSH-R, thyroid stimulating hormone receptor; TG, thyroglobulin; TPO, thyroid peroxidase; TTF1, thyroid transcription factor 1; PAX-8, specific transcriptional factor activated promoters for TG and TPO; PCNA, proliferative cell nuclear antigen; TGF-α, transforming growth factor; VEGF, vascular endothelial growth factor; DPPIV, dipeptidylaminopeptidase IV; NCAM (CD56), neural cell adhesion molecule;CK19, cytokeratin 19; CEA, carcinoembryonic antigen.

Application of prognostic and predictive markers is no use owing to excellent prognosis of well differentiated tumors of follicular cell origin and unique therapy by radioiodine.

## Colorectal Cancer: Natural History and Tumor Markers Applications

Colorectal carcinoma has a worldwide distribution. It represents one of the most common malignancy with persistent high mortality in the United States and Eastern European countries. In spite of improvements of surgical and oncological therapy there has been little change in mortality from colorectal carcinoma during last 40 years. Colorectal cancer shows the increasing incidence and unfortunately the prognosis remains poor for most patiens [Bendardaf 2004].

Colorectal cancer remains asymptomatic for a long time, therefore some cases may be more infiltrated at the time of diagnosis and have poor prognosis. All colorectal carcinomas spread by direct extension into adjacent structures and by metastases through the lymphatic and blood vessels. Most important prognostic indicator of colorectal cancer is the extent of the tumor at the time of diagnosis. In general, the disease has spread beyond the range of curative surgery in 25% to 30% patiens. However, approximately 50% of patiens with „curative“ resection die within five years [Houlston 2001].

Most of cases are sporadic, about 3% of colorectal carcinomas occur in patiens with familiar syndromes (FAP-Familiar Adenomatous Polyposis syndrome, HNPCC-Hereditary Non Polyposis Colorectal Cancer syndrome) or inflammatory bowel disease [Hamilton 2000].

Histological feature of all colonic carcinomas is similar – adenocarcinoma with different grade of differentiation. Sporadically signet-ring appearance of tumorous cells, foci of endocrine differentiation or mucin secretion may be present [Hamilton 2000]. Application of diagnostic tumor markers is required to differentiate anaplastic small cell carcinoma from malignant lymphoma or to determinate endocrine component within tumor. Currently used diagnostic tumor markers are summarized in Table 4 [Bendardaf 2004].

**Table 4. Imunohistochemical markers in differential diagnosis of intestinal tumors**

| Tumor type/ Marker | Carcinoma | Endocrinne tumor | GIST | Malignant lymphoma |
|---|---|---|---|---|
| LCA | - | - | - | + |
| Cytokeratin | + | + | - | - |
| CEA | + | + | - | - |
| EMA | + | + | - | - |
| Chromogranin | - | + | - | - |
| Synaptofyzin | - | + | - | - |
| S100-protein | - | - | +/- | - |
| CD34 | - | - | +/- | - |
| Aktin | - | - | +/- | - |

**Abbreviations**: LCA, common leucocytic antigen; CEA, carcinoembryonic antigen; EMA, epithelial membrane antigen; GIST, gastrointestinal stromal tumor

The identification of patiens with high risk of reccurency is main task in selecting appropriate treatment. Along with traditional prognostic indicators (e.g. age, sex of patient, size of tumor, local and distant spreading, histological type of tumor, pathological staging and grading) prognostic/predictive biochemical and/or tissue molecular markers play recently the important role in determination of biological behavior and treatment. Recommended prognostic markers of colorectal carcinoma comprise [Bendardaf 2004]:

- proliferative markers (MIB-1, topoisomerase-α, PCNA)
- markers of neoplastic transformation (p53, bcl-2, K-ras)
- markers of invasion/metastaziing (matrix metalloproteinases, tissue inhibitors of matrix metalloproteinases, galectin-3 etc.)
- markers of angiogenesis (FVIII, CD31, CD34, VEGF)

Promising predictive tissue markers of colorectal cancer seem to be EGFR-2 and angiogenesis, thymidylate synthase (TS), thymidylate phosphorylase (TP), and dihydropyrimidindehydrogenase (DPD). Levels of last three markers serve as indicator of the sensitivity of tumor cells to fluoritate pyrimidine cytotoxic agents and determine the response of patients with colorectal carcinoma to 5-FU chemotherapy [Bendardaf 2004, Ishibiki 2003, Sakamoto 2003, Tokunaga 2003].

### Aim of Presented Study

In our previous studies of thyroid tumor markers [Kholova 2003, 2004, 2005, Ludvíková 2001] we focused predominantly on proliferative tissue tumor markers, e.g. MIB-1 and topoisomerase-α, angiogenetic markers, and diagnostic marker DPP IV. Recently galectin-3 was proven to be expressed in variety cancer cells including thyroid and colorectal cancer [Bresalier 1997, Brustman 2003, Castronovo 1996, Hermann 2002, Inohara 1999]. This fact provoked us to study this tumor marker in both thyroid tumors and colorectal carcinomas from diagnostic and prognostic point of view. In this study, we describe the expression of galectin-3 in 186 oncocytic and nononcocytic neoplasms of follicular cell origin and in 29 colorectal cancers and their liver metastases. We added galectin-3 to the list of the important thyroid and colorectal tumor markers. Using review of literature, we discuss the diagnostic and prognostic limitations of this marker.

## Material and Method

### Study of Thyroid Neoplams

Studied thyroid neoplasms (186 cases) were retrieved from surgical and consultation files of one autor (M.L.). All specimens (oncocytic follicular adenoma/69 cases; nononcocytic follicular adenoma/40 cases; oncocytic follicular carcinoma/27 cases; nononcocytic follicular carcinoma/7 cases; nononcocytic papillocarcinoma/48 cases; oncocytic papillocarcinoma/24 cases) were histologically classified according to the criteria proposed by the WHO [Hedinger 1988] into six groups clinicopathologic characteristics of them are summarized in Table 5.

**Table 5. Clinicopathologic characteristics of studied groups of tumors**

| Type of tumor | Number of cases | Sex | |
|---|---|---|---|
| | | F | M |
| Oncocytic follicular adenoma (OA) | 69 | 59 | 10 |
| Nononcocytic follicular adenoma (NA) | 40 | 31 | 9 |
| Oncocytic follicular carcinoma (OFC) | 27 | 19 | 8 |
| Nononcocytic follicular carcinoma(FC) | 7 | 5 | 2 |
| Nononcocytic papillocarcinoma (PC) | 48 | 41 | 7 |
| Oncocytic papillocarcinoma (OPC) | 24 | 20 | 4 |

**Abbreviations**: F, female; M, male

Immunohistochemical examination was performed on paraffin sections using SABC (Novostain ABC, Novocastra, Newcastle upon Tyne, UK) immunoperoxidase method with monoclonal antibodies against mitochondrial antigen (clone 113-1, Biogenex; 1:800), and galectin-3 (clone 9C4, Novocastra; 1:100). Endogenous biotin was eliminated by biotin blocking system (DAKO).

Quantitative analysis of galectin-3 was carried out using a light microscope Olympus BX-40 equipped with a 40x magnification objective and special eye-piece 10x10-mm grid. The percentage of galectin-3 positive neoplastic cells (galectin-3 index) was determined by counting at least 1000 tumor cells per slide in randomly selected fields of tumors.

Statistical analysis was performed using the S.A.S. package, releas 8.02. Mean, median, standart deviation and range were counted. The data were analysed by Wilcoxon test; p-values equal or to less than 0.05 were considered as significant.

## Study of Colorectal Cancer

We collected 29 primary colorectal carcinomas (stage IV) with synchronous hepatic metastases. Cancer staging was performed according to TMN classification. Adenocarcinomas were graded on the basis of the extent od glandular appearence into well, moderately and poorly differenciated tumors [Hamilton 2000]. All patiens underwent 2-steps surgery between 1999-2005 ( resection of liver metastases followed surgery of primary tumor in range 1-5 months). All specimen were formalin fixes and paraffin embedded.

Immunohistochemical analysis was performed by standard immunohistochemical method with monoclonal primary antibody again galectin-3 (clone 9C4, Novocastra; 1:100) according to manufacturer′ recomendations. Positivity of endothelial cells served as internal control. Negative controls were made by omitting the primary antibody. Harris′ hematoxylin was used to counterstaining the slides. Futhermore mRNA galectin 3 and housekeeping gene (GAPDH) in 15 liver metastases were quantified using the method of RT real-time PCR.

Quantitative analysis of immunohistochemical expression of galectin-3 was performed as the same manner as analysis in the study of thyroid neoplasms by assessment of percentage of positive tumor cells. Intensity of staining was also been taken into consideration (mild +, moderate ++, strong +++ intensity).

Analysis of galectin-3 mRNA in hepatic metastases was performed in several steps:

*-Tissue samples*

The tumor tissue were obtained from 15 patients with liver metastasis from colorectal carcinoma. All tumor were histologically verified. Tumot tissue samples were taken during surgery, and after surgical resection these were frozen to -70°C and kept at this temperature until used. We examinated 2-3 samples from each tumor .

*-RNA extractions*

Total RNA was isolated from 100 mg of tissue using fastRNA Pro Green Kit (Q BIOgene, USA). The amount of isolated total RNA was assessed spectrophotometrically and kept at -70°C.

*-Reverse-Transcription*

3μg of isolated total RNA were used for reverse transcription (RT), which was performed with Superscript II Reverse Transcriptase (Life Technologies, USA) and oligo $d(T)_{21}$ as a primer.

*-Real-Time Polymerase Chain Reaction*

Primers for Gal-3 were developed in our laboratory (Gal-3: forward primer, 5'-GAA CAA CAG GAG AGT CAT TGT TTG -3'; reverse primer, 5'-TAT GAA GCA CTG GTG AGG TCT ATG-3'), customs synthesis (GeneriBiotech, Czech republic). Primers for GAPDH were synthesized as published in the manual of Corbett Research. PCR fragments of Gal-3 and GAPDH were inserted in to pGEM vector (Promega Corporation, USA) and cloned. PGEM plasmids with cloned fragments of Gal-3 and GAPDH were diluted to concentrations of $10^3$-$10^8$ molecule copies per μl and used as a standards. 1 μl of the RT product of each sample was used for real-time PCR. We performed real-time PCR using a Rotor-Gene apparatus (Corbett Research, Australia). DNA amplification was monitored with 0.5x Sybr-Green I (Molecular Probes, USA). The size of the PCR amplification product for GAPDH was 226 bp, in Gal-3 246 bp. The specificity of the reaction was verified with the melting curve and agarose gel electrophoresis. The quantification was performed as relative, ratio of the number of copies in the assessed gene Gal-3 and GAPDH (Gal-3/GAPDH).

Statistical analysis was conducted by Wilcoxon test and Spearmann correlation coefficient and $p<0,05$ was defined as the level of significance. All statistical analyses were carried out using S.A.S. package, releas 8.02. Statistical analysis of immunohistochemical expression was calculated both without threshold, and with threshold (e.g. immunohistochemical staining was defined as negative if the percentage of positive-staining cancer cells accounted for less than 30% of the total number of cancer cells.)

# Results

## Study of Thyroid Neoplasms

All studied tumors were submitted to galectin-3 immunoanalysis. Immunopositive neoplastic cells showed typical diffuse slightly granular brown cytoplasmic expression (Fig.1). Positivity of endothelial cells as well as macrophages was not considered during semiquantitative analysis, but served as positive internal control. Normal or diseased nonneoplastic thyroid tissue was negative (Fig.1). Galectin-3 indexes were assessed in all cases and were stratified according to intervals 0-10(%), 11-50(%), 51-80(%), 81-100(%) set in advance (review of galectin-3 index values are shown in Table 6 and Chart 1). Oncocytic differentiation was proven by immunohistochemical positivity of mitochondrial antigen.

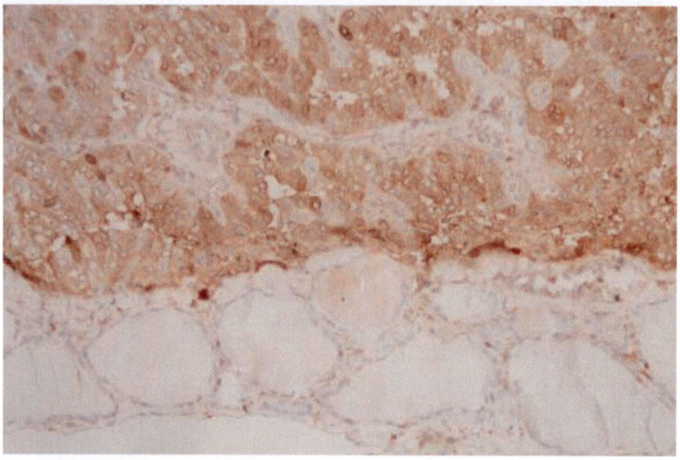

Figure 1. Papillary carcinoma show cytoplasmic galectin-3 positivity. Nonneoplastic thyroid tissue in the bottom is negative (x200).

Comparison of galectin-3 indexes between studied groups of tumors was performed by Wilcoxon test. Galectin-3 was produced in both benign, and malignant thyroid tumors of follicullar cell origin. Significant differences in galectin-3 expression were found between follicular adenomas and papillocarcinomas (oncocytic and nononcocytic)($p<0.0001$), but not between follicullar adenomas and follicular carcinomas ($p=0.0829$; $p=0.6936$). Interestingly, galectin-3 was significantly upregulated in papillary carcinomas in comparison with the other tumors ($p<0.0001$). Noteworthy significant differences were discovered between oncocytic and nononcocytic variants of studied tumors excluding follicular carcinoma. Influence of endogenous biotin (in oncocytic mitochondrion-rich cells) was eliminated before immunohistochemical procedure. Optimal sensitivities and specificities were found for both variants of papillary carcinomas only along with cut-off 50% for discrimination between papillary carcinomas and the other malignant and benign tumors.

**Table 6. Galectin-3 indexes in studied groups of tumors**

| Type of tumor | N | Mean [%] | Med [%] | SD [%] | Range [%] |
|---|---|---|---|---|---|
| NA | 38 | 3,6 | 0 | 10,9 | 0-60 |
| OA | 53 | 6,1 | 1,0 | 9,4 | 0-40 |
| FC | 6 | 1,7 | 0 | 2,6 | 0-5 |
| OFC | 23 | 12,2 | 10,0 | 14,0 | 0-40 |
| PC | 43 | 90,6 | 100,0 | 16,2 | 30-100 |
| OPC | 23 | 83,9 | 90,0 | 18,5 | 25-100 |

N ……. number of cases

SD …..standard deviation

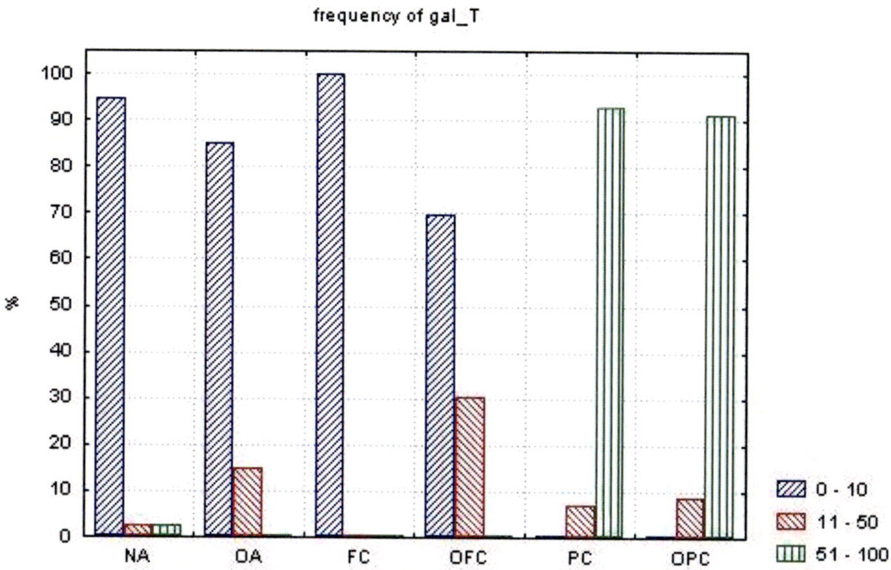


Chart 1. Distribution of galectin-3 in studied groups of tumors considering stratification of indexes (%) into intervals

## Study of Colorectal Cancer

In all specimen of normal colorectal epithelium strongly positive expression was observed. Galectin-3 was stained as granulated forms on nucleus, cytoplasm, apical surface and basal membrane sites. Tumor cells showed granulated cytoplasmic galectin-3 expression. Nuclear expression was not observed in neoplastic cells (Fig. 2).

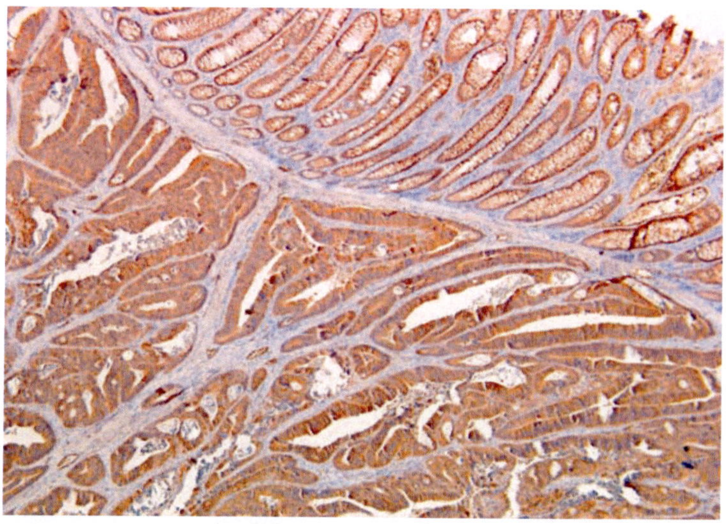

Figure 2. Both colorectal carcinoma, and normal intestinal epithelium (upper right) express galectin-3 (x100).

Galectin-3 cytoplasmic expression was observed in all primary and metastatic colorectal cancer, however 7 cases of primary tumors (7/29; 20,3%) and 6 cases of liver metastase (6/29; 17,5%) were considered as negative using threshold 30%. Five patiens had galectin-3 negativity in both tumors. No differences between both groups of tumors (primary and secondary) were proven ($p<0.0001$). Galectin-3 expression in primary tumors as well as in their metastases significantly correlated regadless of using threshold ($p<0.0001$, $r=0.70695$; $p<0.0001$, $r=0.80889$). Expression of mRNA galectin-3 did not correlate with immunohistochemical analysis of galectin-3 protein in liver metastases ($p=0.4450$). Considerable heterogeneity of intratumoral galectin-3 localization was seen. Grading of primary and secondary tumors did not correspond with galectin-3 expression ($p=0.8864$; $p=0.8155$). Significant correlation was proven between galectin-3 immunoexpression and intensity of staining within primary tumors as well as within metastases, however correlations coefficients were low ($p=0.0003$, $r=0.61990$; $p=0.0016$, $r=0.55880$). Similar low correlation between grading primary and secondary tumors was determined ($p=0.0033$, $r=0.52719$).

## Conclusion

As mentioned above, tissue tumor markers are expected to make diagnostic and prognostic procedure more easier in thyroid tumors as well as in colorectal cancer. Tumor markers can better characterize these tumors than has been possible by classical morphology and traditional prognostic factors. However, to date results of many multi-centric studies were disappointing and studies showed the diagnostic and prognostic limitations of all tissue markers due to the lack of significant specificity, sensitivity or both. No single marker can cover our diagnostic/ prognostic demands, however, the use of the panel of markers increases specificity and predictive value and can be helpful in the diagnostic/prognostic dilemmas [De Leon Mazariegos 2006]. Advances in understanding of the molecular process of cancer will allow identification of new markers and implementatation of them to routine diagnostic/ prognostic procedure. This fact is true not only for tumors rewieved within this chapter.

One of the very promising marker in both thyroid and colorectal tumors seems to be galectin-3 [Ito 2005]. Generally, galectin-3 was proven to play important role in cancerogenesis and pathobiology of tumors, although the detail mechanism of it has not been elucidated yet [Wada 2001]. Galectin-3 expression is affected by neoplastic transformation. Overexpression was found in certain type of gonadal [Devouassoux-Shisheboran 2006], and thyroid tumors [Cvejic 2000, Fernandes 1997] as well as in other types of malignancies such as colorectal [Nakamura 1999], gastric [Mizayaki 2002] brest [Castronovo 1996], and uterine [Brustman 2003] carcinomas. Galectin-3 expression is also supposed to be associated with neoplastic progression and metastatic potential [Endo 2005, Nakamura 1999]. Strong correlation between expression of galectin-3 and the grade and malignant potential of primary brain tumors was presented by Bresalier [1997].

A few different mechanisms of tumor transformation and progression have been proposed with respect to diverse function of galectin-3. Galectin-3 is multifunctional protein implicated in a variety biological processes including cell adhesion, proliferation, differentiation, migration, and apoptosis, and all these processes may result in neoplastic transformation and progression. Nuclear, cytoplasmic, and extracellular galectin-3 seems to be linked with its diverse functions [Davidson 2002]. Shift from nuclear to cytoplasmic expression of galectin-3 during tumor progression may occur and was reported previously in squamous carcinoma of tongue by Lotz [1993]. Galectin-3 exhibits dual role in activation of apoptosis: anti-apoptotic and pro-apoptotic [Nakahara 2005]. Both mechanisms may serve malignant transformation and progression. Intracellular and extracellular galectin-3 demonstrates anti-apoptotic activity in response to various apoptotic stimuli on a wide variety of cells by interaction with different cytoplasmic and nuclear proteins or by increased cell adhesion to an extracellular matrix [Matarrese 2000]. Galectin-3 also prevents T-cell apoptosis through interaction with the bcl-2 family members [Yang 1996]. Resistence to apoptosis is crucial moment for tumor cell survival and spreading. Extracellular galectin-3 exhibiting pro-apoptotic activity on T-cells supports the immune escape mechanism during tumor progression [Yang 1996]. Galectin-3 inhibition of apoptosis involves protection of mitochondrial integrity, inhibition of cytochrome c release and caspase activation [Moon 2001]. Along with anti-apoptotic function of galectin-3, modulation of MUC2 mucin expression at the level of transcription in human colon cancer seems to be important factor of progression [ Dudas 2002, Song 2005 ].

The majority of thyroid tumor markers reflect different processes of neoplastic transformation in follicular and papillary carcinomas. According to multi-step carcinogenesis hypothesis follicular carcinomas are generated from follicular adenomas, while papillary carcinomas are derived from cells generated by normal thyrocytes (Tallini 2002, Takano 2004). Morphological diagnostic approaches do not always consistently and reliably discriminate benign from malignant follicular neoplasms, follicular tumor from follicular variant of papillary carcinoma, and neoplastic papillary structures from hyperplastic, respectively. Therefore lots of molecular markers have been studied in the attempt to improve diagnosis [Lloyd 2001, Papotti 2005]. Available thyroid tissue tumor markers are of limited diagnostic value and can be used routinely only in the panel of markers as an auxiliary diagnostic tool [Mehrotra 2004]. Morphological diagnostic criteria of thyroid tumors remain a golden standard. The „magic biomarker" to segregate thyroid disorders into malignant and benign remains to be discovered.

To the best of our knowledge, this is the first galectin-3 study performed on the largest comprehensive collection of well differentiated benign and malignant thyroid tumors of follicular cell origin with emphasis on its oncocytic and nononcocytic variants. From routine practice point of view we determined or confirmed the important conclusions as follow:

-significant differences of galectin-3 expression were discovered between papillary carcinomas on the one hand and remaining benign and malignant tumors on the other hand only

-galectin-3 seems to be usable tumor marker for papillary carcinomas and its discrimination from papillary hyperplasia and proliferative follicular lesions (cut-off 50%). In agreement with prevoius studies, no significant differences in galectin-3 expression were proven between follicular adenomas and follicular carcinomas [Mehrotra 2004, Nucera 2005].

-galectin-3 showed significant overexpression in oncocytic variants of studied tumors. Overexpression of galectin-3 in oncocytic tumors of thyroid gland seems to be the other argument supporting opinion of being of oncocytic tumors as pathobiologically separate entity. The problem of independence of oncocytic tumorous entities remains to be further eluciated.

-galectin-3 can be add to the list of adjunct tumor markers usable in differential diagnosis of well differentiated thyroid tumors of follicular cell origin (TABLE 4).

**Table 7. Review of basic correlated parameters**

| Type of correlation | p-value | r |
|---|---|---|
| Gal3CRC vs Gal3META | 0.0001 | 0.70695 |
| Gal3CRCx vs Gal3METAx | 0.0001 | 0.80889 |
| Gal3META vs rel mRNAGal3META | 0.4450 | - 0.21346 |
| Gal3METAx vs rel mRNAGal3META | 0.7266 | - 0.09860 |
| Gal3META vs intensityGal3META | 0.0016 | 0.55880 |
| Gal3CRC vs intensityGal3CRC | 0.0003 | 0.61990 |
| Grading CRC vs Grading META | 0.0033 | 0.52719 |
| Gal3CRC vs Grading CRC | 0.8864 | - 0.02775 |
| Gal3META vs Grading META | 0.8158 | 0.04523 |

**Abbreviations:** r, correlation coefficient; Gal3CRC, expression of galectin-3 in primary tumor; Gal3META, expression of galectin-3 in metastasis; Gal3CRCx, expression of galectin-3 in primary tumor with threshold; Gal3METAx, expression of galectin-3 in metastasis with threshold; rel mRNAGal3META, relative amount of mRNA galectin-3 in metastasis; intensityGal3CRC, intensity of expression of galectin-3 in primary tumor; intensityGal3META, intensity of expression of galectin-3 in metastasis; Grading CRC, grade of primary tumor; Grading META, grade of metastasis

Galectin-3 expression was earlier studied in relation to progression of colorectal cancer with contradictory results; down-regulation was published by Lotz [1993] and Castronovo [1992] whereas up-regulation was disclosed by Irimura [1991], Schoeppner [1995] and Nakamura [1999]. Discrepancies in published data should by partly explained by different methods of sample selection, by the use of different antibodies and by different aproaches to interpretation of staining [Itzkowitz 1997, Legendre 2003]. We aimed in present study to determinate galectin-3 involvement in both primary tumor and liver metastasis by immunohistochemistry to explore whether it is related to the tumor progression. Futhermore assessment of galectin-3 mRNA levels in metastatic lesion was performed. Expression of galectin-3 was heterogenous within individual tumors and metastatic nodules therefore seems to be necessary to obtain and examine the large number of samples of each tumor. Liver metastatic lesions showed up-regulated levels of galectin-3 which correlated with the up-regulation in primary tumors. As follows from previous study including that of herein presented, galectin-3 may serve as an important prognostic marker in colorectal cancer and indicate potential propensity of tumor to metastize [ Endo 2005, Sanjuan 1997]. Prevoius studies were curried out on cohort of mixed colorectal lesion with low number of metastaziing colorectal cancers (predominantly lymph nodes metastase) [Endo 2005, Inufusa 2001, Nakamura 1999] and did not show exactly relationship in galectin-3 imunoexpression within primary and metastatic colorectal carcinomas. Number od copies of galectin-3 mRNA does not correlate with immunoprofil of galectin-3 within metastases – this fact remains to be eluciated. Futher studies are required to explain the pathobiological role of galectin-3 in progression of colorectal cancer and its possible predicting value in relationship to anti-galectin-3 therapy.

In conclusion, now and in the future pathologists will play a crucial role in the emerging world of molecular medicine. Pathologists will be expected to provide specific prognostic and predictive information in their diagnostic reports. This may require to work closely with a variety of clinicians. Further investigation is required to better define new tumor-specific biomarkers. Galectin-3 was proven to be useful diagnostic/prognostic marker in thyroid and colorectal tumors, respectively. We recommend to add it to the list of adjunct tumor markers usable in differential diagnosis of well differentiated thyroid tumors of follicular cell origin as well as in predicting prognosis of colorectal cancer.

## References

Asa, SL. The role of immunohistochemical markers in the diagnosis of follicular-patterened lesions of the thyroid. *Endocr Pathol*, 2005, 16, 295-309.

Bendardaf, R; Lamplum, H; Pyrhonen, S. Prognostic and predictive molecular markers in colorectal carcinoma. *Anticancer Research*, 2004, 24, 2519-2530.

Bresalier, RS; Yan, PS; Byrd, JC; Lotan, R; Raz, A. Expression of the endogenous galactose binding protein galectin-3 correlates with the malignant potential of tumors in the central nervous system. *Cancer*, 1997, 80, 776 -787 .

Bronner, MP. Hürthle cell lesions of the thyroid. *Pathol Case Rev,* 1997, 2(5). 200-209.

Brustman, H; Riss, D; Naudé, S. Galectin-3 expression in normal, hyperplastic, and neoplastic endometrial tissues. *Pathol Res Pract*, 2003, 199, 151-158.

Carcangiu, ML; Bianchi, S; Savino, D; Voynick, IM; Rosai, J. Follicular Hürthle cell tumors of the thyroid gland. *Cancer*,1991, 68, 1944-1953.

Castronovo, V; Campo, E; van Der Brule, FA; Claysmith, AP; Cioce, V; Liu, FT. Inverse modulation of steady-state messenger RNA levels of two non-integrin laminin-binding proteins in human colon carcinoma. *J Natl Cancer Inst*, 1992, 84, 1161-1169.

Castronovo, V; Van den Brul, FA; Jackers, P; Clausse, N; Liu, FT; Gillet, O; Sobel, ME. Decreased expression of galectin-3 is associated with progression of human brest cancer. *J Pathol*, 1996, 179, 43 - 47 .

Cvejic, D; Savin, S; Golubovic, S; Paunovic, I; Tatic, S; Havelka, M. Galectin-3 and carcinoembryonic antigen expression in medullary thyroid carcinoma: possible relation to tumor progression. *Histopathology*, 2000, 37, 530-535.

Dabbs DJ: *Diagnostic immunohistochemistry*. Churchill Livingstone 2002.

Davidson, PJ; Davis, MJ; Patterson RJ; Ripoche, MA; Poirier, F; Wang, JL. Shuttling of galectin-3 between the nukleus and cytoplasm. *Glycobiology*, 2002, 12, 329-337.

De-Leon-Mazariegos, R; Canedo-Patzi, M; Perez-Enriquez, B; Candanedo-Gonzalez, F; Saqui-Salces, M; Gamboa-Dominguez, A; Rull-Rodrigo, JA. Low galectin-3 capacity to discriminate thyroid lesions. *Rev Invest Clin*, 2004, 56(5), 623-628. Article in Spanish

Devouassoux-Shisheboran, M; Deschildre, C; Mauduit, C; Berger, G; Mejean-Lebreton, F; Bouvier, R; Droz, JP; Fenichel, P; Benahmed, M. Expression of galectin-3 in gonáda and gonadal sex cord stroma and germ cell tumors. *Oncol Rep*, 2006, 16(2), 335-340.

Dudas, SP; Yunker, CK; Sternberg, LR. Expression of human intestina mucin is modulated by the β-galactoside binding protein galectin-3. Gastroenterology, 2002, 123, 817-826.

Eissa, S; Shoman, S. *Tumor markers*. 1995, Chapman&Hall, London

Endo, K; Kohnoe, S; Tsujita, E; Watanabe, A; Nakashima, H; Baba, H; Maehara, Y. Galectin-3 expression is a potent prognostic marker in colorectal cancer. *Anticancer Research*, 2005, 25, 3117-3122.

Fernandez, PL; Merino, MJ; Gomez, M; Campo, E; Medina, T; Castronovo, V; Cardesa, A; Liu, FT; Sobel, ME. Galectin-3 and laminin expression in neoplastic and non-neoplastic thyroid tissue. *J Pathol*, 1997, 181, 80 -86 .

Fonseca, E; Sobrinho-Simoes, M. Diagnostic problems in differentiated carcinomas of the thyroid. *Path Res Pract*, 1995, 191, 318-331.

Hamilton, SR; Aaltonen, LA. Pathology and genetics of tumours of the digestive system. WHO classification of tumors. *IARC Press*, Lyon, 2000, 103-144.

Hedinger, C; Williams, ED; Sobin, LH. Histological typing of thyroid tumours. *WHO-International Histological Classification of Tumours*. 2nd edn. Berlin: Springer-Verlag, 1988.

Herrmann, ME; LiVolsi, VA; Pasha, T; Roberts, SA; Wojcik, EM; Baloch, ZW. Immunohistochemical expression of galectin-3 in benign and malignant thyroid lesions. *Arch Pathol Lab Med*, 2002, 126, 710-713.

Houlston, RS. What we could do now: molecular pathology of colorectal cancer. J Clin Pathol: Mol Pathol, 2001, 54, 206-214.

Hsu, DK; Hammes SR; Kuwabara I; Greene WC; Liu FT. Human T lymphotropic virus-1 infection of human T lymphocytes induces expression of the β-galactose-binding lecitin, galectin-3. *Am J Pathol*, 1996, 148,1661 - 1670 .

Inufusa, H; Nakanura, M; Adachi, T; Aga, M; Kurimoto, M; Nakatani, Y; Wakano, T; Miyake, M; Okuno, K; Shiozaki, H; Yasutomi, M. Role of galectin-3 in adenocarcinoma liver metastasis. *Int J Oncol*, 2001, 19(5), 913-919.

Irimura, T; Matsushita, Y; Sutton, RC; Carralero, D; Ohannesian, DW; Cleary, KR; Ota, DM; Nicolson, GL; Lotan, R. Increased content of an endogenous lactose-binding lectin in human colorectal carcinoma progressed to metastatic stages. *Cancer Res*, 1991, 51, 387-393.

Ishibiki, Y; Kitajima, M; Sakamoto, K; Tomik, Y; Sakamoto, S; Kaman, M. Intratumoral thymidylate synthese and dihydropyrimidine dehydrogenace activities are good predictors of 5-fluorouracil sensitivity in colorectal cancer. *J Int Med Res*, 2003, 31(3), 181-187.

Ito Y, Yoshida H, Tomoda C, Miya A, Kobayashi K, Matsuzuka F, Yasuoka H, Kakudo K, Inohara H, Kuma K, Miyauchi A. Galectin-3 expression in follicular tumours: an immunohistochemical study of its use as a marker of follicular carcinoma. *Pathology*, 2005, 37(4), 296-298.

Inohara, H; Honjo, Y; Yoshii, T; Akahani, S; Yoshida, J; Hattori, K; Okamoto, S; Sawada, T; Raz, A; Kubo, T: Expression of galectin-3 in fine needle aspirates as a diagnostic marker differentiating benign from malignant thyroid neoplasms. *Cancer* 1999, 85, 2475-2484.

Itzkowitz, SH. Galectins: multipurpose carbohydrate-binding proteins implicated in tumor biology. *Gastroenterology*, 1997, 113, 2003-2005.

Kakudo, K; Katoh, R; Sakamot, A; Asa, S; DeLellis, R; Carney, JA; Naganuma, H; Kameyama, K; Takam, H. Thyroid gland: international case conference. *Endocrine Pathology*, 2002; 13: 131-134.

Katoh, R; Kawaoi, A; Miyag, E; Li, X; Suzuki, K; Nakamur, Y; Kakudo, K. Thyroid transcription factor-1 in normal, hyperpplastic, and neoplastic follicular thyroid cells examinated by immunohistochemistry and nonradioactive in situ hybridization. *Mod Pathol*, 2000, 13, 570-576.

Kholová, I; Ludvíková, M; Ryška, A; Topolčan, O; Pikner, R; Pecen, L; Čáp, J; Holubec, L Jr. Diagnostic role of markers dipeptidyl peptidase IV and thyroid peroxidase in thyroid tumors. *Anticancer Res*, 2003, 23 (2A),871-875.

Kholová, I; Ryška, A; Ludvíková, M; Čáp, J. Thyroid peroxidase in thyroid gland differential diagnosis. The marker of malignancy or differentiation? *Čes-slov Patol*, 2004, 40, 18-21 (in Czech).

Kholová, I; Ryška, A; Ludviková, M; Čáp, J; Pecen, L. Dipeptidyl peptidase IV expression in thyroid cytology: retrospective histologically confirmed study. *Cytopathology*, 2003, 14(1), 27-31.

Legendre, H; Decaestecker, Ch; Nagy, N; Hendlisz, A; Schuring, MP; Salmon, I; Gabius, HJ; Pector, JC; Kiss, R: Prognostic values of galectin-3 and the macrophage migration inhibitory factor (MIF) in human colorectal cancers. *Mod Pathol*, 2003, 16(5), 491-504.

Lotz, MM; Andrews, CW Jr; Korzelius, CA; Lee, EC; Steele GD, Jr; Clarke, A; mercurio AM. Decreased expression of Mac-2 (carbohydrate binding protein 35) and loss of its nuclear localization are associated with the neoplastic progression of colon carcinoma. *Proc Natl Acad Sci USA*, 1993, 90, 3466-3470.

Ludvíková, M; Holubec, L Jr; Ryška, A; Topolčan, O. Proliferative markers in diagnosis of thyroid tumors: a comparative study of MIB-1 and topoisomerase II-α immunostaining. *Anticancer Research*, 2005, 25, 1835-1840.

Ludvíková, M; Ryška, A; Korabečná, M; Rydlová, M; Michal, M. Oncocytic papillary carcinoma with lymphoid stroma (Warthin-like tumour) of the thyroid: a distinct entity with favourable prognosis. *Histopathology* 2001; 39(1): 17-24.

Lloyd, RV. Distinguishing benign from malignant thyroid lesions: galectin-3 as the latest candidate. *Endocrine Patology*, 2001, 12(3), 255-257.

Matarrese,P; Fusco, O; Tinari, N; Natoli, C; Liu, FT; Semeraro, ML; Malorni, W;Iacobelli, S. Galectin-3 overexpression protects from apoptosis by improving cell adhesion properties. *Int J Cancer*, 2000, 85, 545-554.

Mehrotra, P; Okpokam, A; Bouhaidar, R; Johnson, SJ; Wilson, JA; Davies, BR; Lennard, TWJ. Galectin-3 does not reliably distinguish benign from malignant thyroid neoplasms. *Histopathology*, 2004, 45, 493-500.

Moon, BK; Lee, YJ; Battle, P; Jessup, JM; Raz, A; Choi, KHR. Galectin-3 protects human Brest carcinoma cells against nitric oxide – induced apoptosis. *Am J Pathol*, 2001, 159, 1055-1060.

Miyazaki, J; Hokari, R; Kato, S; Tsuzuki, Y; Kawaguchi, A; Nagao, S; Itoh, K; Miura, S. Increased expression of galectin-3 in primary gastric cancer and the metastatic lymph nodes. *Oncol Rep*, 2002, 9, 1307-1312.

Nachtigal,, M; Al-Assaad, Z; Mayer, EP; Kim, K; Monsigny, M. Galectin-3 expression in human atherosclerotic lesions. *Am J Pathol*, 1998, 152, 1199 -1208 .

Nakahara, S; Oka, N; Ray, A. On the role of galectin-3 in cancer apoptosis. *Apoptosis*, 2005, 10, 267 – 275.

Nakamura, M; Inufusa, H; Adachi, T; Aga, M; Kurimoto, M; Nakatani, Y; Wakano, T; Nakajima, A; Hida, JI; Miyake, M; Shindo, K;Yasutomi, M. Involvment of galectin-3 expression in colorectal cancer progression and metastasis. *Int J Oncol*, 1995, 15, 143-148.

Nucera, C; Mazzon, E; Caillou, B; Violi, MA; Moleti, M; Priolo, C; Sturniolo, G; Puyyolo, D; Cavallari, V; Trimarchi, F; Vermiglio, F. Human galectin-3 immunoexpression in thyroid follicular adenomas with cell atypia. *J Endocrinolog Invest*, 2005, 28, 106-112.

Papotti, M; Rodriguez, J; De Pompa, R; Bartolazzi, A; Rosai, J. Galectin-3 and HBME-1 expression in well-differentiated thyroid tumors with follicular architecture of uncertain malignant potential. *Modern Pathology*, 2005; 18: 541-546.

Pugliese, G; Pricci, F; Leto, G; Amadio, L; Iacobini, C; Romeo, G; Lenti, L; Sale, P; Graduji, R; Liu, FT; DiMario, U. The diabetic milieu modulates the advanced glycation and produkt-receptor complex in masangium by inducing or upregulating galectin-3 expression. *Diabetes*, 2000, 49, 1249-1257.

Raphael, SJ. The meanings of markers: anciliary techniques in diagnosis of thyroid neoplasia. *Endocrine Pathology*, 2002, 13: 301-311.

Rosai, J; Carcangiu, ML; DeLellis, RA. Tumors of thyroid gland. Atlas of tumor pathology, 3rd Series, Fascicle 5. Washington, DC: A.F.I.P., 1992.

Rosen, IB; Luk, S; Katz I. Hürthle cell tumor behavior: dilemma and resolution. *Surgery*, 1985, 98, 777-783.

Sakamoto, J; Hamashima, H; Suzuji, H; Ito, K; Mai, M; Saj, S; Fukushi, M; Matsushita, Y; Nakazato, H. Thymidylate synthase expression as a predictor of the prognosis of curatively resected colon carcinoma in patiens registred an adjuvant immunochemotherapy clinical trial. *Oncol Rep*, 2003, 10 (5), 1081-90.

Sanjuan, X; Fernandez, PL; Castells, A; Castronovo, V; Van den Brule, F; Liu, FT; Cardesa, A; Campo, E. Differential expression of galectin 3 and galectin 1 in colorectal cancer progression.*Gastroenterology*, 1997, 113(6),1906-1915.

Sano,H; Hsu, DK; Yu, L; Apgar, JR;, Kuwabara, I; Yamanaka, T; Hirashima, K; Liu, FT. Human galectin-3 is a novel chemoattractant for monocytes and macrophages. *J Immunol*, 2000, 165(4), 2156-2164.

Schoeppner, HL; Raz, A; Ho, SB; Bresalier, RS. Expression of an endogenous galactose-binding lectin correlates with neoplastic progression in the colon. *Cancer*, 1995, 75, 2818-2826.

Song, S; Byrd, JC; Mazurek, N; Liu, K; Koo, JS; Bresalier, RS. Galectin-3 modulates MUC2 mucin expression in human colon cancer cells at the level of transcription via AP-1 activation. *Gastroenterology*, 2005, 5, 129, 1581-1591.

Suster, S. Thyroid tumors with a follicular growth pattern. *Arch Pathol Lab Med*, 2006, 130, 984-988.

Takano, T. Fetal cell carcinogenesis of the thyroid: a hypothesis for better understanding of gene expression profile and genomic alteration in thyroid carcinoma. *Endocrine Journal*, 2004; 51 (6): 509-515.

Tallini, G. Oncocytic tumors. Virchows Arch, 1998, 433, 5-12.

Tallini, G. Molecular pathobiology of thyroid neoplasms. *Endocrine Patology*, 2002, 13, 271-288.

Tesech, M; Shawwa, A; Hendersoon, R. Immunohistochemical determination of estrogen and progesterone receptor status in breast cancer. *Am J Clin Pathol*, 1993, 99, 8-12.

Tokunaga, Y; Malagami, M; Tolika, A; Oshumi, K. Prognostic effects of dihydropyrimidine dehydrogenace in advanced colorectal cancor after surgery: immunohistochemistry using a new monoclonal antibody. *Anticancer Res,* 2003, 23, 1763-1768.

Yang, RY; Hsu, DK; Liu, FT. Expression of galectin-3 modulates t-cell growth and apoptosis. *Proc Natl Acad Sci USA*, 1996, 93, 6737-6742.

Wada, J; Makino, H. Galectins, galactoside-binding mammalian lectins. Clinical application of mulri-functional proteins. *Acta Med Okayama*, 2001, 55(1), 11-17.

Williams, ED. Two proposals regarding the terminology of thyroid tumors. *Int J Surg Pathol*, 2000, 8, 181-183.

In: Tumor Markers Research Focus
Editor: Deborah H. Chang, pp. 241-253
ISBN: 978-1-60021-544-5


*Chapter XIV*

# Cell Population Structure and Tumor Cell Proliferative Indices in Lymphoid Neoplasms

*E.V. Sheval**
A.N. Belozersky Institute of Physico-Chemical Biology, Moscow State University

## Abstract

Uncontrolled cell proliferation is one of the major features of tumor cells. The rate of cell proliferation determines the biologic behavior and, in many cases, the clinical course of a neoplasm. Thus, proliferative indices provide valuable prognostic information in this setting. However, in the case of aggressive human lymphoid tumors, there is an admixture of normal (reactive) cells in all organs infiltrated by neoplastic cells. To ascertain the influence of reactive cell on proliferative index measurements, an approach for detection of tumor cell subpopulation in large cell lymphomas has been developed. The results suggest that proliferative indices calculated for lymphoid neoplasms depend not only on the proliferative activity of the tumor cells, but also on the percentage of cells that are neoplastic. 'Tumor cell proliferative indices' can differ significantly from proliferative indices for the corresponding overall cell populations. We propose that the use of tumor cell proliferative indices results in more accurate assessment of disease prognosis. Also, it seems that the use of different features of cell populations can give valuable information concerning biological behavior of human neoplasms. The complex digital image analysis approach allows us to describe peculiarities in nuclear size distributions (e.g., histogram form, descriptive statistics of overall populations and subpopulations, etc.), morphologic characteristics of cells in different subpopulations, and proliferative rates of cells in overall cell population and different subpopulations. Taken together, these characteristics are referred to as 'the cell population structure'. The significance of the cell population structure investigations for lymphoma diagnostics is discussed.

* E-mail address: sheval_e@genebee.msu.su. Address for correspondence: Eugene V. Sheval, Ph.D., A.N. Belozersky Institute of Physico-Chemical Biology, Moscow State University, GSP-2, 119992 Moscow, Russia

# Introduction

Uncontrolled cell proliferation is one of the most important features of the tumor cells. Based on proliferative activity of the cells forming substrate of lymphoid tumors, all forms could be classified into several separate groups. Thus, all primary (*de novo*) lymphomas are broken up into the cases with low and high proliferative activity [1]. The cells of the tumors falling into the first group are small and are predominantly in $G_0$-phase of the cell cycle. Large cells, most of them in proliferation stage, are typical for the second group. Among the cells belonging to both groups, clones with enhanced biological activity may appear, resulting in higher aggressiveness of the disease. Thus, the rate of the cell proliferation is one of the most important biological characteristics of lymphoma cells, which is determined by the special features of oncogenesis and disease progression.

Within any lymphoid neoplasm, some heterogeneity of cases is observed, which is manifested, in particular, in different response to disease treatment. By the present time, a lot of tumor features (prognostic indicators) have been found, which enable to prognosticate the clinical outcome in each disease entity within the category of lymphoid neoplasm [2, 3]. Proliferative activity of the tumor cells was shown to be one of the predictors determining the course of the disease and treatment response [4]. It should be noted also that many chemotherapy programs are aimed on selective destruction of proliferative cells. In this connection it seems reasonable to consider proliferative characteristics of lymphoma cells in addition to tumor characteristics and the patient's condition when the treatment regimen is selected [5].

Based on these and other considerations, numerous experimental and clinical studies were designed in order to reveal a correlation between proliferative activity of cells forming lymphoid tumors and the course of the disease. *Proliferation indices* – proliferative cell number/total cell number, are used to describe proliferative activity of the tumors. However, just the early studies demonstrated that for non-Hodgkin's lymphoma proliferative activity is a less powerful prognostic indicator than clinical parameters and provide no additional prognostic information [6]. The authors suggested that unexpectedly low prognostic value of proliferative activity could be related with the structure of lymphoma, which are commonly composed of tumor and normal (reactive) lymphocytes [6-8]. Therefore, to determine proliferative activity of the tumor, one should start from isolation of tumor subpopulation, and then determine proliferative activity of the tumor cells. However, no specific methodology for such measurements was suggested.

By present, huge array of knowledge about proliferative activity of cells forming lymphoid tumors has been collected, but the majority of studies still deal with overall cell population, including both tumor and reactive cells. It is quite natural that when the tumor cells comprise overwhelming majority in the affected organs (for example: B-cell chronic lymphoid leukemia, Burkitt lymphoma, etc.) only minimal impact of reactive cells would be expected. However, in the case of large cell lymphomas (diffuse large B-cell lymphoma, anaplastic large cell lymphoma, etc.) it is unreasonable to ignore the impact of normal cells with usually low proliferative activity. In the current paper, we sum up our studies aimed on development of the approaches to segregation of tumor subpopulation from lymphoid tissue infiltrated with malignant cells and determination of its proliferative activity.

## Tumor and Reactive Subpopulations Could Be Separated Based on Their Morphometric Characteristics

The first part of our task – segregation of tumor cell subpopulation from the overall population – requires careful comparative analysis of tumor and reactive cell morphology and the search for quantitative characteristics of these cells. Nuclear size was selected as the simplest quantitative characteristic describing morphology of the tumor cells.

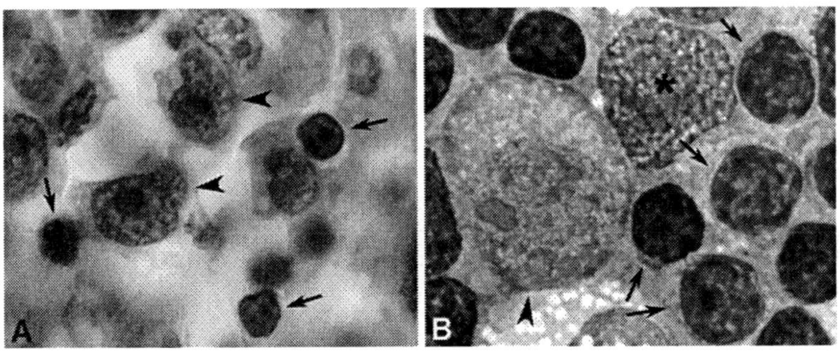


Figure 1. Comparison of cell morphology on paraffin section stained with hematoxylin/eosin (A) and on touch imprints stained with Giemsa solution (B). In the case of diffuse large B-cell lymphoma illustrated, two subpopulations are evident in both preparations. Small reactive lymphocytes (arrows) contain numerous blocks of condensed chromatin; large neoplastic cells (arrowheads) are filled with thin threads of condensed chromatin (so-called chromonemata). All cells on touch imprints are significantly larger than that on histological section. The destructed cells (asterisk in B) are revealed on imprints.

The work was carried out using touch imprints of lymphoid organs of the patients with various lymphomas. Histological section and touch imprint of lymph node of the patient with diffuse large B-cell lymphoma are compared in Figure 1. It is noticeable that in both preparations two cell subpopulations could be found: small reactive lymphocytes and large tumor cells. In the photograph of histological section (Figure 1A), one can see tumor cell nuclei with irregular shape; while in the imprints the nuclei are round and spread (Figure 1B). However, it seems that the imprints are more preferable for the purpose of the assigned task. First, it is difficult to select histological sections (and this is even more difficult an optical section that passes through the exact center of the cell nuclei in the digital images of when the nuclei are with irregular shape, which is typical for the neoplastic cells). On touch imprints, all cells are flattened and positioned in a single optical section, thus reducing error of morphometric analysis. Second, according to published data, image analysis of nuclear features on touch imprints [9], compared with paraffin sections [10], yields more accurate results. It could be suggested that analysis of cell structure using touch imprints will enable to reveal tumor cells in overall cell population more accurately.

Figure 2 shows the images of lymph node imprints obtained from the patients with B-cell chronic lymphoid leukemia (Figure 2A) and Burkitt lymphoma (Figure 2B). Almost all cells in lymph nodes are malignant. Even the visual analysis reveals that nuclei of Burkitt lymphoma cells (Figure 2B) are more heterogeneous is size and on average larger than the nuclei of chronic lymphoid leukemia cells (Figure 2A). This observation is supported also by histograms of the nuclear area distribution (Figure 2A', B'). Both nuclear area distributions are nearly normal. In Burkitt lymphoma case, the histogram base is markedly wider, indicating higher polymorphism of the cells comprising tumor tissue (Figure 2B').

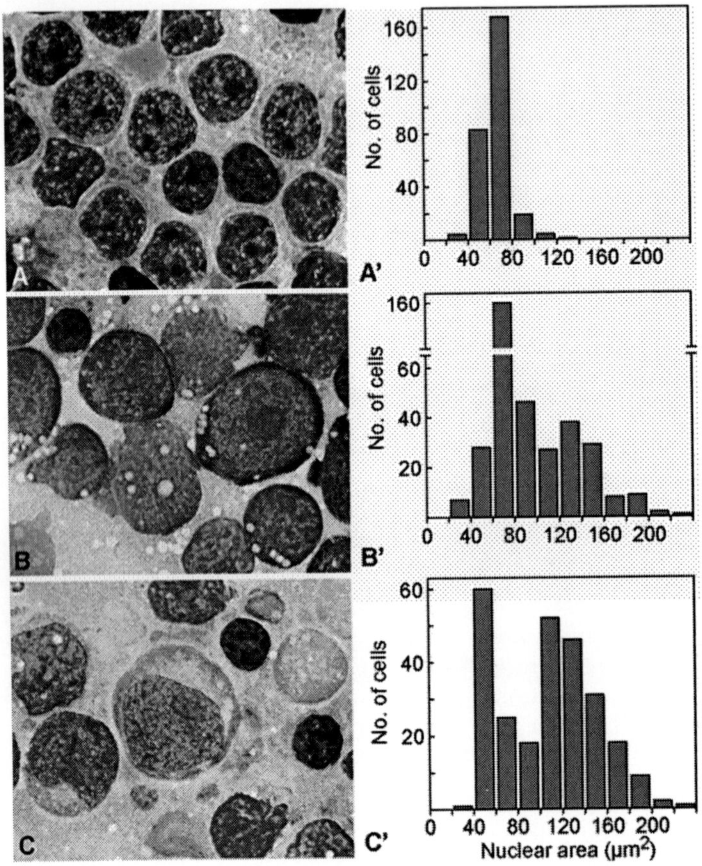


Figure 2. Cell morphology and nuclear area distributions as viewed on touch imprints are shown for B-cell chronic lymphoid leukemia (A, A'), Burkitt lymphoma (B, B'), and diffuse large B-cell lymphoma (C, C'). Neoplastic cells are present in very large proportions in B-cell chronic lymphoid leukemia, and the overall cell population is relatively homogeneous. A nuclear area distribution for B-cell chronic lymphoid leukemia is unimodal, with a sharp peak at 40-80 $\mu m^2$ and a slightly asymmetric distribution about this peak (positive skewness) (A'). Cells with nuclear area <80 $\mu m^2$ are monomorphous, with oval nuclei containing large blocks of condensed chromatin; nucleoli are not visible (A). It should be noted that neoplastic lymphocytes in chronic lymphoid leukemia (A') are larger than reactive lymphocytes in reactive hyperplasia (not illustrated) and in diffuse large cells lymphoma (C'). The nuclear area distribution associated with Burkitt lymphoma is unimodal, with a mean area of 86.1 $\mu m^2$ (B'); neoplastic cells (approximately 95% of all cells) have dispersed chromatin, prominent nucleoli, and highly basophilic cytoplasm with numerous vacuoles (B). In diffuse large B-cell lymphoma, cells with nuclear area <80 $\mu m^2$ are similar in structure to small lymphocytes in reactive lymph nodes, whereas cells with nuclear area >80 $\mu m^2$ have oval nuclei surrounded by abundant blue cytoplasm (C). The nucleoplasm of large cells is filled with thin threads of condensed chromatin arranged in a homogeneous meshwork. Round, pale blue nucleoli surrounded by a thin layer of condensed chromatin also are evident.

In cases of primary large cell lymphomas, the pattern is somewhat different. The analysis of large bulk of diffuse large B-cell lymphoma cases reveals that nuclear area distribution histograms could be divided into two types. In some cases bimodal distribution is found, and the analysis of cell morphology shows that small cells are reactive lymphocytes, while the large ones are tumor cells (Figure 2B, B'). In other cases, asymmetric unimodal nuclear area distribution is found, with asymmetry results from the presence of some amount of large tumor cells (data not shown).

After examination of nuclear area distribution histograms, it became clear that, in cases of large cell lymphomas, tumor population could be segregated based on quite simple morphometric parameter, i.e. the nuclear area. For this purpose, we introduced the threshold value of the nuclear area, which separated small cells (reactive lymphocytes, tumor lymphocytes in patients with B-cell chronic lymphoid leukemia) from large cells (malignant lymphoma cells) [11]. We selected 80 $\mu m^2$ based on the following considerations: 1) some aggressive lymphomas demonstrated bimodal nuclear area distribution with local minimum at ~80 $\mu m^2$; 2) in B-cell chronic lymphoid leukemia cases the nuclear area of majority cells was less than 80 $\mu m^2$. It should be stressed that population separation into large and small cells does not allow to distinguish unambiguously neoplastic cells from reactive cells. More exactly, we speak about segregation of subpopulations enriched with tumor and reactive cells (i.e. population approach).

Thus, we were able to formalize the detection of tumor cell subpopulation, though this approach did not allow us to distinguish tumor cell from normal cell absolutely exactly.

## Tumor Cell Proliferative Indices Can Differ Significantly from Proliferative Indices for the Corresponding Overall Cell Population

When the first part of the assigned task was fulfilled – the tumor cell population was segregated – the opportunity appeared to characterize proliferative activity of neoplastic cells. We used anti-pKi-67 antibodies to detect proliferative cells. This protein is expressed only by proliferative cells making it useful *proliferation marker* [12]. Figure 3 shows the photographs of lymph nodes imprints obtained from the patients with B-cell chronic lymphoid leukemia and Burkitt lymphoma. In case of chronic lymphoid leukemia, only sporadic pKi-67-positive cells are visible in touch imprints, indicating that majority of the cells is in the $G_0$-phase (Figure 3A, B). On the contrary, most Burkitt lymphoma cells are stained with anti-pKi-67 antibodies (Figure 3D, E), i.e. are in the cell cycle ($G_1$, S, $G_2$, and mitosis).

For the assay purposed, morphometric examination of nuclear area for pKi-67-positive and pKi-67-negative cells was performed. Analysis of nuclear area distribution histograms carried out separately for proliferative and non-proliferative cells shows that, in case of B-cell chronic lymphoid leukemia, pKi-67-positive cells form small subpopulation, where average cell size is larger than in subpopulation of pKi-67-negative cells (Figure 2C). In the case of Burkitt lymphoma, proliferative cell subpopulation is not only considerably larger in cell size at the average, but also shows greater area variation compared with non-proliferative cells (Figure 2F). These findings are in agreement with previous observations, which suggested that cell passage through the cell cycle is one of the sources of morphological heterogeneity in cell populations [13].

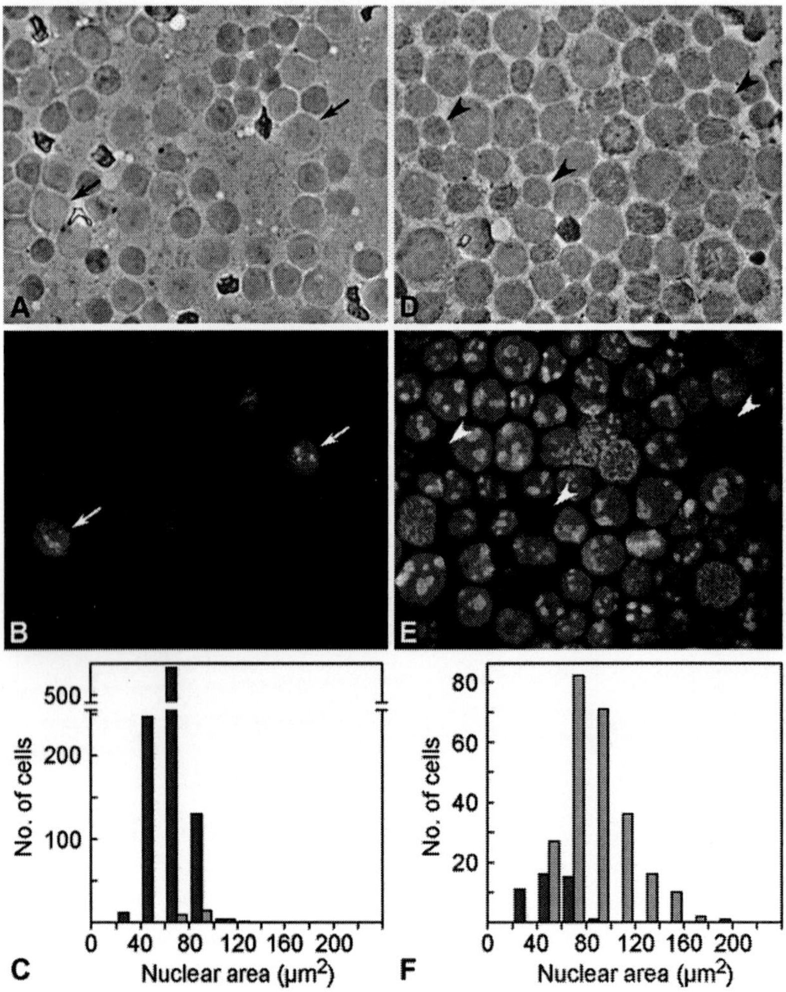


Figure 3. Revealing of pKi-67 in touch imprints of lymph nodes infiltrated with cells of B-cell chronic lymphoid leukemia (A-B) and Burkitt lymphoma (D-E), and histograms depicting nuclear area distributions in the same cases (C and F, respectively). A, D – phase contrast; B, E – immunofluorescent revealing of pKi-67. The arrows indicate pKi-67-positive cells in chronic lymphoid leukemia; the arrowheads indicate pKi-67-negative cells in Burkitt lymphoma. Histograms depict the nuclear area distributions among pKi-67-negative (dark gray bars) and pKi-67-positive cells (pale gray bars).

The majority of human aggressive lymphomas are characterized by considerable admixture of reactive cells in their tissue. Figure 4 shows the photographs of the specimens of two large cell lymphomas (anaplastic large cell lymphoma and diffuse large B-cell lymphoma) stained with anti-pKi-67 antibodies. These specimens differ in proliferative cell percentage (10.2% and 76.2%); however, one could see that most large cells are pKi-67-positive in both cases. This observation is supported by the analysis of the histograms of nuclear area distributions for pKi-67-negative and pKi-67-positive cells. Taking into account that neoplastic cells are larger than reactive lymphocytes, we can suggest that most tumor cells are pKi-67-positive (i.e. they are proliferating). Comparison of these cases indicates that proliferative indices itself could not serve as reliable prognostic indicator, because these indices depend not only on proliferative activity of the tumor cells, but also on their proportion in the tissue.

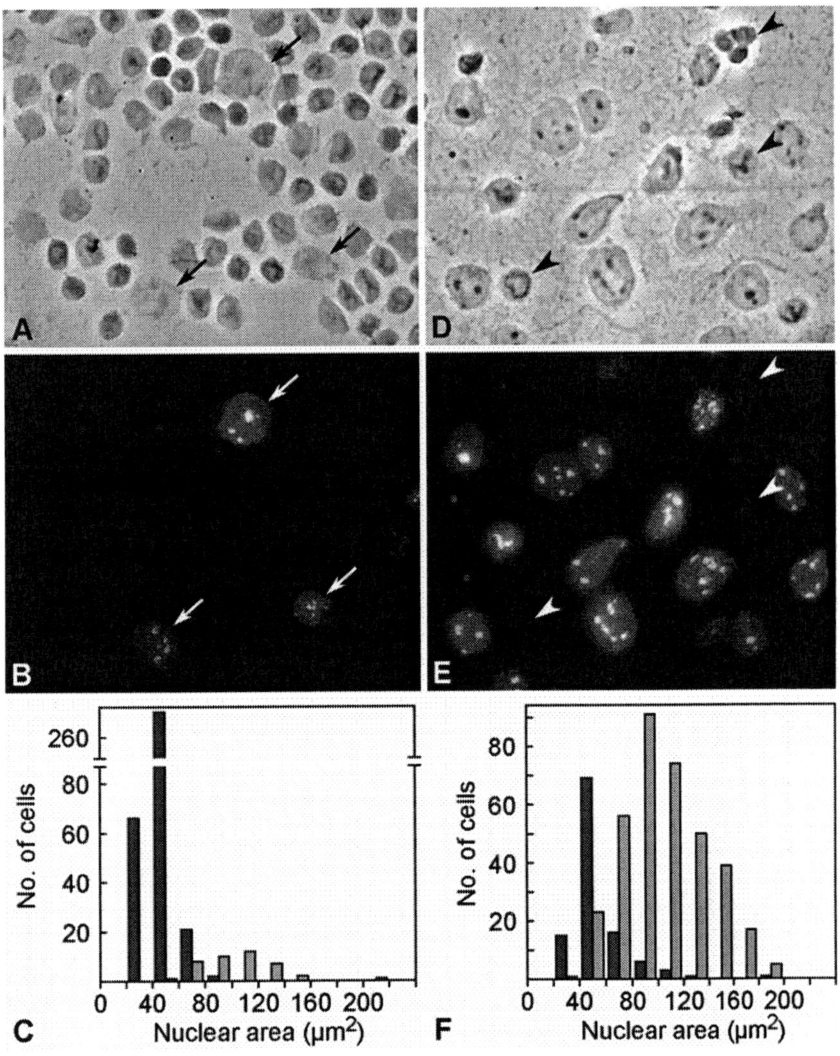


Figure 4. Revealing of pKi-67 in touch imprints of lymph nodes infiltrated with cells of anaplastic large cell lymphoma (A-B) and diffuse large B-cell lymphoma (D-E), and histograms depicting nuclear area distributions in the same cases (C and F, respectively). A, D – phase contrast; B, E – immunofluorescent revealing of pKi-67. In the case of anaplastic large cell lymphoma, a few large pKi-67-positive cells (arrows) are revealed; in the case of diffuse large B-cell lymphoma, the majority of pKi-67-negative cells have small size (arrowheads). Histograms depict the nuclear area distributions among pKi-67-negative (dark gray bars) and pKi-67-positive cells (pale gray bars).

This conclusion is clearly illustrated by a case of diffuse large B-cell lymphoma, shown in Figure 5. In this case, large cells comprise both proliferative and non-proliferative cells, i.e.

this case could be considered as a case with relatively low proliferative activity, though its proliferative index is appreciably higher than in case of anaplastic large cell lymphoma described above (28.8% and 10.2%, respectively).

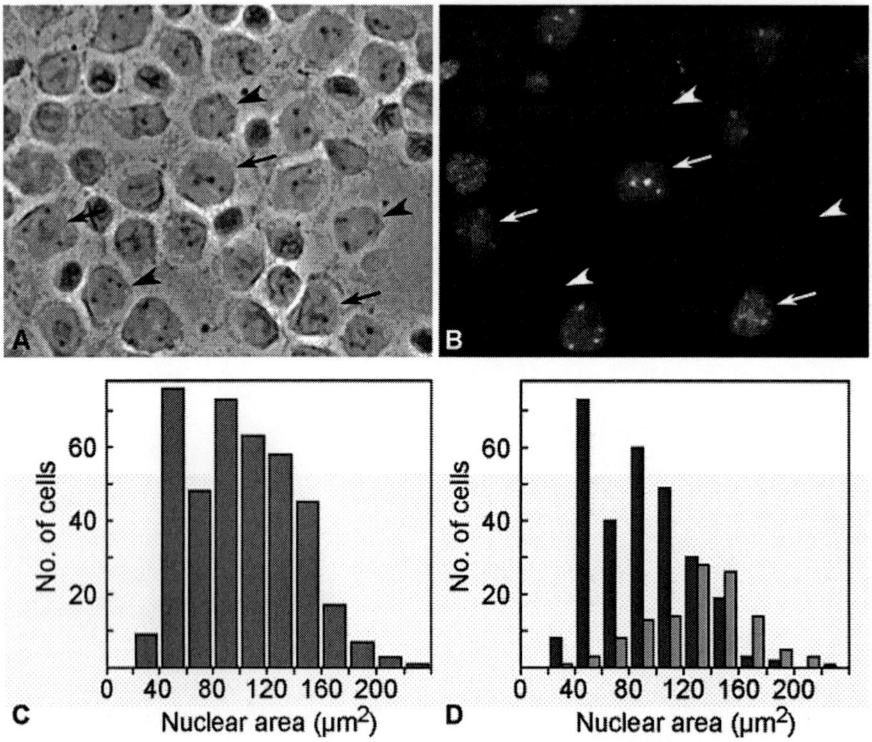


Figure 5. Revealing of pKi-67 in touch imprints of lymph nodes infiltrated with cells of diffuse large B-cell lymphoma (A-B) and histograms depicting nuclear area distributions in the same case (C-D). A – phase contrast; B – immunofluorescent revealing of pKi-67. pKi-67-positive cells (arrows) as well as pKi-67-negative cells (arrowheads) are revealed among large cells. Histograms depict the nuclear area distributions (C) in the overall cell population and (D) among pKi-67-negative (dark gray bars) and pKi-67-positive cells (pale gray bars).

If we assume that proliferative indices of large cells obtained for large cell lymphoma are *tumor cell proliferative indices* in their biological nature, some more conclusions can be made. Thus, we can note that though in anaplastic large cell lymphoma described the proliferative index is low (10.2%), tumor cell proliferative index in this case is extremely high (94.1%) (Figure 4A-C). On the contrary, diffuse large B-cell lymphoma in Figure 5 shows higher proliferative index (28.8%) with relatively low tumor cell proliferative index (38.8%). We should pay attention to one more detail: in both large cell lymphomas in Figure 4, tumor cell proliferative indices exceeds 90%, i.e. proliferation level in these neoplasms approaches to proliferation level of Burkitt lymphoma – the tumor, for which high proliferation index is a diagnostic feature. This suggests that, in Burkitt lymphoma, high content of tumor cells with high proliferative activity in tissue rather than their *per se* high proliferative activity is a more appropriate diagnostic feature.

Thus, proliferative indices, which are traditionally measured for investigation of proliferative activity of the tumor cells, cannot serve as the reliable measure of proliferative activity of lymphoid neoplasms. Prognostic value of this feature could be considerably higher with the use of tumor cell proliferative indices instead.

The morphometric approach suggested enables to describe new variants of proliferative subpopulations arrangement in large cell lymphomas [11]. Flow cytometry could probably appear simpler, but its application will be limited to neoplasms expressing antigens, which are not exposed on the surface of reactive cells. This is not always the case for aggressive lymphomas. On the other hand, analysis of touch imprints (or histological sections) enables to compare the size and morphology of the tumor and reactive cells. In this study, we used only one parameter – nuclear area, for tumor cell segregation. This approach can be developed to involve the use of wider range of parameters, such as ploidy, structure of chromatin, nucleoli, etc. According to published data, the use of image analysis enables to differentiate various neoplasm types (both lymphoid and non-lymphoid) in imprints and in smears [9, 14-18], though to our knowledge these methods have not yet been used for differentiation of the overall population into tumor cells and reactive cells.

# Cell Population Structure is a New Quantitative Characteristic of Lymphoid Tissues Infiltrated with Tumor Cells

Complex analysis of digital images of lymphoid node imprints enables to describe the characteristics of nuclear area distribution (histogram shape, statistics of overall population and isolated subpopulations), morphology of the cells comprising different subpopulations and proliferative activity of the cells from various subpopulations. All together these characteristics describe the *cell population structure*. We suggest that the cell population structure can be considered as the special complex characteristic of tumor tissue. The aim of introduction of this new conception is the demand for detection of tumor population and description of its morphological and functional characteristics. The cell population structure is a population-based characteristic, i.e. it describes the special features of cell population within affected or normal organ, and also determines the impact of separate subpopulations on the overall cell population organization. Using this characteristic one can determine biological properties of the tumor and reactive processes in lymphoid organs more accurately.

It should be noted that this characteristic is very flexible, because different traits and their combinations could be used to describe the cell population structure. To make this idea more understandable, we will describe the analysis of the cell size using flow cytometry as an example [19]. In the cited work, we investigated three cases of lymphoid neoplasms with similar immunophenotype typical for B-cell chronic lymphoid leukemia ($CD19^+/CD5^+$, clonality of the light immunoglobulin chains, $CD23^+$ and $CD10^-$). However, these tumors were classified as different clinical forms based on the analysis of clinical features and tumor cell morphology (B-cell chronic lymphoid leukemia – Case 1, large cell transformation of B-cell chronic lymphoid leukemia – Case 2; CD5-positive diffuse large B-cell lymphoma – Case 3). We tried to determine special morphological features of the tumor cells with the use of flow cytometry. To characterize the tumor cells, their forward (FSC) and side (SSC) light scatterings were analyzed. For this purpose, inverse projection method was used: according to this method, cell subpopulations were isolated based on antigen expression and then projected on FSC/SSC plot. Figure 6A shows FSC/SSC plots for total cell population in the obtained suspensions for all three cases, and a standard lymphocytic region (R1) is marked out. Figure 6B shows the plots of distribution of CD19 and CD5 antigen expression for cell from R1 regions. Coexpressing CD19/CD5 subpopulation (L1) corresponds to tumor cells, subpopulation expressing only CD5 antigen (L2) – to T-lymphocytes, i.e. to reactive cells. In Case 1, the subpopulations of tumor (Figure 6C) and reactive cells (Figure 6D) exhibited similar light scattering characteristics (Table). This suggests that the morphology of the majority of tumor cells is similar to that of normal lymphocytes. In Case 2, the subpopulations of tumor and reactive cells also exhibit similar light scattering characteristics, but for tumor cells average FSC is greater than for reactive T-cells (Figure 6C, D; Table). In this case, the tumor cells and reactive cells have similar SSC values. In Case 3, tumor cell subpopulation exhibit even lower FSC measurements, but two-fold higher SSC compared with reactive T-cells (Figure 6C, D; Table). Therefore, in the cases studied, light scattering analysis enables to suggest morphological differences of the neoplastic cells, which was supported by the microscopic analysis [19].

**Table. Forward (FSC) and side (SSC) light scattering (mean±standard deviation) of reactive T-lymphocytes ($CD19^-/CD5^+$) and neoplastic cells ($CD19^+/CD5^+$). The comparison of FSC and SSC is possible only inside each case (i.e. between tumor and reactive cells, but not between tumor or reactive cells of different cases).**

| | Neoplastic cells | Reactive cells |
|---|---|---|
| FSC | | |
| Case 1 | 78.9±14.9 | 79.9±17.7 |
| Case 2 | 99.0±12.3 | 40.2±25.1 |
| Case 3 | 99.5±24.5 | 105.3±24.0 |
| SSC | | |
| Case 1 | 15.9±23.1 | 19.3±37.0 |
| Case 2 | 20.1±30.3 | 19.7±35.6 |
| Case 3 | 46.6±35.4 | 26.4±35.2 |

This example illustrates the same approach, however in respect to another task solution. We also isolated tumor cell subpopulation and then made attempt to describe its properties. But in this case, we were interested in morphology rather than in proliferation of the tumor cells. Therefore, the cell population structure is not only the additional characteristic of the tumor tissue, but also the special strategy, which can be applied to investigation of different biological properties of tumor cells in the tissue. Formalized segregation of tumor cell subpopulation at the first stage of the study is the essential point of this conception. It is also worth mentioning that we tried to use quantitative characteristics, which enable to fulfill additional statistical analysis of the data obtained, for example, using cluster analysis [11]. Further development of the approach proposed will allow to describe more accurately biological properties of the tumor cells and infiltration of the affected organs.

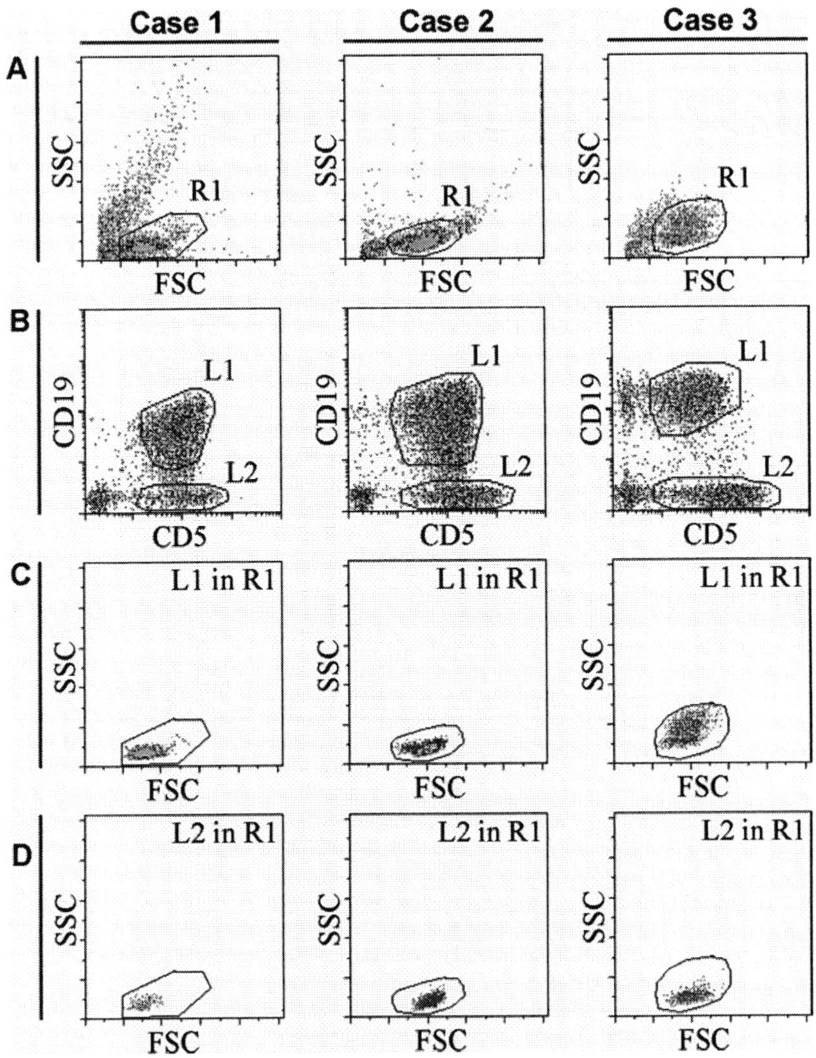


Figure 6. Analysis of forward (FSC) and side (SSC) light scattering of tumor cells and reactive T-lymphocytes. A – distribution by FSC/SSC for total cell population in suspension (R1, lymphocytic region); B – distribution of cells in R1 according to the intensity of CD5 and CD19 fluorescence (L1, tumor cells expressing CD5 and CD19; L2, reactive T-lymphocytes expressing CD5 alone); (C) distribution by FSC/SSC for tumor cell subpopulation (L1 in R1); (D) distribution by FSC/SSC for reactive T-lymphocytes (L2 in R1). When preparing FSC/SSC graphs, the algorithm realized in the cytometer software (z-level) was used, which makes it possible to show the areas of dense cell arrangement [19]. The quantitative analysis of the results of the flow cytometry study is presented in Table.

## Conclusion

Summing up, we state that careless use of the cell parameters (such as proliferative indices) may lead to inaccurate, and, perhaps, even erroneous conclusions. In some cases, the measurement methodology is too formal and does not take biological essence of the described features into account. Rapid development of the cell biology approaches (high resolution videomicroscopy, image analysis, flow cytometry, etc.) enhances the precision of tumor description (even then the old and well-reputed parameters are used).

## References

[1] Sánchez-Beato, M., Sánchez-Aguilera, A., & Piris, M. A. (2003). Cell cycle deregulation in B-cell lymphomas. *Blood*, 101, 1220-1235.

[2] Harris, N. L., Jaffe, E. S., Stein, H., Banks, P. M., Chan, J. K. C., Cleary, M. L., Delsol, G., De Wolf-Peeters, C., Falini, B., Gatter, K. C., Grogan, T. M., Isaacson, P. G., Knowles, D. M., Mason, D. Y., Muller-Hermelink, H.-K., Pileri, S. A., Piris, M. A., Ralfkiaer, E., & Warnke, R. A. (1994). A revised European-American classification of lymphoid neoplasms: a proposal from the International Lymphoma Study Group. *Blood*, 84, 1361-1392.

[3] Jaffe, E. S., Harris, N. L., Stein, H., & Vardiman, J. W.; Eds. World Health Organization classification of tumours: pathology and genetics of tumours of haematopoietic and lymphoid tissues. *IARC Press*: Lyon, 2001.

[4] Leoncini, L., Lazzi, S., Bellan, C., & Tosi, P. (2002). Cell kinetics and cell cycle regulation on lymphomas. *J Clin Pathol*, 55, 648-655.

[5] Holte, H., Suo, Z., Smeland, E. B., Kvaloy, S., Langholm, R., & Stokke, T. (1999). Prognostic value of lymphoma-specific S-phase fraction compared with that of other cell proliferation markers. *Acta Oncol*, 38, 495-503.

[6] Winter, J. N., Andersen, J., Variakojis, D., Gordon, L. I., Fisher, R. I., Oken, M. M., Neiman, R. S., Jiang, S., & Bauer, K. D. (1996). Prognostic implications of ploidy and proliferative activity in the diffuse, aggressive non-Hodgkin's lymphomas. *Blood*, 88, 3919-3925.

[7] Tusenius, K. J., Bakker, P. J., & van Oers, M. N. (1992). Measurement of proliferation indices in non Hodgkin's lymphoma – is it useful? *Leuk Lymphoma*, 7, 181-187.

[8] Spina, D., Leoncini, L., Megha, T., Gallorini, M., Tosi, P., Pileri, S., Kraft, R., Laissue, J. A., & Cottier, H. (1997). Growth patterns of diffuse non-Hodgkin's lymphomas estimated from mitotic and apoptotic indices. *Int J Cancer*, 73, 178–183.

[9] Kneitz, S., Ott, G., Albert, R., Schindewolf, T., Müller-Hermelink, H., & Harms, H. (1996). Differentiation of low-grade non-Hodgkin's lymphomas by means of digital image processing. *Anal Quant Cytol*, 18, 121-128.

[10] Kneitz, S., Ott, G., Albert, R., Müller-Hermelink, H. K., & Harms, H. (1998). Differentiation of low-grade non-Hodgkin's lymphomas using paraffin sections by image processing. *Cytometry*, 34, 75-81.

[11] Sheval, E. V., Churakova, J. V., Dudnik, O. A., & Vorobjev, I. A. (2004). Examination of the proliferative activity of tumor cells in human lymphoid neoplasms using a morphometric approach. *Cancer (Cancer Cytopathol)*, 102, 174-185.

[12] Gerdes, J., Lemke, H., Baisch, H., Wacker, H., Schwab, U., & Stein, H. (1984). Cell cycle analysis of a cell proliferation-associated human nuclear antigen defined by the monoclonal antibody Ki-67. *J Immunol*, 133, 1710-1715.

[13] Weinberg, D. S. (1989). The role of cell cycle activity in the generation of morphologic heterogeneity in non-Hodgkin's lymphoma. *Am J Pathol*, 135, 759-770.

[14] Molnar, B., Szaleczky, E., Pronai, L., Papik, K., Zagoni, T., & Tulassay, Z. (2000). Quantitative DNA and morphometric analysis of gastroscopic brush smears by TV image analysis. *Eur J Gastroenterol Hepatol*, 12, 103-109.

[15] Murata, S., Mochizuki, K., Nakazawa, T., Kondo, T., Nakamura, N., Yamashita, H., Urata, Y., Ashihara, T., & Katoh R. (2002). Detection of underlying characteristics of nuclear chromatin patterns of thyroid tumor cells using texture and factor analyses. *Cytometry*, 49, 91-95.

[16] Nemec, E., Van de Putte, S., Van Pachterbeke, C., Vokaer, R., Budel, V., Deprez, C., Kiss, R., & Decaestecker, C. (2002). Ploidy and chromatin pattern analysis as an aid for cervical smear diagnosis. *Histol Histopathol*, 17, 403-409.

[17] Murata, S.-I., Mochizuki, K., Nakazawa, T., Kondo, T., Nakamura, N., Yamashita, H., Urata, Y., Ashihara, T., & Katoh, R. (2003). Morphological abstraction of thyroid tumor cell nuclei using morphometry with factor analysis. *Microsc Res Tech*, 61, 457-462.

[18] Churakova, Zh. V., Gurevich, I. B., Jernova, I. A., Kharazishvili, D. V., Khilkov, A. V., Nefyodov, A. V., Sheval, E. V., & Vorob'ev, I. A. (2003). Selection of diagnostically valuable features for morphological analysis of blood cells. *Pattern Recognition Image Anal*, 13, 381-383.

[19] Gretsov, E. M., Churakova, J. V., Sheval, E. V., & Vorobjev, I. A. (2004). Comparative characteristics of immunological, clinical and morphological features of human lymphoid tumors in respect with tumor genesis and progression. *Russian J Dev Biol*, 35, 182-190.

In: Tumor Markers Research Focus
Editor: Deborah H. Chang, pp. 255-259
ISBN: 978-1-60021-544-5


*Chapter XV*

# Case Studies on Aberration of Tumor Marker Test in Laboratory Medicine

***Viroj Wiwanitkit***
Department of Laboratory Medicine, Faculty of Medicine, Chulalongkorn University, Bangkok Thailand 10330

## Abstract

Presently, tumor marker is a group of laboratory investigation used in medical laboratory. Laboratory medicine principle is also applied for the tumor marker investigation. Here, the author reports two case studies on aberration of tumor marker test in laboratory medicine. The first case is a female patient with post operative ovarian clear cell carcinoma presented with the unexpected and unexplained high CA125 level due to the immunological alteration from medication. The second case is a male patient with chronic hepatitis B infection presented with abnormal high AFP level due to the macromolecule phenomenon. These two cases are good examples in tumor marker determination in laboratory medicine.

## Introduction

Presently, tumor marker is a group of laboratory investigation used in medical laboratory [1]. Tumor markers are substances related to the presence or progress of a tumor. An ideal tumor marker is (a) detectable only when malignancy is present, (b) specific for the type and site of malignancy, (c) correlates with the amount of malignant tissue present and (b) responds rapidly to a change in tumor size [1]. The predominant contemporary markers are discussed here by chemical class, as follows: glycoprotein markers, including carcinoembryonic antigen (CEA), alpha-fetoprotein (AFP), beta-human chorionic gonadotropin (beta-hCG), and prostate specific antigen (PSA); mucinous glycoproteins, including CA 15-3, CA 19-9, mucinous-like cancer antigen and associated antigens, and CA 125; enzymes, including prostatic acid phosphatase (PAP), neuron specific enolase (NSE), lactic acid dehydrogenase (LDH), and placental alkaline phosphatase (PLAP); hormones and related endocrine molecules, including calcitonin, thyroglobulin, and catecholamines; and, molecules of the immune system, including immunoglobulins and beta-2-microglobulin [2]. However, no tumor marker fulfills all of the above criteria [1 – 2].

Laboratory medicine principle is also applied for the tumor marker investigation. Tumor marker workload is rapidly increasing. Tumor markers are frequently and inappropriately requested, either because they are on patients of the wrong sex, or because they are taken before a cancer diagnosis is reached [3].

The type of oversight applied to tumor markers available for marketing in the U.S.A depends on both the intended use of the test and the manner in which it is being commercialized-whether offered as a test kit or system or as a laboratory testing service [4]. Here, the author reports two case studies on aberration of tumor marker test in laboratory medicine.

# Case studies

## Case 1

The first case was a 56 years old female patient. She was known case of ovarian clear cell carcinoma stage 1C with post operative total hysterectomy and bilateral oophorectomy for 3 years. She had got full course of chemotherapy and had regular following up. On each following up, CA125 monitoring was performed and the results were within normal limit (< 35 U/mL). In this visit, she presented with the unexpected and unexplained high serum CA125 level, upto 250 U/mL. Full investigation for the possible relapse of malignancy was performed. Computerized tomography (CT) for chest and abdomen showed no abnormality.

Further history taking showed that she has regularly taken persantin for antithrombotic purpose and she had just got the drug the day before this visit. The final diagnosis of this case is due to the immunological alteration from medication. After this visit, she is free of disease until present, more than 5 years.

## Case 2

The second case was a 54 male patient with chronic hepatitis B infection. This patient had a regular visit to the sexually transmitted disease (STD) clinic for a long time. He had got normal level of liver function test. However, the physician in charge at the STD clinic found an aberration in his serum AFP results (by immunological assay) in periodically investigation for two years. The patient has got full examination of liver including abdominal ultrasonography as well as CT scan of abdomen and revealed no abnormality. The physician in charge consulted to the laboratory for the possible examination.

In this case, the patient had no additional history on the cause of abnormal high serum AFP level. The laboratory gave a consult to the physician in charge and recommended for the protein electrophoresis examination for this case to investigation the level of immunoglobulin. The result showed that the patient had an abnormal high peak of immunoglobulin. The diagnosis of abnormal high AFP level in this case is due to the macromolecule phenomenon. The new determination of serum AFP level by radioassay showed normal AFP level. After this visit, the patient developed no evidence of hepatocellular carcinoma until present, more than 5 years.

# Discussion

The perfect tumor marker would be one that was produced solely by a tumor and secreted in measurable amounts into body fluids, it should be present only in the presence of cancer, it should identify cancer before it has spread beyond a localized site, its quantitative amount in bodily fluids should reflect the bulk of tumor, and the level of the marker should reflect responses to treatment and progressive disease [1 – 2]. Here, the author reports two case studies on aberration of tumor marker test in laboratory medicine. These two cases are good examples in tumor marker determination in laboratory medicine. Similar to any tests in medicine, false positive of tumor marker determination can be seen.

The first case is a female patient with post operative ovarian clear cell carcinoma presented with the unexpected and unexplained high CA125 level due to the immunological alteration from medication. Basically, a variety of biomarkers have been developed to monitor growth of ovarian cancer and to detect disease at an early interval [5]. CA125 or MUC16 is a new unique tumor marker for epithelial ovarian cancer, and its clinical use has recently increased considerably. CA125 has provided a useful serum tumor marker for monitoring response to chemotherapy, detecting disease recurrence, distinguishing malignant from benign pelvic masses [5]. A rapid fall in CA125 during chemotherapy predicts a favorable prognosis and could be used to redistribute patients on multiarmed randomized clinical trials [5]. However, CA125 lack the sensitivity and specificity to be useful in screening the general population [6]. In this report, CA125 is used as a following up tool of a patient with ovarian cancer after a curative surgery and a complete course of chemotherapy, cisplatin regimen.

Indeed, among patients with ovarian cancer in complete clinical remission, a progressive low-level increase in serum CA-125 levels is strongly predictive of disease recurrence [7].

In this case, the patient show regular normal CA125 level with overall healthy presentation. The problem is the rapid rising of CA125 in a visit without proper explanation. The investigation for the cause of rising was done and shown null finding. Of interest, this case had an interesting history of regular taking persantin believing that it can prevent thrombosis. Pharmacologically, persantin or dipyridamole acts by inhibiting nucleoside transport, which increases adenosine levels leading to inhibition of platelet aggregation and vasodilatation mainly in the coronary tree [8]. It is a vaso-protective drug with proven efficacy in the prevention of strokes [8]. An important adverse effect of persantin is throbbing headache and flu like symptom if a high dose is taken [9 - 10]. These effects are due to the increase in production of immunoglobulin [9 - 11]. In this case, the history of ingestion of persantin the day before this visit indicates the possibility of high level of immunoglobulin as side effect of persantin in this patient. The mentioned high immunoglobulin level is believed to be the cause of the abnormal high CA125 level. Basically, this phenomenon is called macrosubstance phenomenon. It can be seen in determination of many enzymes in laboratory medicine [12], especially for creating kinase, amylase and transaminase. These macrosubstances are the result of the formation of enzyme immunoglobulin complexes; their specific immune character has been demonstrated in some cases [12]. The formation of such immune complexes between the enzyme protein and plasma immunoglobulins seems a rather common phenomenon although neither the mechanism involved nor the pathophysiological significance are known since they have been observed in patients and healthy individuals [12]. Nevertheless, it is important to recognize these macromolecular forms because of the diagnostic uncertainties they may induce during isoenzyme studies and even total enzyme activity measurement [12]. According to this case, not only regular medication but also alternative medicine especially for herb should be investigated in all cancerous patients in following up.

The second case is a male patient with chronic hepatitis B infection presented with abnormal high AFP level due to the macromolecule phenomenon. In general, hepatitis B infection is mentioned as an important cause of hepatocellular carcinoma. Rugge et al noted that screening patients with chronic hepatitis B infection (HBsAg+) for hepatocellular carcinoma by AFP or by AFP plus ultrasound (AFP/US) detected hepatocellular carcinoma tumors at earlier stages and increased resection rates [13]. They proposed that it was unclear whether screening with AFP or AFP/US improves disease-specific or all-cause mortality [13]. However, Wiwanitkit et al recently said that the sensitivity of AFP was insufficient for screening purposes and serum AFP can not be recommended for hepatitis B carriers over standard tests in endemic area [14].

For following up of the patient with chronic hepatitis B, AFP/US is widely practiced.

In this case, the patient was also run in this following up pattern. The problem in this case is the unexplained high AFP level without evidence of malignancy. Similar to the first case, the disturbance from high immmunoglobin can be expected in this case. The high immunoglobulin is believed to be the interference for the determination of serum AFP by immunoassay and can result in aberrant of laboratory result.

## References

[1] Lai LC, Cheong SK, Goh KL, Leong CF, Loh CS, Lopez JB, Nawawi H, Sivanesaratnam V, Subramaniam R; Clinical Practice Guidelines Committee on Tumour Markers of the Academy of Medicine of Malaysia.Clinical usefulness of tumour markers. *Malays J Pathol.* 2003 Dec;25(2):83-105.

[2] Jacobs EL, Haskell CM. Clinical use of tumor markers in oncology. *Curr Probl Cancer.* 1991 Nov-Dec;15(6):299-360.

[3] McGinley PJ, Kilpatrick ES. Tumour markers: their use and misuse by clinicians. *Ann Clin Biochem.* 2003 Nov;40(Pt 6):643-7.

[4] Gutman S. Regulatory issues in tumor marker development. *Semin Oncol.* 2002 Jun;29(3):294-300.

[5] Bast RC Jr, Badgwell D, Lu Z, Marquez R, Rosen D, Liu J, Baggerly KA, Atkinson EN, Skates S, Zhang Z, Lokshin A, Menon U, Jacobs I, Lu K. New tumor markers: CA125 and beyond. *Int J Gynecol Cancer.* 2005 Nov-Dec;15 Suppl 3:274-81.

[6] Fields MM, Chevlen E. Ovarian cancer screening: a look at the evidence. *Clin J Oncol Nurs.* 2006 Feb;10(1):77-81.

[7] Santillan A, Garg R, Zahurak ML, Gardner GJ, Giuntoli RL 2nd, Armstrong DK, Bristow RE. Risk of epithelial ovarian cancer recurrence in patients with rising serum CA-125 levels within the normal range. *J Clin Oncol.* 2005 Dec 20;23(36):9338-43.

[8] Schaper W. Dipyridamole, an underestimated vascular protective drug. *Cardiovasc Drugs Ther.* 2005 Oct;19(5):357-63.

[9] Persantin. Available at www.netdoctor.co.uk/medicines/100002047.html

[10] Lindgren A, Husted S, Staaf G, Ziegler B. Dipyridamole and headache--a pilot study of initial dose titration. *J Neurol Sci.* 2004 Aug 30;223(2):179-84.

[11] Lichtner R, Wedderburn N. Enhancement of the immune response to sheep erythrocytes in mice by phosphodiesterase-inhibiting dipyridamole derivatives.*J Immunopharmacol.* 1984;6(1-2):43-55.

[12] Maire I, Artur Y, Sanderink GJ. Macroenzymes in human plasma. 1: Macroamylase, macrocreatine kinase, macrolactate dehydrogenase. *Ann Biol Clin (Paris).* 1987; 45(3):269-76.

[13] Rugge JB, Lochner J, Judkins D. What is the best surveillance for hepatocellular carcinoma in chronic carriers of hepatitis B? *J Fam Pract.* 2006 Feb;55(2):155-6

[14] Wiwanitkit V. Alpha fetoprotein for screening for hepatocellular cancer in populations with viral hepatitis B: an appraisal of Thai reports. *Asian Pac J Cancer Prev.* 2005 Oct-Dec;6(4):535-6.

In: Tumor Markers Research Focus
Editor: Deborah H. Chang, pp. 261-273

ISBN: 978-1-60021-544-5


*Chapter XVI*

# Impairment of the E-cadherin-Catenin-Complex Unit in Epithelial Ovarian Borderline and Malignant Tumours

***Faleiro-Rodrigues Cristina[1], Macedo-Pinto Isabel and Pereira Deolinda****

Department of Anatomy and Pathology, and Department of Medical Oncology*, Portuguese Institute of Oncology of Francisco Gentil, Centro Regional do Norte, Porto, Portugal

## Abstract

Epithelial (E-) cadherin has a major role in the maintenance of intercellular junction between epithelial cells. The association of the catenins (α-, β- and γ-) to E-cadherin in the formation of the E-cadherin-catenin complex unit (ECCU) is a key step in the function of intact adhesion complexes at the *adherens* junction. Alterations in E-cadherin or any one of the catenin molecules may lead to reduced cell-cell adhesion resulting in tumour cell invasion. In our previous studies, loss and reduced expression of E-cadherin and β-catenin was associated with poor tumour differentiation, peritoneal metastasis, advanced tumour stage, and poor patient prognosis.

**Purpose**: the immunohistochemical expression of E-cadherin and the catenins was examined in a selected group of Epithelial Ovarian Tumours (EOT) in an attempt to evaluate the inter relationship between each of these proteins essential in the formation of the ECCU, and their role in ovarian carcinogenesis.

**Patients and methods**: The series of this study includes 5 borderline tumours and 19 carcinomas selected from a previous studies based on the observation that these tumours showed negative expression for either E-cadherin or β-catenin.

**Results**: Disruption of the E-cadherin–catenin complex was noted in terms of both E-cadherin and catenin loss. Negative expression of E-cadherin and the catenins α-, β-, and γ- was

[1] E-mail address: cristinafaleiro@mail.com, Telephone: +351-22-5084000 Ext 1002 / Fax +351-22-5084001. Correspondence to Faleiro-Rodrigues C., Macedo-Pinto IM, Instituto Português de Oncologia Francisco Gentil, Centro Regional do Norte, Departamento de Anatomia Patológica, Rua Dr. António Bernardino de Almeida, 4200-072 Porto, Portugal.

observed in the majority of the EOT. Some tumours continued to express E-cadherin at the cell membrane, yet showed loss of the catenins, implying that the necessary components to directly interact and associate with E-cadherin are absent and as a result a functional ECCU cannot be formed.

**Conclusion**: Accepting the limitation of our sample size, our results show that loss of E-cadherin or the catenins necessary for strong cell-to-cell adhesion occur in borderline and malignant tumours, implying that the normal function of these molecules is disrupted. Disturbance of the E-cadherin-catenin complex by loss of E-cadherin, or β-catenin, to α-catenin may play a role in ovarian carcinogenesis, since cell movement, proliferation, and tumour cell invasion are key events that would require loss of tight cell-cell adhesion.

**Keywords**: ovarian cancer, cell adhesion, epithelial cadherin, catenins, immunohistochemistry,

# Introduction

Epithelial ovarian carcinoma is the leading cause of death from female genital malignancies, with more than half of the patients diagnosed at an advanced stage of the disease. Intra-abdominal spread of ovarian cancer is common and is a process that theoretically could be closely connected with reduced cellular adhesion between tumour cells, thus facilitating the process of invasion and dissemination [Ozols, 2000].

Epithelial cadherin (E-cadherin, 120 KDa; chromosome 16q22.1) is a transmembrane glycoprotein that mediates calcium-dependent homotypic intercellular adhesion. E-cadherin also plays an important function in maintaining the histological architecture in adult tissues, and in forming the key functional component of adherence junctions between epithelial cells [Gumbiner, 1998]. Although the adhesive activity of E-cadherin resides in its extracellular domain, the function of E-cadherin depends on its ability to form an intracellular complex with the catenin proteins [Ozawa, 1990].

The catenins (from *catena,* the latin word for chain), α- (102 kDa, chromosome 5q21-22) [McPherson, 1994], β- (92 kDa, chromosome 3p21) [Kraus, 1994], and γ-catenin (plakoglobin, 83 kDa, chromosome 17q21) [Aberle, 1995] are a set of peripheral membrane proteins that act as intermediates in the linkage between E-cadherin and the cytoskeleton [Nagafuchi, 1988; Ozawa, 1989].

Several studies have shown that the cadherin-catenin complex is crucial for a cadherin-mediated adhesion at the adherens junction between cells [Morton, 1993; Shimoyama, 1992]. Defective cell adhesion occurs *in vitro* when E-cadherin expression is not paralleled by α-catenin expression [Shimoyama, 1992; Vermeulen, 1995; Breen, 1993]. In functional terms, it is therefore preferable to consider the E-cadherin and the catenins as a complex rather than each separate component [Shiozaki H, 1994; Kadowski, 1994]. The E-cadherin-catenin complex is a functional unit termed here as the E-cadherin-catenin unit (ECCU, Figure 1). At the *adherens* junction, α-catenin links the E-cadherin-β-catenin complex or the E-cadherin-γ-catenin complex to the actin cytoskeleton and thereby forming mutually exclusive complexes [Piepenhagen, 1993]. In this way, the catenins are essential in association with E-cadherin in anchoring, cytoskeleton organization and stabilising cell-to-cell adhesion [Harington, 2000; Kirkpatrick, 1995]. Since the function of E-cadherin is dependent on the catenins for efficient cell-to-cell adhesion, alterations in the catenins are thought to influence tumour behaviour as metastasis and invasion by a process involving loss of cell adherence [Birchmeier, 1995; Jiang, 1996; Shiozaki, 1996; Smith, 1997].

Abnormal and reduced expression of the E-cadherin-catenin complex has been associated with: tumour lack of dedifferentiation, advanced clinical stages, lymph node metastasis and poor prognosis in various carcinomas [Jawhari, 1997; Krishnadath, 1997; Andrews, 1997; Winn, 2002; Yoshida, 2001; Bukholm, 1998; Garcia del Muro, 2000; Shimazui, 1996].

In this chapter we focus on the evaluation of E-cadherin and the catenins (α-, β- and γ-catenin /plakoglobin) in 24 ovarian tumours. These specimens are part of a series of 154 ovarian tumour samples that were previously characterized by the authors [Faleiro-Rodrigues et al, 2005, and earlier papers 2004a, 2004b, 2004c]. The previous work by these authors established that data generated from the series of 154 tumors can be used to draw useful conclusions regarding the role of the cadherin-catenin complex (referred to herein as ECCU) in the progression and prognosis of ovarian cancer since these studies have shown that reduced and loss of E-cadherin or β-catenin expression is associated with markers of disease progression and poor survival.

This chapter therefore attempts to further evaluate the role of the ECCU in ovarian cancer by focusing on the 24 samples selected due to either i) E-cadherin-negative or ii) β-catenin-negative immunohistochemical expression.

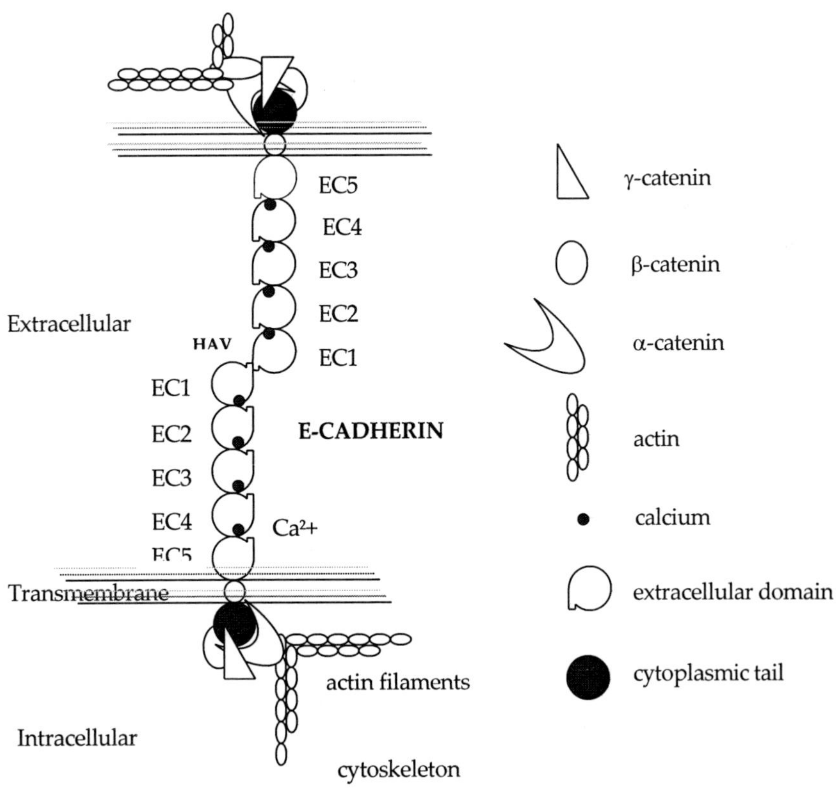


Figure 1. Schematic drawing of a Epithelial Cadherin molecule. The extracellular domain farthest from the membrane is thought to mediate cell-cell adhesion. The cytoplasmic tail interacts with the actin cytoskeleton via a number of intracellular attachment proteins, the catenins.

# Materials and Methods

This study involved a series of 24 primary EOT diagnosed and treated at the Portuguese Institute of Oncology of Francisco Gentil, Porto, Portugal. None of these patients had undergone neo-adjuvant preoperative chemotherapy. The 24 EOT were classified into 5 borderline and 19 malignant tumours. Histological typing was performed according to the World Health Organization (WHO) classification. Differentiation and staging of the malignant tumours were assigned according to the International Federation of Gynaecology and Obstetrics (FIGO) standards that can be seen in Tables 1 and 2.

The malignant tumours were selected from two previous individual studies. In the first study, 7 carcinomas showed negative expression for E-cadherin [Faleiro-Rodrigues, 2004b]. In the second study, 15 carcinomas showed negative expression for β-catenin [Faleiro-Rodrigues, 2004c]. In another study, 3 borderline tumours showed negative expression for E-cadherin and 3 borderline tumours showed negative expression for β-catenin [Faleiro-Rodrigues, 2005]. When these selected epithelial ovarian tumours were brought together, we observed that 1 borderline tumour and 3 carcinomas were the same cases in both these studies, (represented in bold letters and underlined in Table 1 and Table 2) therefore a total of 24 epithelial ovarian tumours were analysed

# Immunohistochemistry

Immunohistochemistry was performed by the avidin-biotin-peroxidase (ABC) complex method with a heat induced antigen retrieval step as previously described [Faleiro-Rodrigues, 2005]. The monoclonal antibodies used were: E-cadherin (C20820), α-catenin (C21620), β-catenin (C19220) and γ–catenin (C26220) (Transduction Laboratories, Lexington, UK).

Visualization of the antigen-antibody reaction was prepared using 3,3-diaminobenzidine tetrahydrochloride with 0.03% hydrogen peroxide. Tissue sections were counterstained with haematoxylin and mounted for microscopic examination.

To ensure accurate and reproducible staining, tissue sections from normal skin epithelium known to be positive for E-cadherin, α-, β- and γ-catenin were used as a positive control. Staining was localized on the cell membrane of epithelial cells, particularly at areas of cell-to-cell contact. The primary antibodies were omitted in the negative controls.

Evaluation and quantification of immunohistopathologically stained specimens was assessed by light microscopy. Negative expression when these proteins were absent at the cell membrane and positive when these proteins were at the cell membrane. The degree of staining at the cell membrane into weak/strong or nuclear/cytoplasmic staining was not taken into account, but has been described elsewhere [Faleiro-Rodrigues et al, 2005].

On a scale of 0-3, the 0 scale consisted of complete absence of expression. Membranous E-cadherin and the catenins were scored semiquantitatively into three categories according to the percentage of tumour cells with immunoreactivity (1=≤10%, 2=11 and ≤ 50%, 3=>51%). We considered that in our series of EOT that membranous staining in ≤10% of a tumour cell population was a very small, insignificant number when compared with a cell population of thousands of cells (in a section of 3μm with approximate dimensions of 1 x2 cm), therefore tumours showing ≤10% of membrane expression were re-classified as negative (observed in Table 1 and 2 as **0** *).

# Results

The clinicopathological characteristics of the patients and the immunohistochemical expression of E-cadherin and the catenins α-, β- and γ- observed in EOT showing negative expression for E-cadherin is shown in Table 1.

Expression of the catenins α-, β- and γ- was observed in 3 borderline and 7 malignant tumours. Negative expression for all the catenins was observed in 1 borderline and 3 malignant tumours (malignant tumours M1, M2 and M3, are the same cases in Table 1 and 2).

The majority of the borderline and malignant tumours also show:

- -Loss of immunoexpression in at least one, two or three of the catenins,
- -Simultaneous negative expression of γ-catenin and α-catenin,
- -Loss of α-catenin most frequently, followed by γ-catenin, and lastly by β-catenin,
- -Negative β-catenin or ≤50% positive membrane staining in tumours also showed negative expression of α-catenin (except for B1 and M4).

When the interrelationship between the catenins was analysed, 2/3 (67%) borderline and 5/7 (71%) malignant tumours showed loss of expression of both α- and γ-catenin in the same tumours.

The patients clinicopathological characteristics and the immunohistochemical expression of E-cadherin, and the catenins α-, β- and γ- observed in epithelial borderline and malignant tumours showing negative expression of β-catenin can be seen in Table 2.

Expression of E-cadherin and the catenins α- and γ- was observed in 3 borderline and 15 ovarian carcinomas. In these tumours, 1 borderline tumour and 6 malignant tumours showed negative expression for E-cadherin and the catenins α-and γ- (M1, M2 and M3, are the same cases in Table 1 and 2).

Borderline and malignant tumours showing E-cadherin immunoreactivity repeatedly showed loss of the catenins α-, β-, γ-.

In general the majority of the borderline and malignant tumours also showed the following:

- -Loss of immunoexpression in at least one, two or three of the ECCU components,
- -Loss of the α-catenin protein,
- -Simultaneous expression of negative γ-catenin and α-catenin,
- -Negative α-catenin expression was observed in all tumours showing negative or positive expression for E-cadherin (except for B1)

When the interrelationship between E-cadherin and the catenins α-and γ- was analysed, 2/3 (67%) borderline and 13/15 (87%) malignant tumours, showed loss of expression of both α- and γ-catenin in the same tumours.

**Table 1. Immunohistochemical expression of α-, β- and γ-catenin in Epithelial Ovarian Tumours negative for E-cadherin expression.**

| Tumours | Case | FIGO stage | Differentiation | Histological type | E-cadherin | α- | β- | γ- |
|---|---|---|---|---|---|---|---|---|
| Borderline | | | | | | | | |
| | <u>B1</u> | Ia | | Mucinous | 0 | 3 | 0 | 3 |
| | B2 | III | | Mucinous | 0 | 0 * | 2 | 0 * |
| | B3 | Ia | | Serous | 0 | 0 | 0 * | 0 |
| Carcinomas | | | | | | | | |
| | <u>M1</u> | IV | Poor | Serous | 0 | 0 | 0 | 0 |
| | <u>M2</u> | III | Poor | Serous | 0 | 0 | 0 | 0 |
| | <u>M3</u> | Ic | Well | Mucinous | 0 | 0 | 0 | 0 |
| | M4 | IV | Poor | Serous | 0 | 2 | 2 | 3 |
| | M5 | IV | Well | Mucinous | 0 | 0 * | 2 | 0 * |
| | M6 | III | Poor | Serous | 0 | 0 * | 2 | 0 * |
| | M7 | Ic | Poor | Clear cell | 0 | 0 * | 2 | 2 |

Bold numbers underlined are the same cases in Tables 1 and 2. . Percentage of positive cells (1=≤10%, 2=11 and ≤ 50%, 3=>51%).
Astrix at 0 *, are tumours that were scored as 0 when they showed ≤10% membrane cell staining.

**Table 2. Immunohistochemical expression of E-cadherin and the catenins α- and γ- in Epithelial Ovarian Tumours negative for β-catenin.**

| Tumours | Case | FIGO stage | Differentiation | Histological type | E-cadherin | α- | β- | γ- |
|---|---|---|---|---|---|---|---|---|
| Borderline | | | | | | | | |
| | <u>B1</u> | Ia | | Mucinous | 0 | 3 | 0 | 3 |
| | B2 | Ia | | Serous | 0 * | 0 | 0 | 0 |
| | B3 | Ia | | Mucinous | 2 | 0 | 0 | 0 |
| Carcinomas | | | | | | | | |
| | <u>M1</u> | IV | Poor | Serous | 0 | 0 | 0 | 0 |
| | <u>M2</u> | III | Poor | Serous | 0 | 0 | 0 | 0 |
| | <u>M3</u> | Ic | Well | Mucinous | 0 | 0 | 0 | 0 |
| | M4 | III | Well | Serous | 0 * | 0 | 0 | 0 * |
| | M5 | Ia | Well | Serous | 0 * | 0 | 0 | 0 * |
| | M6 | III | Well | Serous | 0 * | 0 | 0 | 0 |
| | M7 | III | Moderate | Serous | 0 * | 0 | 0 | 2 |
| | M8 | III | Poor | Serous | 3 | 0 | 0 | 0 * |
| | M9 | Ic | Well | Mucinous | 3 | 0 | 0 | 2 |
| | M10 | IV | Poor | Clear cell | 3 | 0 * | 0 | 0 * |
| | M11 | Ic | Poor | Clear cell | 3 | 0 * | 0 | 0 * |
| | M12 | III | Poor | Clear cell | 3 | 0 * | 0 | 0 * |
| | M13 | IV | Poor | Clear cell | 2 | 0 | 0 | 0 |
| | M14 | Ic | Poor | Clear cell | 2 | 0 | 0 | 0 |
| | M15 | Ia | Poor | Clear cell | 3 | 0 | 0 | 0 |

Bold numbers underlined show the same cases in Tables 1 and 2. Percentage of positive cells (1=≤10%, 2=11 and ≤ 50%, 3=>51%).
Astrix at 0 *, are tumours that were scored as 0 when tumours showed ≤10% membrane cell staining.

Immunoexpression pattern of E-cadherin and the catenins α-, β- and γ-catenin in epithelial ovarian tumours,

When we combined all EOT (Table 1 and 2) we observed:

-A predominant loss of α-catenin,

-Loss of E-cadherin and the catenins in all combinations that make up a functional E-cadherin-catenin complex unit.

## Discussion

Epithelial cadherin is a transmembrane glycoprotein that plays an important role as the primary regulator of cell adhesion in epithelia. It mediates intercellular adhesion and plays an architectural role at the adherence junction between epithelial cells by providing a link between the cell-surface adhesion molecule and the cytoskeleton [Gumbiner, 1998; Shimoyama 1989]. Although the adhesive activity of E-cadherin resides in its extracellular domain, the function of E-cadherin depends on its ability to form an intracellular complex with the catenin proteins [Nagafuchi, 1988; Ozawa, 1989; Takeichi, 1991]. Given the central role of E-cadherin in cell recognition, cell adhesion and morphogenesis, it is important to understand the protein-protein interactions of the catenins involved in the assembly and function of E-cadherin, and the mechanisms by which they exert their affect [Cowin, 1994; Ozawa, 1992]. The E-cadherin–catenin complex begins to form during the passage of E-cadherin from its site of synthesis in the endoplasmic reticulum, through the Golgi complex to the cell membrane [Shore, 1991]. Pulse-chase experiments have shown that the first catenin to interact with E-cadherin is β-catenin or γ-catenin. The initial interaction is then followed by the binding of α-catenin to either β-catenin or γ-catenin, which occurs concomitantly with the arrival of the complex at the cell membrane, resulting in the formation of stable bonds between the complex and the actin cytoskeleton [Hinck, 1994; Kemler, 1993]. The catenins bind to E-cadherin and each other in a specific manner forming a functional E-cadherin-catenin unit [Hinck, 1994; Nathke, 1994]. E-cadherin binds to either β-catenin or γ-catenin, whereas α-catenin binds to β-catenin or γ-catenin, but not E-cadherin. The existence of two distinct E-cadherin-catenin complexes in the same cell, results from specific binding [Mareel, 1997; Piepenhagen, 1993]. It is therefore understandable that cell-cell adhesion is dependent not only on the structural and functional integrity of the E-cadherin molecule, but also on the association of the catenins that mediate it's binding to the cytoskeleton [Ozawa, 1992; Mareel, 1997]. It is essential that all components of the ECCU be present in order to coordinate junction development with cell movement and cell polarization, and for the establishment of tight physical cell-to-cell adhesion [Bracke, 1996; Jiang, 1996].

Disturbance or loss of normal cell-to-cell interactions is of major importance in tumour invasion and appears to be achieved by various mechanisms affecting the E-cadherin–catenin complex [Bracke, 1996; Behrens, 1999; Van Aken, 2001]. In view of the literature on the role of the catenins on E-cadherin function [Gumbiner, 1998; Ozawa, 1990; Nagafuchi, 1988; Ozawa, 1989; Harington, 2000; Kirkpatrick, 1995; Kemler, 1993] we evaluated the inter-relationship between each of the proteins essential in the formation of the ECCU and their possible role in ovarian carcinogenesis in five borderline and nineteen malignant tumours showing negative expression for either E-cadherin or β-catenin [Faleiro-Rodrigues, 2004b; Faleiro-Rodrigues, 2004c]. In view of the fact that cadherin-mediated cell-cell junctions are dependent on the integrity of each of the components in the E-cadherin–catenin complex, we took a closer look at the ECCU in these tumours. This study shows that in the majority of the EOT, negative expression and immunoreactivity of E-cadherin and the catenins α-, β-, and γ- was frequently observed in less than 10% of the tumour cell population. If we take into consideration the protein-protein interactions that make up the E-cadherin-catenin complex by analysing the immunohistochemical expression of the catenins in tumours negative for E-cadherin, and the immunoexpression of E-cadherin and the catenins α- and γ- in those selected tumours negative for β-catenin, we observe the following characteristics in common, (1) Loss of all the proteins essential in the formation of the ECCU in some tumours, (2) loss of immunoexpression in at least one, two or three of the catenins, and (3) loss of α-catenin in the majority of the tumours. When we consider only those EOT negative for E-cadherin and determine the inter-relation between α- and β-catenin, or between α-and γ-catenin, we observe a general loss of α-catenin in these tumours, showing that disturbance of the ECCU by loss of the structural components E-cadherin and α-catenin appear to be are responsible for the deficient cell-cell adhesion complex in these tumours.

Although this investigation does not represent a substancial advance over previously reported data [Faleiro-Rodrigues, 2005] since the main conclusion that loss of E-cadherin and the catenins is enough to alter the function of the others seems obvious, when we focus on only those EOT negative for β-catenin, we observe that the majority of these tumours also show a predominant loss of α-catenin. In these tumours, loss of α-catenin expression was paralleled by the loss of β-catenin in all but one borderline tumour. These two observations suggests that a) the principal complex in this subgroup of tumours was mainly composed of E-cadherin-β-α-catenin, and b) the loss of β-catenin alone in these tumours may be sufficient for the loss of intermolecular binding, given that β-catenin plays a central role in linking E-cadherin to α-catenin [Hinck, 1994; Kemler, 1993].

E-cadherin-mediated linkage of the catenins to the cytoskeleton imparts strong adhesive properties [Kemler, 1993]. The observation that some tumours continued to express E-cadherin at the cell membrane, yet show loss of one, two or three of the catenins that make up the ECCU suggests that the necessary components to directly associate with the cytoplasmic domain of E-cadherin are absent, and consequently a functional ECCU cannot be formed. Together these results highlight that catenins play a central role in the regulation of E-cadherin function.

In spite of the predominant loss of E-cadherin or β-catenin expression in these selected epithelial ovarian tumours, one of the most interesting observations in this study was the loss of α-catenin. Loss of α-catenin was seen in all but two EOT which suggests that α-catenin is dysfunctional in the majority of these tumours. A possible explanation for the loss of α-catenin observed in our series of tumours may be due to the fact that association of α-catenin to either E-cadherin/ β-catenin or E-cadherin/ γ-catenin does not occur due to the loss of the initial components (E-cadherin or β-catenin) that assemble the ECCU complex and therefore α-catenin cannot associate with the actin cytoskeleton to coordinate stable intercellular adhesion. This observation reinforces that E-cadherin and β-catenin, and to a lesser extent, loss of γ-catenin are essential components for the proper functioning of the ECCU and that their loss may directly influence the function of α-catenin [Huber, 2001]. Even though α-catenin has not been as extensively studied as its prominent partner β-catenin which plays an important role in intercellular cell adhesion, and as a nuclear transcriptional co-activator for the lymphoid enhancer-binding factor-1 (LEF1/T-cell specific factor (TCF) family of DNA-binding proteins, new roles have begun to emerge for α-catenin in both cytoskeleton assembly and its dynamic regulation at cell-cell junctions [Kobielak, 2004]. Although α-catenin was previously considered to be solely a structural protein, α-E-catenin gene targeting studies have shown α-catenin in mediating the formation of radial actin cables that are necessary for stabilizing adherens junctions in epithelial cells, sealing membranes and in the assembly of epithelial sheets [Vasioukhin, 2000; Vasioukhin, 2001]. In view of the fact that α-catenin plays a central role in E-cadherin function by connecting E-cadherin to the cytoskeleton, it would follow that loss of α-catenin may perhaps facilitate the process of tumourigenesis and thus contribute to the malignant phenotype [Bullions, 1997; Fuchs, 2004; Oda, 1993; Shimoyama, 1992; Shiozaki, 1994, Vasioukhin, 2000; Vasioukhin, 2001].

Loss and reduced expression of the catenins by immunohistochemistry in various carcinomas has been shown to associate with increased invasiveness, disease progression, and poor prognosis [Andrews, 1997; Bremnes, 2002; Bukholm, 1998; Garcia del Muro, 2000; Jawhari, 1997; Kadowaki, 1994; Krishnadath, 1997; Shimazui, 1996; Shiozaki, 1994; Takayama, 1996; Winn, 2002; Yoshida, 2001], however, the biomolecular studies (gene mutations, hypermethylation, abnormal transcription and translation of the protein) for the loss or reduced expression of the catenins in these tumours were not performed.

The detailed molecular mechanisms for the negative expression of E-cadherin and the catenins that make up the ECCU in our EOT are unclear at this stage. Nevertheless, our results must be interpreted with caution, as the sample size investigated is rather small. Therefore, the E-cadherin–catenin complex in epithelial ovarian tumours should be performed in a larger number of patients. Further investigation in the area of tumour biology may yield greater insight into the early molecular interactions critical to the initiation and progression of tumours.

Accepting our limitation of sample size, the results of our study allow for a number of conclusions:

(1) Loss of E-cadherin and the catenins α-, β- and γ- are necessary for strong cell-to-cell adhesion to occur in borderline and malignant tumours and may play a role in ovarian carcinogenesis,
(2) Loss in only one of the proteins that make up the E-cadherin-catenin complex unit is sufficient to disrupt the function of the others,
(3) The dysfunction of ECCU in our tumours may favour loss of adhesive properties and thus weaker cohesion between epithelial cells, potentially increasing the propensity of tumour cells to invade.

## Acknowledgements

This project was supported by a Ph.D. grant (PRAXIS XXI/BD/9615/96) from the Foundation of Science and Technology (FCT) and a Research Grant n° 250/99 from the Portuguese Ministry of Health, Commission for Investigation in Health Care.

## References

Aberle, H. Bierkamp, C. Torchard, D. Serova, O. Wagner, T. Natt, E. Wirsching, J. Heidkämper, C. Montagna, M. Lynch, H.T. Lenoir, G.M. Schereer, G. Feunteun, J. Kemler, R. (1995). The human plakoglobin gene localizes on chromosome 17q21 and is subjected to loss of heterozygosity in breast and ovarian cancers. *Proc Natl Acad Sci USA* 92, 6384-6388.

Andrews, A. Jones, S. A Helliiwell, T. R Kinsella, A. R. (1997). Expression of the E-cadherin-catenin cell adhesion complex in primary squamous cell carcinomas of the head and neck and their nodal metastases. *Br J Cancer* 75, 1474-1480.

Behrens, J. (1999). Cadherins and catenins: role in signal transduction and tumor progression. *Cancer Metast Reviews* 18, 15-30.

Birchmeier, W. Hulsken, J. Behrens, J. (1995). Adherens junction proteins in tumour progression. *Cancer Surveys* 24, 129-140.

Bracke, M. E. Van Roy, F. M. Mareel, M. M. (1996). The E-cadherin /catenin complex in invasion and metastases. *Curr Top Microbiol Immunol* 213, 123-161.

Breen, E. Clarke, A. Steele, G. Mercurio, A. M. (1993). Poorly differentiated colon carcinoma cell lines deficient in α-catenin expression express high levels of surface E-cadherin but lack Ca2+ -dependent cell-cell adhesion. *Cell Adhesion and Commun* 1, 239-250.

Bremnes, R. M. Veve, R. Hirsch, F. R. Franklin, W. A. (2002). The E-cadherin cell-cell adhesion complex and lung cancer invasion, metastasis, and prognosis. *Lung Cancer* 36, 115-124.

Bukholm, I. K. Nesland J M, Karesen R, Jacobsen U, Borresen-Dale A L (1998). E-cadherin and α-, β-catenin and γ-catenin protein expression in relation to metastasis in human breast carcinoma. *J Pathol* 185, 262-266.

Bullions, L. C. Notterman, D. A. Chung, L. S. Levine, A. J. (1997). Expression of wild-type α-catenin protein in cells with a mutant α-catenin gene restores both growth regulation and tumor suppressor activities. *Mol Cell Biol* 17, 4501-4508.

Cowin, P. (1994). Unraveling the cytoplasmic interactions of the cadherin superfamily. *Proc Natl Acad Sci* 91, 10759-10761.

Faleiro-Rodrigues, C. Macedo-Pinto, I. Pereira, D. Ferreira, V. M. Lopes, C. S. (2004a). Association of E-cadherin and β-catenin immunoexpression with clinicopathologic features in primary ovarian carcinomas. *Human Pathol* 35,663-669.

Faleiro-Rodrigues, C. Macedo-Pinto, I. Pereira, D. Lopes, C. S. (2004b). Prognostic value of E-cadherin immunoexpression in patients with primary ovarian carcinomas. *Ann of Oncology 15*(10), 1532-1542.

Faleiro-Rodrigues, C. Macedo-Pinto, I. Pereira, D. Lopes, C. S. (2004c). Loss of β-catenin, is associated with poor survival in ovarian carcinomas. *Int J Gynecol Pathol* 23(4),337-346.

Faleiro-Rodrigues, C. Macedo-Pinto, I. Maia, S. S. Vieira, R. H. Lopes, C. S (2005). The biological relevance of the E-cadherin-catenin complex proteins in primary epithelial ovarian tumours. *Gynecologic and Obstetric Investigation* 60, 75-83.

Kobielak, A. Fuchs, E. (2004) Alpha catenin: at the junction of intercellular adhesion and actin dynamics. *Nature Reviews Molec Cell Biol* 5, 614-625.

Garcia del Muro, X. Torregosa, A. Munoz, J. Catellsague (2000). Prognostic value of expression of E-cadherin and β-catenin in bladder cancer. *Eur J Cancer* 36, 357-362.

Gumbiner, B. Stevenson, B. Grimaldi, A. (1988). The role of the cell adhesion molecule ovumorulin in the formation and maintenance of the epithelial junctional complex. *J Cell Biol* 107, 1575-1587.

Harington, K. J. Syrigos, K. N. (2000). The role of E-cadherin -catenin complex, more than an intercellular glue? *Annals of Surgical Pathol* 7, 783-788.

Hinck, L. Näthke, I. S. Papkoff, J. Nelson, W. J. (1994). Dynamics of cadherin/catenin complex formation: novel protein interactions and pathways of complex assembly. *J Cell Biol* 125, 1327-1340.

Huber, A. H. Stewart, D. B. Laurents, D. V. Nelson, W. J. Weis, W. I. (2001). The cadherin cytoplasmic domain is unstructured in the absence of β-catenin. *J Biol Chem* 276, 12301-12309.

Jawhari, A. Jordan, S. Poole, S. Browne, P. Pignatelli, M. Farthing, M. J. G. (1997). Abnormal immunoreactivity of the E-cadherin-catenin complex in gastric carcinoma: relationship with patient survival. *Gastroenterology* 112, 46-54.

Jiang, W. G. (1996). E-cadherin and its associated protein catenins, cancer invasion and metastasis. *Br J Surgery* 83, 437-446.

Kadowaki, T. Shiozaki, H. Inoue, M. Tamura, S. Oka, H. Doki, Y. Iihara, K. Matsui, S. Iwazawa, T. Nagafuchi, A. et al_(1994). E-cadherin and α-catenin expression in human oesophageal cancer. *Cancer Res* 54, 291-296.

Kemler, R. (1993). From cadherins to catenins: cytoplasmatic protein interactions and regulation of cell adhesion. *Trends Genetics* 9, 317-321.

Kirkpatrick, C. Peifer, M. (1995). Not just glue: cell-cell junctions as cellular signaling centers. *Curr Opin Genetics Development* 5, 56-65.

Kraus, C. Liehr, T. Hulsken, J. Behrens, J. Birchmeier, W. Grzeschik, K-H. Ballhausen, W. (1994). Localization of the human β-catenin gene (CTNNB1) to 3p21: a region implicated in tumour development. *Genomics* 23, 272-274.

Krishnadath, K. K. Tilanus, H. W. van Blankenstein, M. Hop, W. C. J. Kremers, E. D, Dinjens , W. N. M. Bosman, F. T. (1997). Reduced expression of the cadherin-catenin complex in oesophageal adenocarcinoma correlates with poor prognosis. *J Pathol* 182, 331-338.

Mareel, M. Boterberg, T. Noë, L. Van Hoorde, L. Vermeulen, S. Bruyneel, E. Bracke, M. (1997). E-cadherin/catenin/Cytoskeleton complex: A regulator of cancer invasion. *J Cellular Physiol* 173, 271-274.

McPherson, J. D. Morton, R. A. Ewing, C. M. Wasmuth, J. J. Overhauser, J. Nagafuchi, A. Tsukita, S. Isaacs, W. B. (1994). Assignment of the human α-catenin gene (CTNNA1) to chromosome 5q21-q22. *Genomics* 19, 188-190.

Morton, R. A. Ewing, C. M. Nagafuchi, A. Tsukita, S. Isaacs, W. B. (1993). Reduction of E-cadherin levels and deletion of the α-catenin gene in human prostate cancer cells. *Cancer Res* 53, 3585-3590.

Nagafuchi, A. Takeichi, M. (1988). Cell binding function of E-Cadherin is regulated by the cytoplasmic domain. *EMBO J 7,* 3679-3684.

Näthke, I. S. Hinck, L. Swedlow, J. R. Papkoff, J. Nelson, W. J. (1994). Defining interactions and distributions of cadherin and catenin complexes in polarized epithelial cells. *J Cell Biol* 125; 1341-1352.

Oda, M. Kanai, Y. Shimoyama, Y. Nagafuchi, A. Tsukita, S. Hirohashi, S. (1993). Cloning of the human α-catenin cDNA and its abberant mRNA in a human cancer cell line. *Biochem Biophys Res* Commun 193, 897-904.

Ozawa, M. Baribault, H. Kemler, R. (1989). The cytoplasmic domain of the cell adhesion molecule ovumorulin associates with three independent proteins structurally related in different species. *EMBO J.* 8. 1711-1717.

Ozawa, M. Ringwald, M. Kemler, R. (1990). Uvomorulin-catenin complex formation is regulated by a specific domain in the cytoplasmic region of the cell adhesion molecule. *Proc Natl Acad Sci USA* 87, 4246-4250.

Ozawa, M. Kemler, R. (1992). Molecular organization of the Uvomorulin-catenin complex. *J Cell Biol* 116, 989-996.

Ozols, R. F. Rubin, S. C. Thomas, G. M. Robboy, S. J. Epithelial ovarian cancer: In Hoskins, W. J. Perez, C. A. Young RC (eds): *Principles and Practice of Gynecologic Oncology*, 3rd edition: Philadelphia: PA: Lippincott Williams & Wilkins 2000; 981-1058.

Piepenhagen, P. A. Nelson, W. J. (1993). Defining E-cadherin -associated protein complexes in epithelial cells: plakoglobin, β-and γ-catenin are distinct components. *J Cell Scien*ce 104, 751-762.

Shimazui, T. Schalken, J. A. Giroldi, L. A. Jansen, C. F. J, Akaza, H. Koiso, K. Debruyne, F. M. J. Bringuier, P. P. (1996). Prognostic value of cadherin -associated molecules (α-, β-, γ-catenins and p120cas) in bladder tumors. *Cancer Res* 56, 4154-4158.

Shimoyama, Y. Hirohashi, S. Hirano, S. Noguchi, M. Shimosato, Y. Takeichi, M. Abe, O. (1989). Cadherin cell -adhesion molecules in epithelial tissues and carcinomas. *Cancer Res* 49, 2128-2133.

Shimoyama, Y. Nagafuchi, A. Fujita, S. Gotoh, M. Takeichi, M. Tsukita, S. Hirohashi, S. (1992). Cadherin dysfunction in a human cancer cell line: possible involvement of loss of α-catenin expression in reduced cell-cell adhesiveness. *Cancer Res* 52, 770-5774.

Shiozaki, H. Lihara, K. Oka, H. Kadowaki, T. Matsui, S. Gofuku, J. Inou, M. Nagafuchi, A. Tsukita, S. Mori, T. (1994). Immunohistochemical detection of α-catenin in human cancers. *Am J Pathol* 144 ,667-674.

Shiozaki, H. Oka, H. Inoue, M. Tamura, S. Monden, M. (1996). E-cadherin mediated adhesion system in cancer cells. *Cancer* 77, 1605-1613.

Shore, E. M. Nelson, W. J. (1991). Biosynthesis of the cell adhesion molecule uvomorulin (E-cadherin) in Madin-Darby canine kidney epithelial cells. *J Biol Chem* 266, 19672-19680.

Smith, M. E. Pignatelli, M. (1997). The molecular histology of neoplasia: the role of the cadherin/catenin complex. *Histopathol* 31, 107-111.

Takayama, T. Shiozaki, H. Shibamoto, S. Oka, H. Kimura, Y. Tamura, S. Inoue, M. Monden, T. Ito, F. Monden, M. (1996). β-catenin expression in human cancers. *Am J Pathol* 148, 39-46.

Takeichi, M. (1991). Cadherin cell adhesion receptors as a morphogenetic regulator. *Science* 251, 1451-1455.

Van Aken, E. De Wever, O. Correia da Rocha, A. S. Mareel, M. (2001). Defective E-cadherin/catenin complexes in human cancer. *Virchows Arch* 439, 725-751.

Vasioukhin, V. Bauer, C. Yin, M. Fuchs, E. (2000). Directed actin polymerization is the driving force for epithelial cell-cell adhesion. *Cell* 100, 209-219.

Vasioukhin, V. Bauer, C. Degenstein, L. Wise, B. Fuchs, E. (2001). Hyperproliferation and defects in epithelial polarity upon conditional ablation of α-catenin in skin. *Cell* 104, 605-617.

Vermeulen, S. J. Bruyneel, E. A. Bracke, M. E. de Bruyne, G. K, Vennekens, K. M, Vleminckx, K. L. Berx, G. J. Van Roy, F. M. Mareel, M. M. (1995). Transition from the noninvasive to the invasive phenotype and loss of α-catenin in human colon cancer cells. *Cancer Res* 55, 4722-4728.

Winn, R. A, Bremnes, R. M, Bemis, L. Franklin, W. A. Miller, Y. E. Cool, C. Heasley, L. E. (2002). γ-catenin expression is reduced or absent in a subset of human lung cancers and re-expression inhibits transformed cell growth. *Oncogene* 21, 7497-7506.

Yoshida, R. Kimura, N. Harada, Y. Ohuchi, N. (2001). The loss of E-cadherin, α- and β-catenin expression is associated with metastasis and poor prognosis in invasive breast cancer. *Int J Oncology* 18, 513-520.

In: Tumor Markers Research Focus
Editor: Deborah H. Chang, pp. 275-282

ISBN: 978-1-60021-544-5


*Chapter XVII*

# Tumor Biomarkers in Personalized Medicine

***Elzbieta Izbicka*[*] *and Tadeusz Izbicki***

Institute for Drug Development, Cancer Therapy and Research Center, San Antonio, Texas, USA, and Department of Surgical Oncology, National Research Institute of Mother and Child, Warsaw, Poland

## Abstract

To attain a goal of personalized medicine, we need to improve our understanding of cancer at the molecular level to implement effective primary and secondary prophylaxis, early diagnosis, and optimize drug treatment for each individual. With help from biomedical sciences we can start answering vital questions regarding inheritance of cancer risk, biology and treatment of individual patient: Am I at risk for cancer? Is family history an important factor? Have I inherited and/or can I pass my predisposition to cancer? Is there anything I can do to alter the risk? If the cancer already exists, we want to know if it responds to a particular therapy and whether it will respond over time. Genomic (DNA), transcriptional (RNA) and translational (protein) research alone will not be sufficient to provide answers to these questions, which are likely to come from concerted efforts in these disciplines with a focus on early stages of cancer. Proteomics has potential for discovering new practical biomarkers for primary prophylaxis (avoidance of risk factors), secondary prophylaxis (mass screening), and early detection. Emerging tools for sensitive, high resolution and high throughput proteomic analysis including protein arrays, multiplexed immunoassays and mass spectral body fluids (blood, cerebrospinal fluid, urine) and tissue analyses are now yielding new putative proteomic biomarkers and protein signature patterns that need to be validated in the clinic. Recently discovered dramatic gender-specific differences in expression of thousands of genes further underline needs for analysis of the proteome in health and disease. These novel

[*] E-mail address: eizbicka@idd.org web www.idd.org, Tel 210.450.3879, fax 210.450.0058. Corresponding author: Elzbieta Izbicka, PhD, CTRC Institute for Drug Development, 14960 Omicron Drive, San Antonio, TX 78245

approaches to prophylaxis, early detection and therapy are expected to change the ways how cancer is diagnosed and treated.

## Personalized Medicine

Our goal is to provide personalized medicine geared to individual needs. To attain this goal, we need to improve current understanding of cancer at the molecular level and optimize drug treatment for each individual, so that these vital questions can be answered: Am I at risk for cancer? Is family history an important factor? Have I inherited and/or can I pass my predisposition to cancer? Is there anything I can do to alter the risk? Will my cancer respond to therapy? Is my cancer responding to therapy? Once the presence of cancer is confirmed, we should account for heterogeneity of the disease because it often increases over time due to accumulation of cellular mutations through cancer progression.

The patients would greatly benefit from detection of the disease as early as possible. If drug treatment is an option, profiling for the presence of cancer targets should be done before the therapy is initiated and through the drug treatment. Many currently used anticancer drugs are also toxic to normal cells, and some patients do not respond favorably or suffer adverse drug effects (1). Furthermore, standard endpoints used in evaluation of drug efficacy such as tumor shrinkage do not always apply to novel targeted therapies so alternative methods for demonstrating drug efficacy are needed. We want to develop effective screens that will allow for selection of the best individualized therapy, either conventional or experimental, including the most effective drug combinations. Overall, molecular diagnostics with integration of diagnosis and therapy will play an important role in the development of personalized medicine.

## What Is a Biomarker?

We will adapt a definition of biomarker as a "characteristic that is objectively measured and evaluated as an indicator of normal biologic process, pathogenic process, or pharmacologic responses to a therapeutic intervention (2). In this review, we will focus on the subset of molecular biomarkers that may be discovered using new high throughput "omic" proteomic technologies.

## Genomic Biomarkers

The information database on genomic biomarkers is growing exponentially and many reviews are available on the subject. Recent publications (3-5) stress the fact that global gene expression analysis is moving from the basic research to clinical trials. Several studies have shown the utility of gene expression profiles for the classification of tumors into defined, clinically relevant subtypes and the prediction of clinical outcomes with a "biosignature" profile of human cancer.

In the personalized medical approach, genotype-based selection of patients for effective cancer therapy may select for the individuals who are most likely to benefit from the therapy with the least undesirable side effects. Several technologies that are being currently used include single nucleotide polymorphism genotyping, haplotyping, and gene expression studies by biochip/microarrays (1). In addition, the analysis of mitochondrial genome is gaining more recognition. Recent studies demonstrated the presence of sequence variants in mitochondrial DNA (mtDNA). Heteroplasmic and homoplasmic sequence variants occur in the mitochondrial genome in patient tumors. Increase in mtDNA content and decline in mitochondrial function occurs in response to therapy (6-8), suggesting that mtDNA is an important pharmacodynamic marker.

Implementation of genomic biomarkers presents many challenges, which include analytical, bioinformatics, bioethical, interpretation and commercialization issues. The tasks are rather complex, considering the needs to rapidly detect, analyze and identify many different biomarkers in a short time period, with adequate standards and quality controls for the tests.

## Proteomic Biomarkers

In simplistic terms, genome analysis at the DNA level may tell what could happen, and at the RNA level- what might happen in the cell. Finally, it is the proteins doing the actual work that can tell the story on what is actually happening in that cell. Approximately 30,000 genes present in the human genome are thought to encode at least ten times more proteins. According to some estimates, the number of different protein molecules expressed by the human genome is probably closer to a million than to the hundred thousand generally considered (9). These forms may represent multiple types of post-translational modifications and proteolytic fragments of larger proteins with potentially different biological activities that the parent proteins. This vast proteome reflects dynamic changes in protein structure and function that occur in real time. Some researchers believe human serum contains every protein produced by the body. So far, only a small fraction of serum proteome has been identified. A limiting factor is dynamic range of protein concentrations (somewhere in the order of $10^{12}$), which complicates the analysis of low-abundance proteins in the presence of the six highly abundant proteins that represent 90% of the total protein mass in human serum (10).

A recent report on analysis of gene expression differences between sexes in multiple somatic tissues of mice in a microarray analysis of over 20,000 transcripts revealed that the extent of sexual dimorphism in gene expression was much greater than previously recognized. Thousands of genes showed sexual dimorphism and exhibited highly tissue-specific patterns of expression (11). With virtually the same genetic code and genome differences of less than 2% between men and women, these dramatic gender-specific differences in expressions of thousands of mammalian genes further underline needs for analysis of tumor biomarkers at the proteome level in health and disease.

The analysis of the proteome may reveal what actually happens in the cell and its milieu in the body. Easier said than done... Proteomics is considered technically challenging because of sheer numbers of discrete protein forms and their tremendous dynamic range of concentrations. Tools for protein analysis lack an equivalent of polymerase chain reaction, which revolutionized gene analysis. No wonder, proteomic biomarkers are relatively “new kids on the block”. Only the most sensitive and high resolution methods can fathom the “deep proteome", where some of the most interesting, low abundance biomarkers are likely to be found. Recent progress in mass spectrometry combined with methods for selective proteome enrichment may overcome the technical limitations of non-amplified signal detection and address the most relevant questions for diagnosis and therapy biomarkers.

# Proteomic Biomarkers at Different Stages of Cancer

Cancer is not a single disease but an accumulation of several events, genetic and epigenetic, arising in a single cell over long time. Conventional approaches seek biomarkers for events that distinguish a cancer cell from a normal cell, but the process of cancer pathology may start even earlier. Individual stages and biomarkers for diagnosis and therapy are discussed. For the purpose of this review, we will narrow further discussion to proteomic biomarkers.

## Pre-initiation

Pre-initiation is a recognized early step in carcinogenesis. We propose to define yet another stage, which we refer to as pre-pre-initiation. At that stage, damage occurs to natural barriers, which protect a cell from the undesirable effects of external environment. Cell membranes that normally ward off invasion of xenobiotics or pathogens may undergo oxidation of phospholipids or modifications of glycoproteins. Thus, occasional chemical changes of the membrane proteins may signal the first very early changes.

Pre-initiation is usually defined as impairment of detoxification, removal of toxins, and DNA repair. Defective oxygen metabolism results in generation of free radicals and is in part responsible for DNA mutations, enhancement of mutagen action, and degradation of proteins.

There is not yet a cancer cell as such. Blood biomarkers may reflect the inflammatory and immune responses of the host. Trace blood metabolites of abnormal cells may signal some abnormalities at these early stages. Primary and secondary prophylaxis and early detection will be very challenging. Non-specific therapeutic intervention might be feasible through changes in diet and lifestyle to enhance immune defense.

## Initiation and Promotion

At this stage, a pre-cancerous cell "goes to the dark side" and shows signs of escaping from control of local and long-distance signals. Incoming messages are disrupted by changes of function of membrane receptors and appearance of new tumor-specific receptors.

Theoretically, sampling of cancer cells is now possible but because of low numbers of these, blood biomarkers are more likely to be analyzed. Blood biomarkers are likely to be of the host origin (inflammatory and immune response). Cancer-specific proteins may also be present in blood, but their detection may be challenging. The validity of established cancer biomarkers (e.g., PSA) has been questioned for early detection efforts. Therapeutic interventions may target abnormal receptors and signaling pathways, and boost immune defense mechanisms.

### Progression

This is the phase when cancer cells display the genetic program with some features of embryonic cells, including invasion of surrounding tissue and formation of metastases. The attack on the tissue becomes an attack on a whole organism.

Tumors at that stage are often pathologically detectable and may be sampled for biopsies. Diverse blood biomarkers signaling the presence of cancer are likely to be either actively secreted by cancer cells to blood, result from breakdown of cancer cells, or may be a host response to tumor. The number of validated blood cancer biomarkers is limited. Most anticancer therapies to date are designed to treat cancer at that late stage, when the chances for successful treatment are diminished in comparison with less advanced stages.

## What Are We Doing Today?

What can we do today to answer patients' questions related to early detection and diagnosis and treatment of the disease?

Discovery and actual identification of proteomic biomarkers is intimately linked to the type of tissue used for the analysis. Tumor tissue is a preferred source for biomarker studies (this is the site where the action is!) but the access to tumor biopsies is often limited. Surrogate tissue such as blood or other body fluids is more readily accessible and easier to sample, but biomarker discovery and origin tracing (for tumor or host) is not simple. Blood biomarkers are difficult to measure because they are obscured by six highly abundant proteins carried in human serum or plasma (10). Removing the high-abundance proteins from serum samples can increase the visibility of low-abundance proteins and enable precise analysis of possible biomarkers. Unfortunately, serum and plasma screens have too often resulted in identification of high-abundance proteins indicative of inflammatory response of the host (12-14).

The methods of tissue preservation also affect biomarker discovery process. Most proteomic analysis relies on relatively unstable material (fresh or frozen blood preparations-serum or plasma, tissue biopsies) and is incompatible with formalin-fixed, paraffin-embedded (FFPE) tissue. FFPE specimens represent the vast majority of tissue available for pathological assessment, and efforts are being made to develop protocols for recovery of proteins from FFPE prior to mass spectrometry analysis (15).

To date, mass spectral blood and tissue analysis has yielded new putative biomarkers. Clinical trials are now testing tissue samples prior to and during therapy with molecularly targeted agents. However, these efforts are not problem-free (5). Despite a visible increase in numbers of publications on biomarkers, the number of approved protein tests for plasma proteins has actually declined over the past decade (10).

Concerted efforts of the Early Detection Research Network (EDRN) at the National Cancer Institute (NCI) is bringing together scientific expertise from leading national and international institutions to identify and validate biomarkers for the detection of precancerous and cancerous cells in determining risk for developing cancer (16). Protein signature patterns derived from mass spectrometry are moving into validation (17, 18). However, the process of biomarker validation is rather lengthy and one should not anticipate numerous approvals granted by the Food and Drug Administration in the nearest future.

In the meantime, more efforts are needed to provide much needed personalized touch for patients with cancer to help with selection of customized drug treatment. Historically, tumor cells from individuals have been evaluated in tumor clonogenic assays (TCA) for evaluation of drug response and selection of optimal drug treatment. The pluripotent cancer stem cell fraction, a minute percentage of the total cells, is considered a key player in the development of metastases and recurrences. These cells can divide and form colonies in a semi-sold matrix. TCA has been used for chemosensitivity testing of tumors and xenografts, and in drug discovery and development efforts. In a recent comparison of the response of human tumors established as xenografts in nude mice, the highest correct predictive values were found when the clinical response of tumors was compared to their explants established in the nude mouse and treated in vivo, reaching 97% correct predictions for tumor resistance and 90% for tumor sensitivity. The TCA with established human tumor xenografts has proven predictive value in the chemosensitivity testing of standard and experimental anticancer drugs (19).

To identify biomarkers for drug sensitivity of tumors from individual donors and aid in selection of the best therapy for the patients, future efforts may include evaluation of human tumor implants in vivo. Tumor model establishment and maintenance may require evaluation of phenotypic stability of tumors in consecutive passages, for example through analysis of mitochondrial DNA and assessment of changes in expression and circulation of standard blood markers. With established tumors, effects of drugs as monotherapies and combinations on tumor growth rates may be combined with identification of proteomic biomarkers for drug response in serum and tumor xenograft tissue, which will lead to selection of the most efficacious drug treatment for the patient.

## Future, Hopefully Not too Distant

In the future we need to put together information derived from comprehensive studies of genes, gene products and signaling pathways, which will employ specialized high-throughput platforms. Each of these approaches on its own may not be enough to get relevant information needed for an efficient individualized diagnostics (20). Therefore, an integrated approach combining the analysis of DNA, RNA, and protein may be necessary to detect the cancer as early as possible, functionally classify tumors and find best therapies for each individual.

## References

[1] Jain, K. K. Personalized medicine. *Curr Opin Mol Ther*, 4: 548-558, 2002.

[2] Biomarkers and surrogate endpoints: preferred definitions and conceptual framework. *Clin Pharmacol Ther*, 69: 89-95, 2001.

[3] Ross, J. S., Schenkein, D. P., Kashala, O., Linette, G. P., Stec, J., Symmans, W. F., Pusztai, L., and Hortobagyi, G. N. Pharmacogenomics. *Adv Anat Pathol*, 11: 211-220, 2004.

[4] Ginsburg, G. S. and Haga, S. B. Translating genomic biomarkers into clinically useful diagnostics. *Expert Rev Mol Diagn*, 6: 179-191, 2006.

[5] Ludwig, J. A. and Weinstein, J. N. Biomarkers in cancer staging, prognosis and treatment selection. *Nat Rev Cancer*, 5: 845-856, 2005.

[6] Jakupciak, J. P., Wang, W., Markowitz, M. E., Ally, D., Coble, M., Srivastava, S., Maitra, A., Barker, P. E., Sidransky, D., and O'Connell, C. D. Mitochondrial DNA as a cancer biomarker. *J Mol Diagn*, 7: 258-267, 2005.

[7] Mambo, E., Chatterjee, A., Xing, M., Tallini, G., Haugen, B. R., Yeung, S. C., Sukumar, S., and Sidransky, D. Tumor-specific changes in mtDNA content in human cancer. *Int J Cancer*, 116: 920-924, 2005.

[8] Jiang, W. W., Rosenbaum, E., Mambo, E., Zahurak, M., Masayesva, B., Carvalho, A. L., Zhou, S., Westra, W. H., Alberg, A. J., Sidransky, D., Koch, W., and Califano, J. A. Decreased mitochondrial DNA content in posttreatment salivary rinses from head and neck cancer patients. *Clin Cancer Res*, 12: 1564-1569, 2006.

[9] Bairoch, A. and Apweiler, R. The SWISS-PROT protein sequence database and its supplement TrEMBL in 2000. Nucleic Acids Res, *28:* 45-48, 2000.

[10] Anderson, N. L. and Anderson, N. G. The human plasma proteome: history, character, and diagnostic prospects. Mol Cell Proteomics, *1:* 845-867, 2002.

[11] Yang, X., Schadt, E. E., Wang, S., Wang, H., Arnold, A. P., Ingram-Drake, L., Drake, T. A., and Lusis, A. J. Tissue-specific expression and regulation of sexually dimorphic genes in mice. *Genome Res*, 16: 995-1004, 2006.

[12] Tolson, J., Bogumil, R., Brunst, E., Beck, H., Elsner, R., Humeny, A., Kratzin, H., Deeg, M., Kuczyk, M., Mueller, G. A., Mueller, C. A., and Flad, T. Serum protein profiling by SELDI mass spectrometry: detection of multiple variants of serum amyloid alpha in renal cancer patients. *Lab Invest*, 84: 845-856, 2004.

[13] Fung, E. T., Yip, T. T., Lomas, L., Wang, Z., Yip, C., Meng, X. Y., Lin, S., Zhang, F., Zhang, Z., Chan, D. W., and Weinberger, S. R. Classification of cancer types by measuring variants of host response proteins using SELDI serum assays. *Int J Cancer*, 115: 783-789, 2005.

[14] Rai, A. J., Stemmer, P. M., Zhang, Z., Adam, B. L., Morgan, W. T., Caffrey, R. E., Podust, V. N., Patel, M., Lim, L. Y., Shipulina, N. V., Chan, D. W., Semmes, O. J., and Leung, H. C. Analysis of Human Proteome Organization Plasma Proteome Project (HUPO PPP) reference specimens using surface enhanced laser desorption/ionization-time of flight (SELDI-TOF) mass spectrometry: multi-institution correlation of spectra and identification of biomarkers. *Proteomics*, 5: 3467-3474, 2005.

[15] Hood, B. L., Darfler, M. M., Guiel, T. G., Furusato, B., Lucas, D. A., Ringeisen, B. R., Sesterhenn, I. A., Conrads, T. P., Veenstra, T. D., and Krizman, D. B. Proteomic analysis of formalin-fixed prostate cancer tissue. *Mol Cell Proteomics*, 4: 1741-1753, 2005.

[16] Verma, M. and Srivastava, S. New cancer biomarkers deriving from NCI early detection research. *Recent Results Cancer Res*, 163: 72-84; discussion 264-266, 2003.

[17] Semmes, O. J., Feng, Z., Adam, B. L., Banez, L. L., Bigbee, W. L., Campos, D., Cazares, L. H., Chan, D. W., Grizzle, W. E., Izbicka, E., Kagan, J., Malik, G., McLerran, D., Moul, J. W., Partin, A., Prasanna, P., Rosenzweig, J., Sokoll, L. J., Srivastava, S., Thompson, I., Welsh, M. J., White, N., Winget, M., Yasui, Y., Zhang, Z., and Zhu, L. Evaluation of Serum Protein Profiling by Surface-Enhanced Laser

Desorption/Ionization Time-of-Flight Mass Spectrometry for the Detection of Prostate Cancer: I. Assessment of Platform Reproducibility. *Clin Chem*, 51: 102-112, 2005.

[18] Simpkins, F., Czechowicz, J. A., Liotta, L., and Kohn, E. C. SELDI-TOF mass spectrometry for cancer biomarker discovery and serum proteomic diagnostics. *Pharmacogenomics*, 6: 647-653, 2005.

[19] Fiebig, H. H., Maier, A., and Burger, A. M. Clonogenic assay with established human tumour xenografts: correlation of in vitro to in vivo activity as a basis for anticancer drug discovery. *Eur J Cancer*, 40: 802-820, 2004.

[20] Bast, R. C., Jr., Lilja, H., Urban, N., Rimm, D. L., Fritsche, H., Gray, J., Veltri, R., Klee, G., Allen, A., Kim, N., Gutman, S., Rubin, M. A., and Hruszkewycz, A. Translational crossroads for biomarkers. *Clin Cancer Res*, 11: 6103-6108, 2005.

# Index

## A

## B

## C

## D



## E

## F

## G



## H

## I

## J



## K



## L

## M

## N

## O



## P

## S

## T

## U



## V

## W



## X



## Y